Visual Diagnosis in
PEDIATRICS

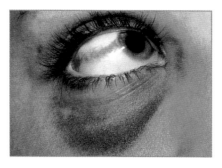

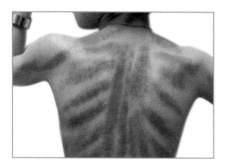

Visual Diagnosis in
PEDIATRICS

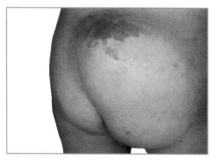

Editor-in-Chief
Esther K. Chung, MD, MPH
Assistant Professor
Department of Pediatrics
Jefferson Medical College of Thomas Jefferson University
Jefferson Pediatrics/duPont Children's Health Program
Philadelphia, Pennsylvania
Alfred I. duPont Hospital for Children
Wilmington, Delaware

Associate Editors
Julie A. Boom, MD
Assistant Professor
Department of Pediatrics
Baylor College of Medicine
Director
Immunization Project
Texas Children's Hospital
Houston, Texas

George A. Datto, III, MD
Instructor
Department of Pediatrics
Jefferson Medical College of Thomas Jefferson University
Philadelphia, Pennsylvania
Pediatrician
Department of Pediatrics
Alfred I. duPont Hospital for Children
Wilmington, Delaware

Paul S. Matz, MD
Assistant Professor
Department of Pediatrics
Drexel University College of Medicine
Attending Physician
Department of Pediatrics
St. Christopher's Hospital for Children
Philadelphia, Pennsylvania

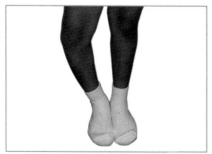

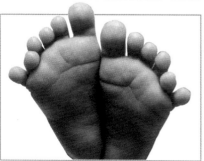

 Lippincott Williams & Wilkins
a Wolters Kluwer business
Philadelphia · Baltimore · New York · London
Buenos Aires · Hong Kong · Sydney · Tokyo

Acquisitions Editor: Anne M. Sydor/Sonya Seigafuse
Managing Editor: Nicole T. Dernoski
Project Manager: Nicole Walz
Senior Manufacturing Manager: Ben Rivera
Creative Director: Doug Smock
Cover Designer: Karen Kappe
Production Services/Compositor: Schawk, Inc.
Printer: Quebecor World Bogota

Library of Congress Cataloging-in-Publication Data

Visual diagnosis in pediatrics / editor-in-chief, Esther K. Chung ; associate editors, Julie A. Boom, George A. Datto, III, Paul S. Matz.
    p. ; cm.
  Includes bibliographical references and index.
  ISBN-13: 978-0-7817-5652-5
  ISBN-10: 0-7817-5652-9
  1. Children—Diseases—Diagnosis—Handbooks, manuals, etc. 2. Children—Medical examinations—Handbooks, manuals, etc. I. Chung, Esther K. II. Title.
  [DNLM: 1. Pediatrics—Handbooks. 2. Child. 3. Diagnosis, Differential—Handbooks. 4. Medical History Taking—Handbooks. 5. Physical Examination—Handbooks. WS 39 V834 2006]
RJ50.V57 2006
618.92'075—dc22
        2006002392

---

9 8 7 6 5 4

We dedicate this book to:

Marc, Kathryn, John and Janie and to Gloria for her help
—*Julie*

My wife, Catherine and my son, Gregory
—*George*

Miriam and Rebecca
—*Paul*

My parents, Drs. Ed Baik Chung and Okhyung Kang, and Dennis, Marissa, and little Emma
—*Esther*

Special thanks go to:
- George Datto, whose photographs make up approximately one-quarter of our collection
- Steve Handler, who generously contributed photographs from his slide collection and book
- Daniel Lerner, JMC, Class of 2006, for volunteering his time to assist with this book
- Dave Super and the Medical Media Services at Thomas Jefferson University for their quality work

Photo Credits

Joyce Adams, MD
Clinical Professor of Pediatrics
Division of Adolescent Medicine
University of California, San Diego
San Diego, California

Ben Alouf, MD
Department of General Pediatrics
Alfred I. duPont Hospital for Children
Wilmington, Delaware

M. Douglas Baker, MD
Pediatric Emergency Medicine
Yale-New Haven Children's Hospital
New Haven, Connecticut

Douglas A. Barnes, MD
Shriners Hospitals for Children
Houston, Texas

John P. Barrett, MD
Private Practitioner
Pittsburgh, Pennsylvania

Mary L. Brandt, MD
Baylor College of Medicine
Houston, Texas

Gerardo Cabrera-Meza, MD
Baylor College of Medicine
Houston, Texas

Sophia M. Chung, MD
Associate Professor
Department of Ophthalmology
St. Louis University School of Medicine
St. Louis, Missouri

Jayme Coffman, MD
Medical Director, C.A.R.E. Team
Cook Children's Medical Center
Fort Worth, Texas

Steven P. Cook, MD
Chief
Division of Pediatric Otolaryngology
Alfred I. duPont Hospital for Children
Wilmington, Delaware

Carrie Ann Cusack, MD
Department of Dermatology
Drexel University College of Medicine
Philadelphia, Pennsylvania

Christopher D. Derby, MD
Cardiothoracic Surgeon
Nemours Cardiac Center
Alfred I. duPont Hospital for Children
Wilmington, Delaware

Ellen Deutsch, MD
Division of Otolaryngology
Alfred I. duPont Hospital for Children
Wilmington, Delaware

Jan E. Drutz, MD
Baylor College of Medicine
Houston, Texas

Christine Finck, MD
Section of General Surgery
St. Christopher's Hospital for Children
Philadelphia, Pennsylvania

Brian Forbes, MD
The Children's Hospital of Philadelphia
Philadelphia, Pennsylvania

Martin Fried, MD
Jersey Shore Medical Center
Neptune, New Jersey

John A. Germiller, MD, PhD
Assistant Professor
Division of Pediatric Otolaryngology
The Children's Hospital of Philadelphia
Philadelphia, Pennsylvania

Bettina M. Gyr, MD
Staff Orthopaedic Surgeon
Shriners Hospitals for Children—
Twin Cities Unit
Minneapolis, Minnesota

Steven D. Handler, MD, MBE
Division of Pediatric Otolaryngology
The Children's Hospital of Philadelphia
Philadelphia, Pennsylvania

Fernando L. Heinen, MD
Deutsches Hospital of Buenos Aires
Buenos Aires, Argentina

Martin Herman, MD
Section of Orthopedic Surgery
St. Christopher's Hospital for Children
Philadelphia, Pennsylvania

Larry H. Hollier, Jr, MD
Baylor College of Medicine
Houston, Texas

Glenn Isaacson, MD
Temple University Health System
Temple University Children's Medical Center
Philadelphia, Pennsylvania

Douglas Katz, MD
Section of General Surgery
St. Christopher's Hospital for Children
Philadelphia, Pennsylvania

Kevin P. Lally, MD
University of Texas Medical Sciences Center
Houston, Texas

Michael Lemper, DDS
Department of Pediatric Dental Medicine
St. Christopher's Hospital for Children
Philadelphia, Pennsylvania

Moise L. Levy, MD
Baylor College of Medicine
Houston, Texas

Joseph Lopreiato, MD
Uniformed Services University of the Health Sciences
Bethesda, Maryland

Steven Manders, MD
Department of Dermatology
Cooper University Hospital
Cherry Hill, New Jersey

Gary Marshall, MD
University of Louisville
Louisville, Kentucky

Tony Olsen, MD
Senior Consultant
Department of Pediatrics
Naestved Hospital
Naestved, Denmark

William Phillips, MD
Baylor College of Medicine
Houston, Texas

Joseph Piatt, MD
Section of Neurosurgery
St. Christopher's Hospital for Children
Philadelphia, Pennsylvania

Kenneth Rosenbaum, MD
Children's National Medical Center
Children's Hospital
Washington, DC

Amy Ross, MD
Department of Dermatology
Drexel University College of Medicine
Philadelphia, Pennsylvania

Shriners Hospitals for Children
Houston, Texas

Philip Siu, MD
Chinatown Pediatric Services
Philadelphia, Pennsylvania

Sidney Sussman, MD
Department of Pediatrics
Cooper University Hospital
Cherry Hill, New Jersey

Tom Thacher, MD
Department of Family Medicine
Jos University Teaching Hospital
Jos, Nigeria

Scott T. VanDuzer, MD
Section of Plastic Surgery
St. Christopher's Hospital for Children
Philadelphia, Pennsylvania

Mark A. Ward, MD
Baylor College of Medicine
Houston, Texas

Seth Zwillenberg
Department of Otolaryngology
St. Christopher's Hospital for Children
Philadelphia, Pennsylvania

Contributors

Angela Allevi, MD
Assistant Professor
Department of Pediatrics
Thomas Jefferson University
Philadelphia, Pennsylvania
Staff Pediatrician
Department of Pediatrics
Alfred I. duPont Hospital for Children
Wilmington, Delaware

Lee R. Atkinson-McEvoy, MD
Assistant Clinical Professor
Department of Pediatrics
University of California, San Francisco
UCSF Children's Hospital
San Francisco, California

Robert L. Bonner, Jr., MD
Assistant Professor
Division of Ambulatory Pediatrics
Drexel University College of Medicine
Department of Pediatrics
St. Christopher's Hospital for Children
Philadelphia, Pennsylvania

Dean John Bonsall, MD, MS, FACS
Assistant Professor
Department of Ophthalmology
University of Cincinnati
Division of Pediatric Ophthalmology
Cincinnati Children's Hospital Medical Center
Cincinnati, Ohio

Julie A. Boom, MD
Assistant Professor
Department of Pediatrics
Baylor College of Medicine
Director
Immunization Project
Texas Children's Hospital
Houston, Texas

Mariam R. Chacko, MD
Professor
Pediatrics/Adolescent and Sports Medicine
Baylor College of Medicine
Attending Physician
Adolescent Medicine
Texas Children's Hospital
Clinical Care Center
Houston, Texas

Esther K. Chung, MD, MPH
Assistant Professor
Department of Pediatrics
Jefferson Medical College of Thomas Jefferson University
Jefferson Pediatrics/duPont Children's Health Program
Philadelphia, Pennsylvania
Alfred I. duPont Hospital for Children
Wilmington, Delaware

Kathleen Cronan, MD
Associate Professor
Department of Pediatrics
Jefferson Medical College of Thomas Jefferson University
Philadelphia, Pennsylvania
Chief
Division of Emergency Medicine
Alfred I. duPont Hospital for Children
Wilmington, Delaware

George A. Datto, III, MD
Instructor
Department of Pediatrics
Jefferson Medical College of Thomas Jefferson University
Philadelphia, Pennsylvania
Pediatrician
Department of Pediatrics
Alfred I. duPont Hospital for Children
Wilmington, Delaware

Allan R. De Jong, MD
Clinical Professor
Department of Pediatrics
Jefferson Medical College of Thomas Jefferson University
Philadelphia, Pennsylvania
Director
Children at Risk Evaluation Program
Alfred I. duPont Hospital for Children
Wilmington, Delaware

Gary A. Emmett, MD, FAAP
Clinical Associate Professor
Department of Pediatrics
Thomas Jefferson University
Director of General Pediatrics
Thomas Jefferson University Hospital
Philadelphia, Pennsylvania

T. Ernesto Figueroa, MD, FAAP, FACS
Clinical Associate Professor
Department of Urology
Thomas Jefferson University
Philadelphia, Pennsylvania
Chief
Division of Pediatric Urology
Alfred I. duPont Hospital for Children
Wilmington, Delaware

Vani V. Gopalareddy, MD
Attending Physician
Division of Pediatric Gastroenterology and Hepatology
Alfred I. duPont Hospital for Children
Wilmington, Delaware

William R. Graessle, MD
Assistant Professor
Department of Pediatrics
UMDNJ-Robert Wood Johnson Medical School, Camden
Director
Pediatric Medical Education
Department of Pediatrics
Cooper University Hospital
Camden, New Jersey

Maryellen E. Gusic, MD
Associate Dean for Clinical Education
Associate Professor
Division of General Pediatrics
Department of Pediatrics
Penn State College of Medicine
Penn State Children's Hospital
Hershey, Pennsylvania

Karina Irizarry, MD
Fellow
Department of Pediatric Gastroenterology,
Hepatology and Nutrition
University of Colorado at Denver and
Health Sciences Center
The Children's Hospital
Denver, Colorado

Aviva L. Katz, MD
Assistant Professor of Pediatrics
Department of General Surgery
Jefferson Medical College of Thomas Jefferson University
Philadelphia, Pennsylvania
Attending Pediatric Surgeon
Department of General Surgery
Alfred I. duPont Hospital for Children
Wilmington, Delaware

Shareen F. Kelly, MD
Assistant Professor
Department of Pediatrics
Drexel University College of Medicine
Ambulatory Pediatrics
St. Christopher's Hospital for Children
Philadelphia, Pennsylvania

Brandi M. Kenner, MD
Resident Physician
Department of Pediatrics
Baylor College of Medicine
Texas Children's Hospital
Houston, Texas

Hans B. Kersten, MD
Assistant Professor of Pediatrics
Division of Ambulatory Pediatrics
Drexel University College of Medicine
Department of Pediatrics
St. Christopher's Hospital for Children
Philadelphia, Pennsylvania

Aida Zarina Khanum, MD
Fellow
Academic General Pediatrics
Baylor College of Medicine
Texas Children's Hospital
Houston, Texas

Shirley P. Klein, MD, FAAP
Clinical Assistant Professor
Department of Pediatrics
Jefferson Medical College of Thomas Jefferson University
Philadelphia, Pennsylvania
Director
Pediatric Practice Program
Wilmington Hospital Health Center
Christiana Care Health System
Wilmington, Delaware

Susanne Kost, MD, FAAP
Associate Professor
Department of Pediatrics
Thomas Jefferson University
Philadelphia, Pennsylvania
Attending Physician
Division of Emergency Medicine
Alfred I. duPont Hospital for Children
Wilmington, Delaware

Kelly R. Leite, DO
Assistant Professor
Department of Pediatrics
Penn State College of Medicine
Division of General Pediatrics
Department of Pediatrics
Penn State Children's Hospital
Hershey, Pennsylvania

Paul S. Matz, MD
Assistant Professor
Department of Pediatrics
Drexel University College of Medicine
Attending Physician
Department of Pediatrics
St. Christopher's Hospital for Children
Philadelphia, Pennsylvania

Devendra I. Mehta, MBBS, MS, MRCP
Assistant Professor
Department of Pediatrics
Thomas Jefferson University
Philadelphia, Pennsylvania
NCMP/Pediatric Gastroenterologist
Department of Pediatrics
Nemours Children's Clinic—Orlando
Orlando, Florida

Shoshana Melman, MD
Associate Professor
Department of Pediatrics
Drexel University College of Medicine
Attending Physician
General Pediatrics
St. Christopher's Hospital for Children
Philadelphia, Pennsylvania

Denise W. Metry, MD
Assistant Professor
Departments of Dermatology and Pediatrics
Baylor College of Medicine
Clinic Chief
Departments of Dermatology and Pediatrics
Texas Children's Hospital
Houston, Texas

Colette C. Mull, MD
Assistant Professor
Departments of Emergency Medicine and Pediatrics
Drexel University College of Medicine
Director
Pediatric Emergency Medicine Fellowship
St. Christopher's Hospital for Children
Philadelphia, Pennsylvania

Heather E. Needham, MD
Assistant Professor
Department of Pediatrics
Baylor College of Medicine
Department of Pediatrics
Ben Taub General Hospital
Houston, Texas

Julieana Nichols, MD, MPH
Assistant Professor
Community and General Pediatrics
The University of Texas Health Science Center
at Houston
Clinical Staff
Department of Pediatrics
Memorial Hermann Hospital
Houston, Texas

Teresia O'Connor, MD
Clinical Postdoctoral Fellow
Department of Pediatrics
Baylor College of Medicine
Texas Children's Hospital
Houston, Texas

Christopher O'Hara, MD
Assistant Professor
Department of Pediatrics
Drexel University College of Medicine
Attending Pediatrician
Pediatric Generalist Service
St. Christopher's Hospital for Children
Philadelphia, Pennsylvania

Parul B. Patel, MD, FAAP
Fellow
Department of Pediatric Emergency Medicine
Thomas Jefferson University
Philadelphia, Pennsylvania
Alfred I. duPont Hospital for Children
Wilmington, Delaware

Charles A. Pohl, MD
Clinical Associate Professor
Department of Pediatrics
Jefferson Medical College of Thomas Jefferson University
Pediatrician
Jefferson Pediatrics/duPont Children's Health Program
Philadelphia, Pennsylvania

Erin Preston, MD
Instructor
Department of Pediatrics
Thomas Jefferson University
Philadelphia, Pennsylvania
Alfred I. duPont Hospital for Children
Wilmington. Delaware

Amy Renwick, MD
Attending Physician
General Pediatrics
Alfred I. duPont Hospital for Children
Wilmington, Delaware

Denise A. Salerno, MD, FAAP
Associate Professor
Department of Pediatrics
Temple University School of Medicine
Attending Physician
Department of Pediatrics
Temple University Children's Medical Center
Philadelphia, Pennsylvania

Harold V. Salvati, MD
Assistant Professor
Department of Pediatrics
Drexel University College of Medicine
Attending Pediatrician
Department of Pediatrics
St. Christopher's Hospital for Children
Philadelphia, Pennsylvania

Steven M. Selbst, MD
Professor
Department of Pediatrics
Jefferson Medical College of Thomas Jefferson University
Philadelphia, Pennsylvania
Vice Chair of Education
Pediatric Residency Program Director
Department of Pediatrics
Alfred I. duPont Hospital for Children
Wilmington, Delaware

Nicholas B. Slamon, MD
Fellow
Pediatric Critical Care
Department of Anesthesiology and Critical Care
Alfred I. duPont Hospital for Children
Wilmington, Delaware

Laura E. Smals, MD
Assistant Professor
Department of Pediatrics
Drexel University College of Medicine
Director of Medical Student Education
St. Christopher's Hospital for Children
Philadelphia, Pennsylvania

Nancy D. Spector, MD
Assistant Professor
Department of Pediatrics
Drexel University College of Medicine
Associate Residency Program Director
Department of Pediatrics
St. Christopher's Hospital for Children
Philadelphia, Pennsylvania

Sujata R. Tipnis, MD, MPH
Voluntary Faculty
Department of Pediatrics
University of Miami Miller School of Medicine
Miami, Florida
Staff Pediatrician
Department of Pediatrics
Sheridan Children's Healthcare Services
Parkway Regional Medical Center
North Miami, Florida

David E. Tunkel, MD
Associate Professor
Departments of Otolaryngology-Head and Neck
Surgery and Pediatrics
Johns Hopkins University School of Medicine
Director
Division of Pediatric Otolaryngology
Department of Otolaryngology-Head and
Neck Surgery
Johns Hopkins Hospital
Baltimore, Maryland

Renee M. Turchi, MD, MPH
Assistant Professor
Department of Pediatrics
Drexel University College of Medicine
Associate Director
Center for Children with Special Health Care Needs
Department of Pediatrics
Philadelphia, Pennsylvania

Cynthia Collier Warren, MD, FAAP
Assistant Professor
Department of Pediatrics
Drexel University College of Medicine
Medical Director
St. Christopher's Pediatric Associates,
Child and Adolescent Practice
St. Christopher's Hospital for Children
Philadelphia, Pennsylvania

Evan J. Weiner, MD, FAAP
Fellow
Department of Pediatric Emergency Medicine
University of Florida Health Science Center
Jacksonville, Florida

English D. Willis, MD
Associate Professor
Department of Pediatrics
Temple University School of Medicine
Philadelphia, Pennsylvania
Director
Pediatric Residency Program
Department of Pediatrics
Crozer Chester Medical Center
Upland, Pennsylvania

Michael J. Wilsey, Jr., MD
Clinical Assistant Professor
Department of Pediatrics
University of South Florida College of Medicine
Tampa, Florida
Attending Physician
Department of Pediatric Gastroenterology
All Children's Hospital
St. Petersburg, Florida

Jeoffrey K. Wolens, MD
Assistant Professor
Academic Medicine Section
Department of Pediatrics
Baylor College of Medicine
Chief of Pediatric Services
Department of Pediatrics
Shriners Hospitals for Children
Houston, Texas

Serena Yang, MD, MPH
Assistant Professor
Department of Pediatrics
Baylor College of Medicine
Attending Physician
Department of Pediatrics
Texas Children's Hospital
Houston, Texas

Terri L. Young, MD
Professor
Departments of Ophthalmology and Pediatrics
Duke University Medical Center
Duke University Hospital
Duke University Eye Center
Durham, North Carolina

Robert L. Zarr, MD, MPH, FAAP
Assistant Clinical Professor
School of Medicine and Health Sciences
George Washington University
Washington, DC

Ilia Zeltser, MD
Chief Resident
Department of Urology
Thomas Jefferson University
Chief Resident
Department of Urology
Thomas Jefferson University Hospital
Philadelphia, Pennsylvania

Foreword

Two lessons from the educators worth remembering but frequently overlooked apply to the development of a new venture: consider the audience and follow the objectives of the project. International visitors frequently remark how the United States is overtaken by the express concept whether it is fast foods, cable news trailers, or literature searches, we want information in a concise form that is readily accessible. Health care is no exception. The office visits are compressed by demands of both patients requesting appointments and health systems requiring more productivity. These cultural realities have influenced book designs—organize the material for rapid access and present the essential material.

To reach these goals, the editors considered the doctor or nurse in primary care who sees a patient's physical finding which he or she cannot identify or for which he or she seeks confirmation of a diagnosis. The editors first collected a comprehensive photo gallery and then organized the material by location, such as face, lower extremity, or skin. The reader can rapidly search that section to match a picture with a patient's problem. Then the authors created clarifying text to assist in differentiating between conditions that may have similar appearances. The suggestions of additional history, physical findings, and differential diagnoses guide the reader towards defining the patient's problem. This initial step may be sufficient or may then lead to consultation with other texts that contain more information about specific disease.

Since the objective of the book is to provide information rapidly to assist in making a visual diagnosis, the written material needs to be limited. The authors have succeeded in keeping focused on the assessment of the patient. The temptation to expand beyond the original objective of visual diagnosis haunted the developmental meetings but the editors held firm, changing the discussion to how to organize the material in a way that would be most useful to the readers.

This book succeeded in accomplishing the original goals of the editors and publishers to create a fresh and focused visual compendium of pediatric conditions that allows the reader to enter into the diagnostic process in an efficient way. The organization and contents of this book succeeds in the objective of improving the health of the patients. The editors and authors of the chapters are to be congratulated in producing this important reference. This volume is an important addition to the basic library of a primary care office, helping the patient get the best care possible.

—M. William Schwartz, MD
Professor Emeritus
Department of Pediatrics
University of Pennsylvania School of Medicine

Preface

Visual Diagnosis in Pediatrics is meant to provide clinicians with a rapid diagnostic tool composed of pearls or "key points" to the history and physical examination, and to offer an array of photographs not typically found in one written source. The organization of the **Table of Contents** progresses from head to toe, just as a clinician would approach the patient. **Sections** represent major parts of the body, and are made up of **Chapters** that reflect patients' chief complaints and problems. As an example, if a child presents with a swollen, red eye, the clinician might turn to the "Eye Swelling" and the "Red Eye" chapters to find clinical pearls and a collection of side-by-side photographs of potential diagnoses. To distinguish diagnoses that appear to be similar, each chapter contains a **Table** that highlights distinguishing characteristics for the most common diseases. In these differential diagnoses tables, we also alert clinicians to potential disease complications of missed or delayed diagnoses. For those interested in less common diseases, the **Other Diagnoses to Consider** section offers the reader a list of entities not shown or discussed in the chapter. **Suggested Readings** are provided at the end of each chapter.

Special recognition goes to the chapter authors and photographers, all seasoned clinicians, ranging from general pediatricians to pediatric subspecialists. Numerous contributors, representing medical institutions from across the country, have provided new and old photographs. This book would not have been possible without the generosity of so many—parents who allowed photographs to be taken of their children; clinicians with intellectual curiosity, motivation, and the desire to share their experiences; and experts who willingly shared CDs and who trustingly parted with irreplaceable slides and books. Phone calls and emails were exchanged at all hours of the day—at home, in restaurants, and even on vacation. What began as a mere conversation among colleagues blossomed into a unique collection of photographs and clinical pearls that we hope will help you in caring for your patients.

My special thanks goes to the Associate Editors, Julie Boom, George Datto, and Paul Matz, who carried out their responsibilities of finding authors, taking and gathering photographs, and completing the project on schedule, even when this meant sacrificing valuable time with family and friends. Dennis Lee, my husband, deserves particular thanks for his moral support, understanding, and selflessness. What an honor it has been to have Bill Schwartz as a consultant. His advice is always filled with wisdom, and his work is a true inspiration. The talented group at LWW—including Tim Hiscock, Anne Sydor, Nicole Dernoski, and Nicole Walz—facilitated the conceptual development of the book and organized the voluminous material that went into the making of this book. Thanks to Bridget Nelson and Liz Clemmons at Schawk for their frequent correspondence and unrelenting effort in producing this volume.

Our goal was to produce a book that will be a visual guide to clinicians as they encounter and care for pediatric patients, who bring new challenges to our days and show us many of life's lessons. SEE for yourself!

Table of Contents

Sections

ONE   General Appearance   1

1   General Appearance   3
Evan J. Weiner

TWO   Head   9

2   Scalp Swellings in Newborns   11
Hans B. Kersten

3   Newborn Physical Findings: Facial Lesions   16
Laura E. Smals

4   Abnormal Head Shape   22
Laura E. Smals

5   Hair Loss   28
George A. Datto, III

6   White Specks in the Hair   35
Hans B. Kersten

7   Lumps on the Face   40
Kelly R. Leite and Kathleen Cronan

THREE   Eyes   47

8   Red Eye   49
Parul B. Patel and Steven M. Selbst

9   Swelling of/Around the Eye   57
English D. Willis and Terri L. Young

10   Discoloration of/Around the eye   65
Maryellen E. Gusic and Dean John Bonsall

11   Pupil, Iris, and Lens Abnormalities   71
Renee M. Turchi and Esther K. Chung

12   Misalignment of the Eyes   79
Maryellen E. Gusic and Dean John Bonsall

FOUR **Ears** 85

13   Abnormalities in Ear Shape and Position   87
Charles A. Pohl

14   Ear Swelling   93
Kathleen Cronan

15   Ear Pits and Tags   99
Renee M. Turchi and David E. Tunkel

16   Ear Canal Findings   105
Lee R. Atkinson-McEvoy and Esther K. Chung

17   Tympanic Membrane Abnormalities   110
Charles A. Pohl

FIVE **Nose** 117

18   Nasal Bridge Swelling   119
Shoshana Melman

19   Nasal Swelling, Discharge, and Crusting   125
Shareen F. Kelly

SIX **Mouth** 131

20   Mouth Sores and Patches   133
Robert L. Bonner, Jr.

21   Focal Gum Lesions   139
Nancy D. Spector

22   Discoloration of the Teeth   145
Harold V. Salvati

23   Oral Clefts and Other Variants   150
Cynthia Collier Warren and Paul S. Matz

24   Tongue Discoloration and Surface Changes   157
Christopher O'Hara

25   Swellings Within the Mouth   163
Nancy D. Spector

26   Throat Redness   169
Robert L. Bonner, Jr.

SEVEN **Neck** 175

27   Neck Masses and Swelling   177
Serena Yang

EIGHT   Chest   185

28   Abnormal Chest Shape   187
     Amy Renwick

29   Breast Swelling and Enlargement   193
     Heather E. Needham and Mariam R. Chacko

30   Chest Lumps   198
     George A. Datto, III

NINE   Abdomen   205

31   Abdominal Midline Bulge   207
     Aviva L. Katz

32   Enlarged/Distended Abdomen   213
     Vani Gopalareddy and Devendra I. Mehta

TEN   Back   219

33   Curvature of the Back   221
     Shareen F. Kelly

34   Midline Back Pits, Skin Tags, Hair Tufts, and Other Lesions   227
     Paul S. Matz

ELEVEN   Extremities   233

35   Nail Abnormalities   235
     Denise W. Metry and Brandi M. Kenner

36   Arm Displacement   241
     Jeoffrey K. Wolens

37   Arm Swelling   246
     Teresia O'Connor

38   Hand Swelling   253
     Serena Yang

39   Finger Abnormalities   259
     Robert L. Zarr

40   Fingertip Swelling   265
     Julieana Nichols

41   Newborn Physical Findings: Lower Extremity Abnormalities   270
     Serena Yang

42   Leg Asymmetry   275
     Jeoffrey K. Wolens

43   Leg Bowing and Knock Knees   281
     Sujata R. Tipnis

44   Intoeing   287
Sujata R. Tipnis

45   Knee Swelling   293
Julie A. Boom

46   Foot Deformities   301
Sujata R. Tipnis

47   Foot Swelling   307
Aida Zarina Khanum

48   Foot Rashes and Lumps   313
Denise W. Metry and Brandi M. Kenner

TWELVE   Genital and Perineal Region   319

49   Female Genitalia—Variations   321
Colette C. Mull

50   Penile Abnormalities   329
T. Ernesto Figueroa and Ilia Zeltser

51   Penile Swelling   337
T. Ernesto Figueroa and Ilia Zeltser

52   Perineal Red Rashes   345
Kathleen Cronan

53   Perineal Sores and Lesions   351
Allan R. De Jong

54   Vulvar Swelling and Masses   359
Allan R. De Jong

55   Scrotal Swelling   365
William R. Graessle

THIRTEEN   Perianal Area and Buttocks   371

56   Perianal and Buttock Swelling   373
Karina Irizarry and Michael J. Wilsey, Jr.

57   Perianal and Buttock Redness   379
Robert L. Zarr

58   Imperforate Anus   384
Julieana Nichols

FOURTEEN   Skin   389

59   Newborn Physical Findings: Skin Abnormalities   391
Denise A. Salerno

60   Facial Rashes   399
Gary A. Emmett

61   Diffuse Red Rashes   407
Susanne Kost

62   Red Patches and Swellings   413
Nicholas B. Slamon

63   Linear Red Rashes   419
Erin Preston

64   Focal Red Bumps   425
George A. Datto, III

65   Raised Red Rashes   431
Kathleen Cronan

66   Vesicular Rashes   439
Shirley P. Klein

67   Nonblanching Rashes   445
William R. Graessle

68   Scaly Rashes   451
Esther K. Chung

69   Fine, Bumpy Rashes   459
George A. Datto, III

70   Hypopigmented Rashes   464
George A. Datto, III

71   Hyperpigmented Rashes   471
George A. Datto, III

72   Bullous Rashes   477
Angela Allevi

Index   485

General Appearance

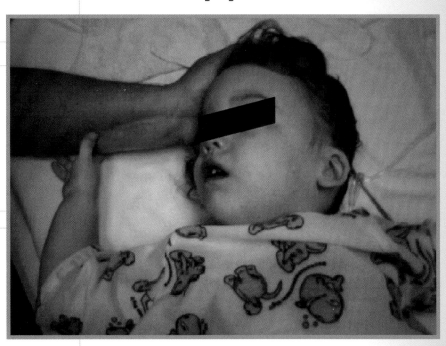

EVAN J. WEINER

General Appearance

APPROACH TO THE PROBLEM

A patient's general appearance is considered one of the most important elements of the physical examination. It represents a subjective observation of the patient's physical appearance and demeanor that allows for an assessment of his or her overall state of being. This observation consists of a general impression—ill-appearing, developmentally appropriate, and so forth—that is accompanied by detailed information, including the patient's degree of alertness, activity level, cry/phonation, respiratory effort, coloring, position/posture, nutritional status, hygiene, facial expression, body/facial morphology, movement/gait, stature, growth, development, intellect, ability to interact with others, and behavior.

KEY POINTS IN THE HISTORY

- Knowing whether the patient's general appearance on presentation reflects that noted by the parents is essential.

- When evaluating a febrile child, response to and timing of antipyretics, consolability, and willingness to feed are components of the history that help to distinguish severity of illness. Reevaluation after defervescence is also helpful.

- When pain is present, quantifying the degree of pain with the use of facial or numerical pain scales is preferred to subjective descriptions of pain.

- Knowing the child's baseline medical and developmental status will help guide the clinician's assessment, and is particularly helpful in assessing children with development delays or physical impairments.

- In the case of a critically ill or injured patient, elicit an AMPLE history—as described by Advanced Trauma Life Support (ATLS)—Allergies, Medications, Past medical history, Last meal, and preceding Events.

- A changing or inconsistent story, or one that is incompatible with the physical findings, raises the suspicion of child maltreatment.

- Loss of consciousness, seizure activity, fainting, cyanosis, nonresponsiveness, lethargy, pallor, night sweats, bilious emesis, and bleeding suggest increased severity and warrant further investigation.

KEY POINTS IN THE PHYSICAL EXAMINATION

- Elements of a very ill appearance include grunting; a weak or persistent cry; pale, cyanotic, or mottled skin; sunken eyes; dry mucous membranes; dulled social response; and depressed sensorium.

- A social smile is frequently present in patients with occult bacteremia, but it is rarely present in a young child with meningitis or other serious bacterial infections.

- Absent tears, dry mucus membranes, ill general appearance, and delayed capillary refill time are reliable external clues of dehydration.

- Irritability in an infant moved from an upright to a supine position may indicate congestive heart failure or esophagitis. Extreme irritability in an infant picked up from a lying position may indicate meningeal irritation or meningitis.

- Rapid breathing, nasal flaring, accessory muscle use, and apprehensive affect are signs of *respiratory distress*. Depressed sensorium and cyanosis are signs of *respiratory failure*.

- Children with epiglottitis classically appear toxic, and position themselves in a "tripod" position with the neck hyperextended. Muffled voice, drooling, and stridor may indicate an upper airway obstruction such as a retropharyngeal abscess or foreign body. Torticollis and trismus suggests a parapharyngeal process.

- A shock state can be clinically diagnosed by the presence of an altered sensorium, pale or mottled skin, peripheral cyanosis, tachypnea, or other evidence of poor organ perfusion. In septic shock, the skin may appear flushed.

- A patient with peritoneal irritation classically lies flat and still and does not want to be examined. A patient with colicky abdominal pain frequently appears restless and unable to find a comfortable position. Paroxysms of extreme irritability and drawing up of the legs, interspersed with periods of lethargy, may signify intussusception in a young child.

- Although pain is best assessed by patient self-reporting, observer clues to pain include moaning, crying, grimacing, whining, clinging, squirming, drawing up legs, arching, and shivering. In newborns, additional clues include brow bulging, eye squeezing, or nasolabial furrowing.

- A flattened affect may signify developmental delay, autism, sensory impairment, psychiatric disorders, or neglect.

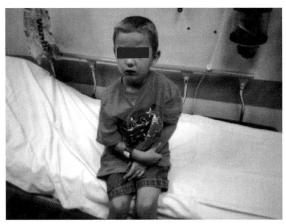

Figure 1-1 Well-appearing child with left supracondylar fracture. This well-appearing, but apprehensive, child's positioning informs of his supracondylar fracture of the left humerus. (Courtesy of Evan J. Weiner, MD.)

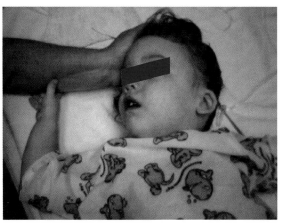

Figure 1-2 Ill-appearing child. This child appears weak and clingy, but alert and reactive. Her ill appearance is the result of a mucocutaneous form of mycoplasma infection. (Courtesy of Evan J. Weiner, MD.)

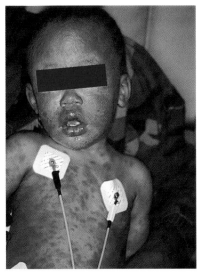

Figure 1-3 Ill-appearing child with Stevens-Johnson syndrome. (Courtesy of Joseph Lopreiato, MD.)

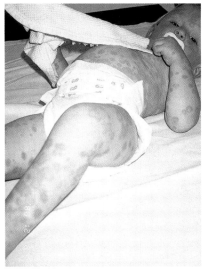

Figure 1-4 Ill-appearing child with urticaria. (Used with permission from Fleisher GR, Ludwig S, Baskin MN. *Atlas of pediatric emergency medicine.* Philadelphia: Lippincott Williams & Wilkins; 2004:88.)

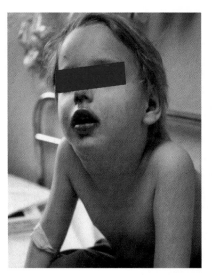

Figure 1-6 Epiglottitis and tripod positioning. This child's "tripod" positioning is indicative of epiglottitis. Note the child's toxic appearance. (Photo courtesy of M. Douglas Baker, MD.)

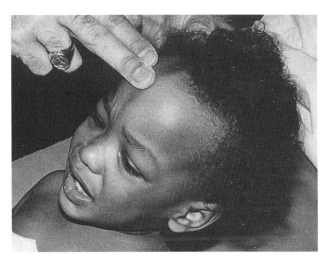

Figure 1-5 Meningitis. (Used with permission from Fleisher GR, Ludwig S, Baskin MN. *Atlas of pediatric emergency medicine.* Philadelphia: Lippincott Williams & Wilkins; 2004:183.)

DIFFERENTIAL DIAGNOSIS

DIAGNOSIS	ICD-9	DISTINGUISHING CHARACTERISTICS	DURATION/ CHRONICITY
Bacterial Meningitis	320.9	Altered sensorium Toxic appearance	Acute to subacute
Dehydration	276.5	Dry mucous membranes Absent tears Sunken eyes Lethargy	Acute to subacute
Congestive Heart Failure	428.0	Orthopnea Jugular venous distension Hepatomegaly Cyanosis	Subacute
Increased Intracranial Pressure	742.3 Hydrocephalus 959.01 Head injury	Depressed sensorium Bulging fontanelle Cushing's triad	Acute to subacute
Acute Abdomen	789.0 560.0 Intussusception	Abdominal tenderness Irritability	Acute
Respiratory Failure	518.81	Wheezing Stridor retractions Tachypnea cyanosis	Acute to subacute
Toxic Ingestion	960–989	Toxidrome Evidence of substance ingested	Acute

ASSOCIATED FINDINGS	COMPLICATIONS	PREDISPOSING FACTORS
Petechiae Nuchal rigidity Kernig/Brudzinski signs Emesis Seizures	Septic shock Multisystem organ failure Hearing loss	Immunocompromised individuals Immunization delay
Peripheral cyanosis Poor perfusion	Electrolyte disturbance Acidosis Renal failure Shock	Vomiting Diarrhea Hemorrhage Anorexia Polyuria
Growth failure Associated malformations Respiratory distress Edema Mottling/poor perfusion	Cardiac arrest Renal failure Hypoxia Shock	Congenital heart disease Cardiomyopathy Myocarditis Hypertension
Emesis Seizures Focal neurologic signs Apnea Sundowning	Cardiopulmonary arrest Traumatic brain injury	Trauma Hydrocephalus Tumor
Vomiting Dry mucous membranes Tachypnea	Sepsis Bowel perforation	Appendicolith Intestinal obstruction For intussusception: • Meckel's diverticulum • Viral illness
Apnea Depressed sensorium	Cardiopulmonary arrest	Infection Bronchospasm Upper airway obstruction Foreign body
Vomiting Depressed sensorium Aspiration/respiratory distress/apnea	Liver failure Aspiration Arrhythmia Neuronal injury	Lack of child-proofing/supervision Suicidality

OTHER
DIAGNOSES TO
CONSIDER

- Hepatic encephalopathy

- Toxic shock syndrome

- Severe anemia

- Uremia

- Adrenal crisis

- Inborn error of metabolism

- Neoplasm

- Failure to thrive

SUGGESTED READINGS

Athreya B, Silverman B. Subjective observations. In: *Pediatric physical diagnosis*. Norwalk, CT: Appleton-Century Crofts; 1985:58–70.

Barness L. General appearance, skin, and lymph nodes. In: *Manual of pediatric physical diagnosis*. 6th ed. Philadelphia: Mosby–Year Book; 1991:17–20.

Bass JW, Wittler RR, Weisse ME. Social smile and occult bacteremia. *Pediatr Infect Dis J*. 1996;15(6):541.

Fleisher GR, Ludwig S, Baskin MN. *Atlas of pediatric emergency medicine*. Philadelphia: Lippincott Williams & Wilkins; 2004:88,183.

Gorelick M, Shaw K, Murphy K. Validity and reliability of clinical signs in the diagnosis of dehydration in children. *Pediatrics*. 1997;99(5):E6.

McCarthy P, Sharpe M, Spiesel S, et al. Observation scales to identify serious illness in febrile children. *Pediatrics*. 1982;70(5):802–809.

Terndrup T. Pediatric pain control. *Ann Emerg Med*. 1996;27(4):466–470.

Section
TWO

Head

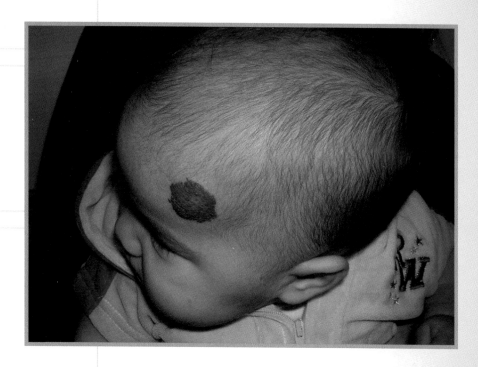

HANS B. KERSTEN

Scalp Swellings in Newborns

APPROACH TO THE PROBLEM

Most scalp swellings unique to newborns are related to the forces exerted on the head during the infants' passage through the birth canal. These problems are usually self-limited, and they resolve within a couple of days to weeks, although some may require close monitoring. Fixed abnormalities in skull shape may represent synostosis (see Abnormal Head Shape Chapter).

KEY POINTS IN THE HISTORY

- Molding and caput succedaneum are usually evident right after birth, but a cephalohematoma and subgaleal hemorrhage may take hours to form or become evident.

- Caput succedaneum results from local subcutaneous edema and fluid collection most commonly in the occipitoparietal region following a vaginal birth.

- Caput succedaneum and molding usually resolve in the first few days of life.

- Cephalohematoma is a hemorrhage that occurs between the periosteum and the skull bone.

- Cephalohematoma may take weeks to resolve.

- Five percent to twenty-five percent of patients with cephalohematoma have an accompanying skull fracture.

- Subgaleal hemorrhage is bleeding under the galea aponeurotica that may occur with significant birth trauma.

- There is an increased incidence of subgaleal hemorrhage with vacuum extraction.

KEY POINTS IN THE PHYSICAL EXAMINATION

- The swelling in caput succedaneum crosses suture lines because it is above the cranium in the subcutaneous tissue.

- Caputs, unlike cephalohematomas, tend to have pitting edema.

- Cephalohematomas are boggy and do not extend across suture lines because they are limited by the boundaries of the periosteum.

- There is no discoloration of the scalp with a cephalohematoma unless there is an overlying caput or bruising in the subcutaneous tissue.

- Subgaleal hematomas are considered fluctuant masses that cross suture lines, may be associated with a fluid wave or ecchymoses behind the ear, and may extend to other areas of the scalp.

- Infants with subgaleal hemorrhages must be observed in an intensive care nursery for progressive enlargement because the bleeding may be massive and associated with severe anemia and neonatal mortality.

- The ecchymoses that may be associated with caput succedaneum and the bleeding seen with cephalohematomas and subgaleal hematomas may contribute to neonatal jaundice.

DIFFERENTIAL DIAGNOSIS

DIAGNOSIS	ICD-9	DISTINGUISHING CHARACTERISTICS	DISTRIBUTION	ASSOCIATED FINDINGS	COMPLICATIONS
Molding	767.3	Overlapping bones along suture lines	Along suture lines	Caput succedaneum	Hemorrhage Fracture
Caput Succedaneum	767.1	Soft swelling that crosses suture lines	Occipitoparietal or diffuse swelling May see dependent edema on one side	Scalp ecchymoses Vertex delivery Vacuum suctioning	Hemorrhage Fracture Jaundice
Cephalohematoma	767.1	Swelling that does not cross suture lines Boggy feeling	Focal swelling Usually parietal area May be bilateral	Palpable rim Vacuum suctioning	Hemorrhage Skull fracture Jaundice Calcification
Subgaleal Hematoma	767.11	Fluctuant to tense swelling that crosses suture lines	Focal or diffuse swelling Ecchymoses behind ear Fluid wave	Vacuum suctioning	Hemorrhage Shock Severe anemia Death

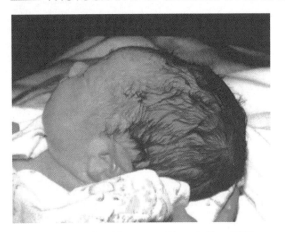

Figure 2-1 Molding. (Courtesy of Joseph Piatt, MD.)

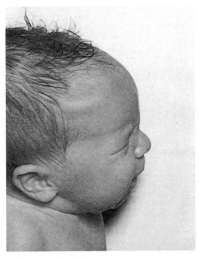

Figure 2-2 Caput succedaneum. Caput succedaneum shows pitting on pressure. (Used with permission from O'Doherty N. *Atlas of the newborn.* Philadelphia: JB Lippincott Co.; 1979:136.)

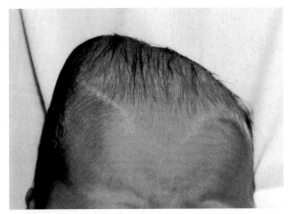

Figure 2-3 Cephalohematoma over the right parietal bone. (Used with permission from Fletcher, MA. *Physical diagnosis in neonatology.* Philadelphia: Lippincott–Raven Publishers, 1998:185.)

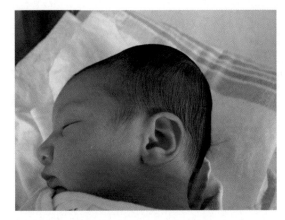

Figure 2-4 Cephalohematoma. Note the prominence of the left parieto-occipital area in this newborn with a cephalohematoma. (Courtesy of Esther K. Chung, MD.)

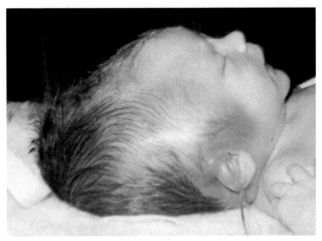

Figure 2-5 Subgaleal hematoma. A discoloration and swelling extends across suture lines onto the neck, even onto the ear, causing protuberance of the pinna. (Used with permission from Fletcher, MA. *Physical diagnosis in neonatology.* Philadelphia: Lippincott–Raven Publishers; 1998:185.)

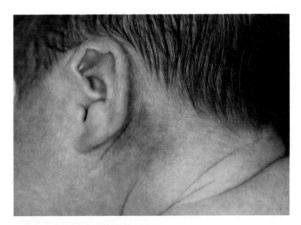

Figure 2-6 Ecchymosis after subgaleal hemorrhage. The bilateral location of this blood collection away from the site of application of forceps and crossing suture lines suggests a wide area of involvement typical of a moderately large subgaleal hematoma. (Used with permission from Fletcher, MA. *Physical diagnosis in neonatology.* Philadelphia: Lippincott–Raven Publishers; 1998:128.)

OTHER
DIAGNOSES TO
CONSIDER

- Plagiocephaly

- Skull fractures

- Porencephalic or leptomeningeal cyst

- Cranial meningocele

SUGGESTED READINGS

Bates B, ed. *A guide to physical examination and history taking.* 5th ed. Philadelphia: JB Lippincott Co; 1991:586–589.

Behrman RE, Kliegman RM, Jenson HB, eds. *Nelson textbook of pediatrics.* 16th ed. Philadelphia: WB Saunders; 2000:488–489.

Fletcher MA. *Physical diagnosis in neonatology.* Philadelphia: Lippincott–Raven Publishers; 1998:128,173–185.

McMillan JA, DeAngelis CD, Feigin RD, Warshaw JB, eds. *Oski's pediatrics: principles and Practice.* 3rd ed. Philadelphia: Lippincott Williams & Wilkins; 1999;163:610–611.

O'Doherty N. *Atlas of the newborn.* Philadelphia: JB Lippincott Co, 1979:136.

Rudolph CD, Rudolph AM, Hostetter MK, Siegel NJ, eds. *Rudolph's pediatrics.* 21st ed. New York: McGraw-Hill, 2003;87:186–187.

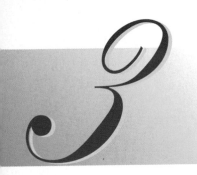

LAURA E. SMALS

Newborn Physical Findings: Facial Lesions

**APPROACH TO
THE PROBLEM**

Lesions on the face of a newborn may be the result of congenital malformations, birthmarks, or common skin rashes such as seborrhea and neonatal acne. These lesions are usually benign, but at times, they may represent underlying pathology. Familiarity with the appearance of various newborn facial lesions will enable the physician to allay parental fears and to provide appropriate recommendations.

**KEY POINTS IN
THE HISTORY**

- A reddish lesion that has been present since birth indicates a congenital lesion such as a nevus simplex (salmon patch, stork bite, angel's kiss) or nevus flammeus (port-wine stain).

- Pruritus suggests infantile eczema.

- When assessing lesions that have been present since birth, it is essential to ask about the infant's delivery to determine whether incidental trauma or trauma from the use of forceps may be contributing factors.

- A rash that spreads from the scalp to the face in early infancy may indicate seborrhea (also known as *cradle cap*).

KEY POINTS IN
THE PHYSICAL
EXAMINATION

- An erythematous patch on the forehead, eyelids, or nape of the neck is likely to be a nevus simplex.

- A deeply red-purplish patch is most likely to be a nevus flammeus, or port-wine stain.

- Erythematous pustules on the cheeks at 2 to 4 weeks of life suggest neonatal acne.

- Yellowish, shiny plaques on the scalp and face, particularly involving the brow, are most likely seborrhea.

- Dry, scaly pustules, papules, and plaques are seen in infantile eczema.

- In young infants with eczema, a circular collection of papules may be seen and, at times, be mistaken for tinea corporis.

- Multiple small, yellow papules on the nose of a newborn are likely sebaceous hyperplasia, a self-limited benign finding often mistaken for milia.

- Eczema tends to spare the nasolabial folds and skin folds behind the ear, but seborrhea does not.

DIFFERENTIAL DIAGNOSIS

DIAGNOSIS	ICD-9	DISTINGUISHING CHARACTERISTICS	DISTRIBUTION	ASSOCIATED FINDINGS	COMPLICATONS
Nevus Simplex (Salmon Patch)	757.38	Erythematous macular patch present at birth that generally fades with time Represents dilated capillaries	Nape of neck, forehead, and eyelids	Will darken in color with Valsalva (crying, etc.) maneuver	None
Nevus Flammeus (Port-Wine Stain)	757.32	Begins as pink-red macular patch that darkens and becomes more purple (port-wine colored) with time Dilated superficial and deep capillaries	Most commonly face and neck, but may occur anywhere Typically unilateral	TB-BL • If involving the ophthalmic branch (V1) of the trigeminal nerve, must evaluate for Sturge Weber syndrome • Ipsilateral glaucoma • Port-wine stains may be seen in other syndromes, including: Klippel-Trenaunay, Beckwith-Wiedemann, and Cobb syndromes	None
Neonatal Acne	706.1	Closed comedomes, occasionally open comedomes, pustules, and papules Rarely requires treatment—usually resolves within 1–3 months	Forehead, nose, and cheeks	Secondary to maternal hormone stimulation	None
Sebaceous Hyperplasia	706.9	1–2 mm yellow papules Resolves spontaneously within 4–6 months	Nose and cheeks of young infants	Secondary to hormonal stimulation	None
Infantile Eczema	690.12	Erythematous papules, pustules, plaques, with crusting and scale	Face, scalp, anywhere on the body—tends to spare the diaper area	Pruritus and excoriation	Superinfection
Forceps Marks	763.2	Linear or curvilinear marks	Sides of face and skull	Indentation Abrasion	Very rarely may be associated with skull fracture
Seborrhea	706.3	Yellowish, greasy plaques with scale Erythematous papules	Scalp, face, behind ears, and in folds of neck	Irritation	Superinfection

PHOTOGRAPHS OF SELECTED DIAGNOSES

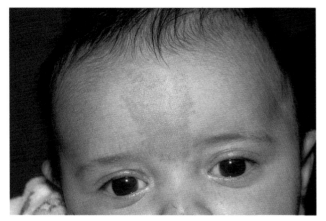

Figure 3-1 Nevus simplex (salmon patch). (Used with permission from Goodheart HP. *Goodheart's photoguide of common skin disorders.* 2nd ed. Philadelphia: Lippincott Williams & Wilkins; 2003:1.)

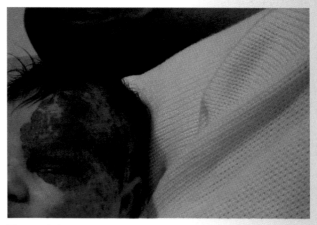

Figure 3-2 Nevus flammeus (port-wine stain). (Courtesy of Brian Forbes, MD.)

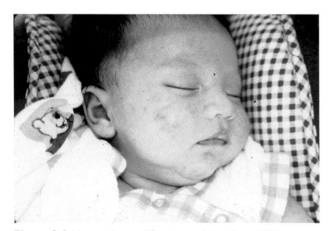

Figure 3-3 Neonatal acne. (Courtesy of Amy Ross, MD.)

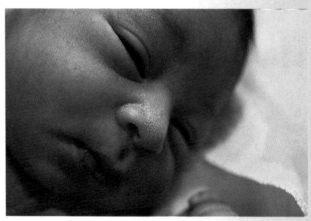

Figure 3-4 Sebaceous hyperplasia. (Courtesy of George A. Datto, III, MD.)

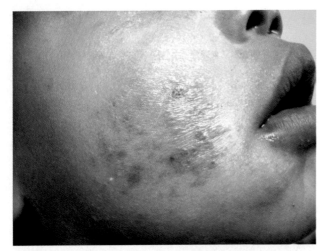

Figure 3-5 Infantile eczema. (Courtesy of Paul S. Matz, MD.)

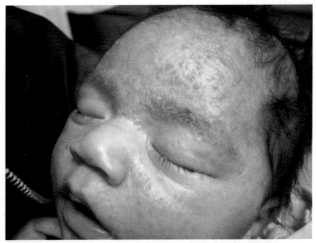

Figure 3-7 Seborrhea. (Courtesy of Paul S. Matz, MD.)

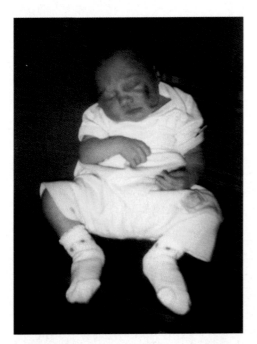

Figure 3-6 Forceps marks. (Courtesy of John P. Barrett, MD.)

OTHER
DIAGNOSES TO
CONSIDER

- Milia

- Miliaria rubra or crystallina

- Herpes simplex virus

- Telangiectasia

SUGGESTED READINGS

Cohen B. *Pediatric dermatology*. London: Mosby-Wolfe; 1993:2.6–2.9.

Conlon JD, Drolet BA. Skin lesions in the neonate. *Pediatr Clin North Am*. 2004;51:863–888.

Goodheart HP. *Goodheart's photoguide of common skin disorders*. 2nd ed. Philadelphia: Lippincott Williams & Wilkins; 2003:1.

Habif TP. *Clinical dermatology: a color guide to diagnosis and therapy*. 4th ed. St. Louis: C.V. Mosby; 2003:819–823.

Hurwitz S. *Clinical pediatric dermatology: a textbook of skin disorders of childhood and adolescence*. 2nd ed. Philadelphia: WB Saunders; 1993:12–17, 45–60, 247–249.

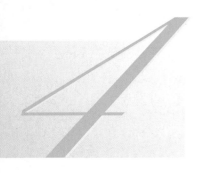

LAURA E. SMALS

Abnormal Head Shape

APPROACH TO THE PROBLEM

Abnormal head shape may be the result of genetic disorders, metabolic abnormalities, or improper positioning of the head. The shaping of the skull can be disrupted by internal, external, or intrinsic forces. *Internal* forces include abnormalities of the brain and surrounding tissues such as hydrocephalus or a Dandy-Walker malformation. *External* forces include intrauterine compression or abnormal positioning of the head secondary to torticollis. *Intrinsic* forces include craniosynostosis or premature closure of one or more cranial sutures. Any disruption in these forces can lead to an abnormal head shape, and possibly, abnormal neurological development.

KEY POINTS IN THE HISTORY

- Prematurity may lead to dolichocephaly because of positional molding in the hospital.

- Perinatal injury or trauma may cause intracranial bleeding and can lead to hydro-cephalus.

- Prolonged labor can result in severe molding of the skull.

- History of intrauterine fibroids or oligohydramnios can lead to cranial compression and abnormal head shape at birth.

- An abnormal developmental history may indicate abnormal brain development.

- History of vomiting and poor head control can be signs of increased intracranial pressure.

- History of head tilt to one side and flattening of one side of the head may be a sign of congenital torticollis.

- Positional plagiocephaly, along with a history of the child lying in the crib for a majority of the day, may indicate neglect.

KEY POINTS IN THE PHYSICAL EXAMINATION

- When assessing the head shape, it is best to look at the top of the head from above.

- Measure head circumference to see whether macrocephaly or microcephaly is present in addition to abnormal head shape.

- Alopecia along a "flattened" area of the skull may be seen.

- In craniosynostosis, the smaller or flattened side of the skull is where the suture has prematurely fused (Fig. 4.1). Cloverleaf skull occurs as the result of multiple suture synostosis and is rare (Fig. 4.10).

- Dysmorphic features may indicate a genetic syndrome as the cause of a craniosynostosis.

- Facial asymmetry may be noted in plagiocephaly or craniosynostosis.

DIFFERENTIAL DIAGNOSIS

DIAGNOSIS	ICD-9	DISTINGUISHING CHARACTERISTICS	DISTRIBUTION	ASSOCIATED FINDINGS	COMPLICATIONS
Positional Plagiocephaly	754.0	Flattened area of skull with history of lying with head in one position routinely	Usually posterior occiput Can be on one side of skull, especially when associated with torticollis	Alopecia in area of flattening	Facial asymmetry Poor cosmetic appearance
Brachycephaly	756.0	Broad head with recessed forehead secondary to premature closure of coronal suture	Shortened anterior-posterior (AP) diameter	More common in girls	If untreated, can compromise orbits and globe resulting in loss of vision
Craniosynostosis	756.0	Abnormal head shape secondary to premature closure of one or more cranial sutures	Will vary with type	Mental retardation when complete (all sutures affected) May be associated with certain syndromes (e.g., Apert syndrome)	Increased ICP, mental retardation, visual and hearing deficits if complete craniosynostosis is not detected
Dolichocephaly	754.0	Long and narrow skull secondary to premature closure of sagittal suture	Elongation of AP diameter	More common in boys. May occur in premature infants without synostosis because of positional molding	Poor cosmetic appearance
Trigonocephaly	756.0	"Keel shaped" or triangular shaped head secondary to premature closure of metopic suture	Frontal forehead area	Hypertelorism	May also be associated with mental retardation, urinary tract abnormalities, cleft palate, coloboma, and holoprosencephaly

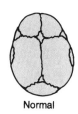

Normal

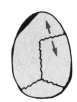

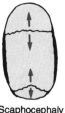

Trigonocephaly
(metopic)

Brachycephaly
(coronal, metopic)

Frontal plagiocephaly
(unilateral coronal)

Occipital plagiocephaly
(unilateral lambdoid)

Scaphocephaly
(sagittal)

Figure 4-1 Skull shapes associated with craniosynostosis. The heavy line denotes the area of maximal flattening. The arrows indicate the direction of continued growth across the sutures that remain open. (Used with permission from Fletcher MA. *Physical diagnosis in neonatology.* Philadelphia: Lippincott–Raven; 1998:186.)

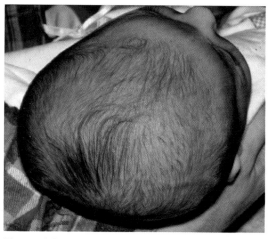

Figure 4-2 Positional plagiocephaly. (Courtesy of Joseph Piatt, MD.)

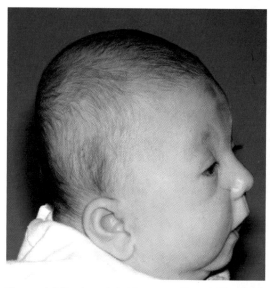

Figure 4-3 Brachycephaly. (Courtesy of Joseph Piatt, MD.)

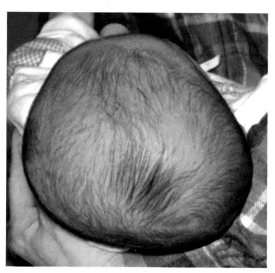

Figure 4-4 Lambdoid synostosis. (Courtesy of Joseph Piatt, MD.)

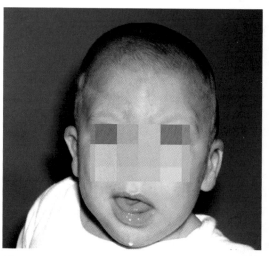

Figure 4-5 Metopic synostosis. (Courtesy of Joseph Piatt, MD.)

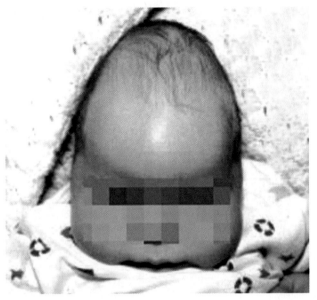

Figure 4-6 Sagittal synostosis. (Courtesy of Joseph Piatt, MD.)

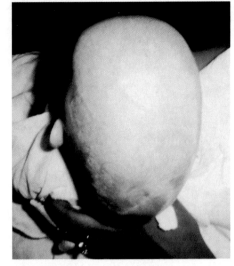

Figure 4-8 Dolichocephaly (scaphocephaly), top view. Marked increase in head length with narrowed width resulting from premature fusion of sagittal suture. Premature infants allowed to remain with the head in a side-lying position develop scaphocephalic changes but with more flattening of the sides or sides of the skull. (Used with permission from Fletcher MA. *Physical diagnosis in neonatology.* Philadelphia: Lippincott–Raven; 1998:186.)

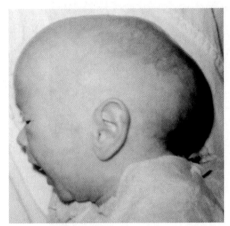

Figure 4-7 Dolicocephaly (scaphocephaly), side view. (Used with permission from Fletcher MA. *Physical diagnosis in neonatology.* Philadelphia: Lippincott–Raven; 1998:188.)

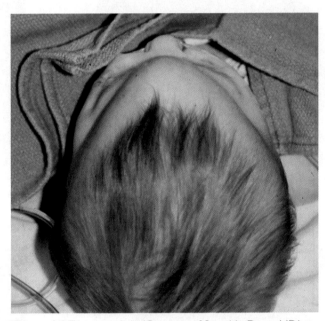

Figure 4-9 Trigonocephaly. (Courtesy of Scott VanDuzer, MD.)

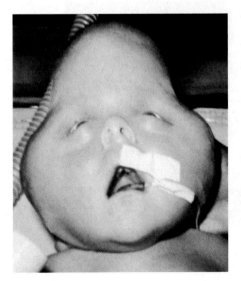

Figure 4-10 Cloverleaf skull (kleeblattschadel) caused by craniosynostosis of all sutures forcing brain growth through the anterior and temporal fontanels. This most severe form of restricted skull growth has the poorest prognosis because of a combination of craniostenosis and hydrocephalus. (Used with permission from Fletcher MA. *Physical diagnosis in neonatology.* Philadelphia: Lippincott–Raven; 1998:186.)

- Dandy-Walker malformation

- Cerebral agenesis

- Hydrocephalus

Diseases associated with craniosynostosis:

- Ataxia-telangiectasia

- Hyperthyroidism

- Mucopolysaccharidoses

- Sickle cell disease

- Thalassemia major

Syndromes associated with craniosynostosis:

- Antley Bixler

- Apert

- Baller Gerold

- Carpenter

- Crouzon

SUGGESTED READINGS
Fletcher MA. *Physical diagnosis in neonatology*. Philadelphia: Lippincott–Raven;1998:186.
Gartner JC, Zitelli BJ. *Common and chronic symptoms in pediatrics*. St. Louis: C.V. Mosby; 1997:102–109.
Peitsch WK, Keefer CH, LaBrie RA, Mulliken JB. Incidence of cranial asymmetry in healthy newborns. *Pediatrics*. 2002;110:72.
Ridgway EB, Weiner HL. Skull deformities. *Pediatr Clin North Am*. 2004;51(2):359–387.
Rohan AJ, Golombek SG, Rosenthal AD. Infants with misshapen skulls: when to worry. *Contemp Pediatr*. 1999;16:47–70.

GEORGE A. DATTO, III

Hair Loss

APPROACH TO THE PROBLEM

Hair loss may result from several disorders such as metabolic abnormalities, infectious processes, inflammatory conditions, and hair shaft defects. Though hair loss may occur in isolation, it may be a sign of a more widespread systemic illness. Any process that disrupts the growth cycle of the hair or causes structural damage to the follicle or shaft may result in hair loss. Hair loss can be quite distressing to both the parent and child.

KEY POINTS IN THE HISTORY

• Tight braiding of a child's hair is a common reason for hair loss (traction alopecia).

• Tinea capitis, though uncommon in white children, is the leading cause of hair loss in African American children.

• The presence of scale in the scalp may not be appreciated if the parents are using hair grease or other oily preparations.

• Significant illness in the past 3 months may cause the hair to enter the telogen phase, resulting in diffuse hair loss that becomes most evident when combing or washing.

• Children with systemic symptoms may have hair loss as a manifestation of more serious disease.

• Children with anxiety or obsessive-compulsive symptoms may manifest their disease by pulling at their hair when under psychological stress.

KEY POINTS IN THE PHYSICAL EXAMINATION

- The geographic distribution of hair loss is often a clue to its etiology.

- Diffuse hair loss is often associated with systemic disease.

- Significant scalp erythema in the area of hair loss is unusual in pediatrics and should prompt a referral to a dermatologist.

- Tinea capitis does not always present as hair loss and, at times, may present as scalp dryness. A fungal scalp culture can help to distinguish tinea capitis from other dry scalp lesions.

- Seborrhea dermatitis is not a common disease in a prepubertal child outside of early infancy.

- The black dot sign refers to the breakage of hair shafts close to the scalp.

- Hair shafts that have broken away from the scalp may be caused by braiding and hair pulling or intrinsic hair shaft defects.

- Scalp pustules, sterile abscesses, and kerions are host inflammatory responses to tinea and usually do not represent bacterial superinfection.

- Wood's lamp examination will produce a yellow-green fluorescence for Microsporum dermatophyte species but not Trichophyton (species accounting for 90% of tinea capitis.)

- The oval areas of hair loss in alopecia areata are often located in the parietal or occipital area of the scalp.

- A telogen hair has a depigmented bulb at its base.

DIFFERENTIAL DIAGNOSIS

DIAGNOSIS	ICD-9	DISTINGUISHING CHARACTERISTICS	DISTRIBUTION
Tinea Capitis	110.0	Scaly scalp with alopecia Black dot sign	Focal Diffuse—may appear similar to seborrhea
Traction Alopecia	704.0	Thinned hair at braid margins	Focal Most pronounced at margins of braids
Telogen Effluvium	704.02	Sudden loss of hair with brushing or washing	Diffuse
Alopecia Areata	704.01	Smooth scalp in areas of hair loss Sharp borders Peach hue to scalp	Parietal Occipital
Trichotrillomania	312.39	Broken hair shafts of varying lengths Irregular borders	Crown of head Occipital Parietal
Sebaceous Nevus of Jadassohn	706.9	Waxy orange nevus Congenital	Focal
Cutis Aplasia	709.3	Congenital Oval area of hair loss	Midline of scalp near sagittal suture
Discoid Lupus	695.4	Erythematous scalp with adherent scale	Focal

ASSOCIATED FINDINGS	COMPLICATIONS	PREDISPOSING FACTORS
Occipital and postauricular adenopathy Id reaction that may become more prominent with treatment	Kerion	*Trichophyton tonsurans* African American and Hispanic children
Small inflammatory papules Regional lymphadenopathy	Scarring of hair follicles	Tight braids or ponytails
N/A	N/A	Acute illness 6 weeks to 3 months prior to hair loss
Eyebrow hair loss Nail changes Can be associated with autoimmune disease	N/A	Autoimmune pathogenesis Atopy
Anxious child Obsessive-compulsive disorder	Trichophagy with associated bezoars	Expression of underlying psychiatric disorder
N/A	Potential for basal cell carcinoma	N/A
Can be seen with a wide variety of congenital anomalies	Permanent scarring with hair loss	N/A
Similar lesions on sun-exposed skin	Scarring leading to permanent hair loss	Autoimmune pathogenesis

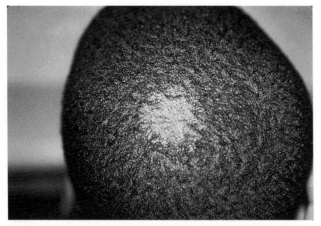

Figure 5-1 Tinea capitis. Circumscribed area of hair loss with scaliness of scalp. (Courtesy of George A. Datto, III, MD.)

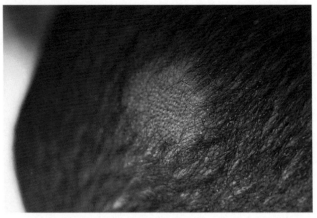

Figure 5-2 Black dot sign. Broken hair shafts at scalp give appearance of black dots on scalp. (Courtesy of George A. Datto, III, MD.)

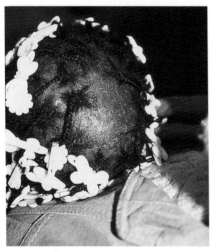

Figure 5-3 Kerion. Intense inflammatory response to tinea capitis. Significant hair loss with inflammatory pustules of scalp. (Courtesy of George A. Datto, III, MD.)

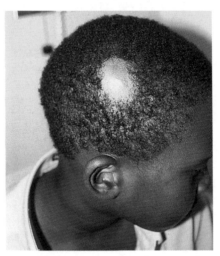

Figure 5-4 Alopecia areata. (Courtesy of George A. Datto, III, MD.)

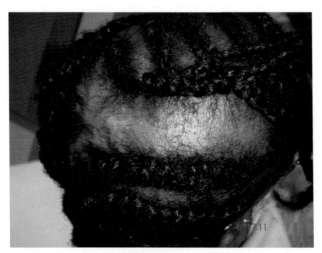

Figure 5-5 Traction alopecia. Alopecia where traction has been applied in association with hair brading. (Courtesy of Carrie Ann Cusack, MD.)

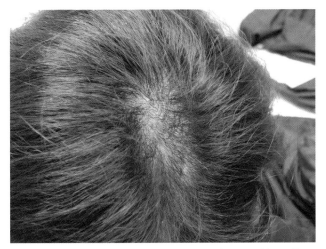

Figure 5-6 Trichotrillomania. Broken hair shafts caused by pulling at hair. (Courtesy of George A. Datto, III, MD.)

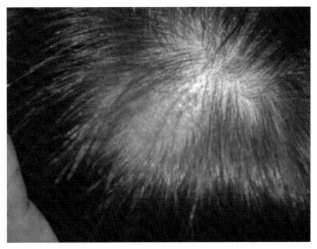

Figure 5-7 Sebaceous nevus of Jadassohn. (Courtesy of Department of Dermatology, Drexel University College of Medicine.)

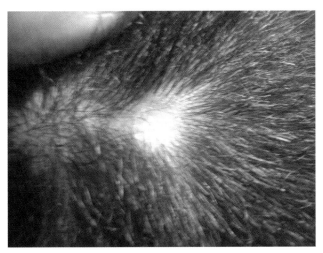

Figure 5-8 Cutis aplasia. Scar on vertex of scalp with complete hair loss secondary to cutis aplasia. (Courtesy of Paul S. Matz, MD.)

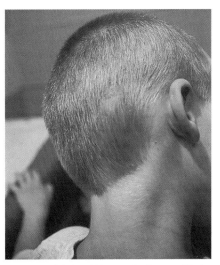

Figure 5-9 Discoid lupus. Oval area of hair loss associated with scalp erythema, scaling, and follicular plugging. (Courtesy of George A. Datto, III, MD.)

OTHER
DIAGNOSES TO
CONSIDER

- Monilethrix

- Pili torti

- Menkes syndrome

- Trichorrhexis nodosa

SUGGESTED READINGS

Al Soagir S, Hay JR. Fungal infection in children: tinea capitis. *Clin Dermatol.* 2000;18(6):679–685.

Harrison S. Optimal management of hair loss (alopecia) in children. *Am J Clin Dermatol.* 2003;4(11):757–770.

Wade MS. Disorders of hair in infants and children other than alopecia. *Clin Dermatol.* 2002;20(1):16–28.

HANS B. KERSTEN

White Specks in the Hair

APPROACH TO THE PROBLEM

White specks in the hair often are a manifestation of diseases involving the scalp, although they may result from infestations in the hair. White specks in the hair do not usually occur in isolation, so it is important to identify involvement of the disease process on the scalp and other parts of the body. Once properly identified, white specks in the hair can be treated effectively.

KEY POINTS IN THE HISTORY

- Seborrheic dermatitis is common in infants and may also occur during puberty.

- Seborrheic dermatitis in infants usually resolves by 7 to 8 months of age and is not typically itchy.

- Children with atopic dermatitis often have a family history of atopy.

- Tinea capitis is a common cause of white specks in the hair and/or alopecia in African American children, but it is uncommon in white children.

- Tinea capitis is acquired through personal contact with spores from the lesion.

- Head lice infestation is usually a disease of school-aged children, particularly girls.

- Head lice and atopic dermatitis cause itching of the scalp.

- Head lice are acquired through close contact with an infested person or contact with infested items such as hats, headsets, combs, brushes, and bed sheets.

KEY POINTS IN THE PHYSICAL EXAMINATION

- Seborrheic dermatitis is characterized by greasy, scaly, yellowish, or salmon-colored lesions on the scalp. Lesions may also appear on the face, eyebrows, neck, shoulders, intertriginous areas, flexural areas of the extremities, or diaper area.

- Atopic dermatitis may also involve the face and trunk, but the rash usually has popliteal and antecubital involvement that can help distinguish it from seborrheic dermatitis.

- With tinea capitis, round patches of inflammation with scale and alopecia are typical.

- Occipital lymphadenopathy is commonly seen with tinea capitis.

- Diffuse tinea capitis may resemble seborrheic dermatitis.

- Wood's lamp examination will produce a yellow-green fluorescence for Microsporum *dermatophyte* species but not Trichophytan species (which accounts for 90% of tinea capitis).

- The nits from head lice are attached firmly to the hair shaft, are difficult to remove by hand, and may be confused with dandruff.

- The lesions of atopic dermatitis usually merge into the surrounding skin, whereas the lesions of seborrheic dermatitis usually are well circumscribed.

- With head lice, the scalp is normal in appearance. With atopic dermatitis, seborrheic dermatitis, and tinea capitis, there is scaling on the scalp.

- Scales on the scalp may not be appreciated if family members are applying hair grease or other oily preparations to the scalp.

DIFFERENTIAL DIAGNOSIS

DIAGNOSIS	ICD–9	DISTINGUISHING CHARACTERISTICS	DISTRIBUTION	ASSOCIATED FINDINGS	COMPLICATIONS
Tinea Capitis	110.0	Scaly scalp Black dot sign	Focal or diffuse	Adenopathy Id reaction—papulovesicular rash on trunk	Kerion—a boggy, edematous inflammatory reaction to tinea capitis Hair loss
Seborrhea	706.3	Greasy, yellowish scale Young infants and adolescents Well-circumscribed lesions Rash on scalp, diaper, or intertriginous areas Generally not itchy Localized cradle cap	Focal or diffuse	Rash involving the face, eyebrows, neck, shoulders, flexural and intertriginous areas of the extremities, and/or diaper area	Candidal infections in intertriginous areas
Eczema	692.9	Always itchy Fluctuating course Rash distribution changes with age Generally worse in the winter time	Diffuse	Diffusely dry skin Lichenification Dermatographism Atopic diseases Hyperaccentuated palmar creases	Secondary infection Bleeding Lichenification
Head Lice (Pediculosis Capitis)	132.0	Difficult to dislodge from hair shaft Nits right next to scalp Lice on scalp Normal scalp	Diffuse nits in hair Nape of neck	Lice on scalp or in hair Normal scalp	None

PHOTOGRAPHS OF SELECTED DIAGNOSES

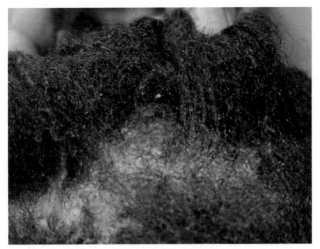

Figure 6-1 Tinea capitis. (Courtesy of Paul S. Matz, MD.)

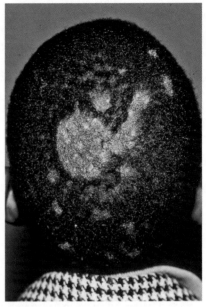

Figure 6-2 Tinea capitis. (Courtesy of Paul S. Matz, MD.)

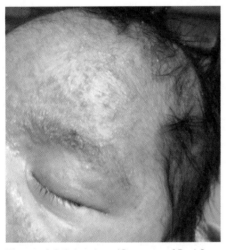

Figure 6-3 Seborrhea. (Courtesy of Paul S. Matz, MD.)

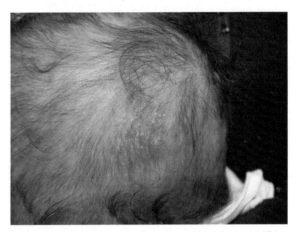

Figure 6-4 Scalp eczema. (Courtesy of Paul S. Matz, MD.)

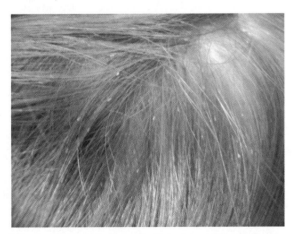

Figure 6-5 Pediculosis capitis. Note the whitish nits found along the hair shafts. (Courtesy of Hans B. Kersten, MD.)

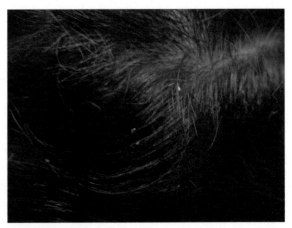

Figure 6-6 Pediculosis capitis. (Courtesy of Hans B. Kersten, MD.)

OTHER
DIAGNOSES TO
CONSIDER

- Acrodermatitis enteropathica

- Wiskott Aldrich syndrome

- Letterer-Siwe disease

- Psoriasis

- Impetigo

SUGGESTED READINGS

Ahuja A, Land K, Barnes CJ. Atopic dermatitis. *South Med J.* 2003;96:1068–1072.

Chen BK, Friedlander SF. Tinea capitis update: a continuing conflict with an old adversary. *Curr Opin Pediatr.* 2001;13:331–335.

Gupta AK, Bluhm R. Seborrheic dermatitis. *J Eur Acad Dermatol Venereol.* 2004;18:13–26.

Paller AS, Mancini AJ. *Hurwitz Clinical pediatric dermatology: a textbook of skin disorders of childhood and adolescence.* 3rd ed. Philadelphia: Elsevier Saunders; 2006:49–64, 67–69, 451–455, 488–491.

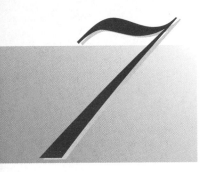

KELLY R. LEITE AND KATHLEEN CRONAN

Lumps on the Face

APPROACH TO THE PROBLEM

Lumps on a child's face may provoke anxiety in the child and the child's parents. Many of these diagnoses do not require immediate therapy, but it is important to correctly identify lesions that require urgent medical attention. The more common pediatric facial lesions include dermoid cysts, epidermoid cysts, hemangiomas, buccal cellulitis, panniculitis, fat necrosis, pyogenic granuloma, mumps, and suppurative parotitis.

KEY POINTS IN THE HISTORY

- Hemangiomas and dermoid cysts are present at birth or appear during early infancy.

- Epidermoid cysts can appear at any age but more commonly appear after puberty.

- Associated constitutional symptoms, such as fever and malaise, may suggest mumps, suppurative parotitis, or buccal cellulitis.

- A lump without pain or other symptoms is likely to be a dermoid cyst, epidermoid cyst, fat necrosis, or a hemangioma.

- A history of bleeding after minor trauma suggests a pyogenic granuloma.

- Patients with a pyogenic granuloma or fat necrosis may report a history of trauma.

- A lesion that enlarges during the first year of life then involutes supports the diagnosis of hemangioma.

- Recent prolonged exposure to cold objects suggests (popsicle) panniculitis.

- A history of recurrent parotid swelling or a family history of parotid swelling may indicate juvenile recurrent parotitis, nonsuppurative parotid inflammation of unknown etiology.

- Mumps should be suspected in an unimmunized child with parotid inflammation.

- Chronic, nonpainful swelling of the parotid gland may be seen in patients with human immunodeficiency virus (HIV) infection.

KEY POINTS IN THE PHYSICAL EXAMINATION

- Tenderness to palpation is seen with buccal cellulitis, panniculitis, and parotitis/mumps.

- Swelling that obscures the angle of the jaw suggests parotid inflammation or parotitis.

- Children with mumps are rarely toxic appearing.

- Suppurative parotitis, most commonly caused by *Staphylococcal aureus,* is associated with an ill-appearing child with purulent discharge from Stensen's duct.

- Nodules or papules with normal overlying skin suggest dermoid cysts, epidermoid cysts, or deep (cavernous) hemangiomas.

- Swelling associated with erythema of the overlying skin suggests buccal cellulitis, panniculitis, fat necrosis, or suppurative parotitis.

DIAGNOSIS	ICD-9	DISTINGUISHING CHARACTERISTICS	DISTRIBUTION
Epidermoid Cyst	706.2	Well-demarcated, solitary nodule or papule	Face, scalp, neck, trunk
Dermoid Cyst	709.8	Firm, skin-colored nodule	Often midline, forehead, periorbital, or lateral eyebrow
Hemangioma	228.01	Superficial or "strawberry" lesions (pink/red) Deep or cavernous lesions (blue/skin colored)	Head and neck most commonly May occur on trunk, oral, or genital mucosa
Parotitis	072.9 (mumps) 527.2	Painful swelling of parotid that obscures the angle of the mandible	Parotid gland Mumps is usually bilateral; suppurative parotitis is unilateral
Buccal Cellulitis	682.0	Tender to palpation Salmon or violaceous color of the cheek	Subcutaneous and dermal layers of cheek Unilateral
Popsicle Panniculitis	729.3	Painful erythematous nodules	Perioral subcutaneous fat Angle of mouth Often bilateral
Fat Necrosis	778.1—newborn 709.3	Single or multiple erythematous nontender nodules	Cheeks, buttocks, thighs Sites of recent trauma
Pyogenic Granuloma	686.1	Bright-red, moist-appearing, exophytic lesion	60% occur on head or neck Usually solitary

DURATION/CHRONICITY	ASSOCIATED FINDINGS	COMPLICATIONS
Slow growing Persists for life	Normal overlying skin May have a central dimple	Recurrent inflammation Lesions may rupture
Congenital	Intracranial extension in midline lesions Spinal cord defects in sacral lesions	Meningitis/infection when there is communication with underlying structures
Rapidly enlarge during first year of life	Multiple lesions associated with visceral hemangiomas Rapidly enlarging lesions seen in Kasabach Merritt syndrome or PHACE syndrome	Bleeding after trauma Obstruction of airway, vision, or GU tract
Viral type is seen in childhood Suppurative type can be seen in neonates or older children	A brief prodrome seen with mumps Increased amylase level in 70% of cases	Rare complications of mumps: encephalitis, pancreatitis, deafness, nephritis, myocarditis
Acute onset with a peak incidence at 9–12 months Resolves with treatment	Acute otitis media often seen Toxic appearance	Bacteremia, meningitis, intracranial extension, cavernous sinus thrombosis
Lesions not apparent immediately Lesions persist 2 to 3 weeks	Nontoxic appearing child	None
Appear 1–6 weeks of age Resolves spontaneously	Associated trauma	Calcification Ulceration Infection
Most commonly occurs in childhood Persists unless excised	Associated trauma	Profuse bleeding Infection Satellite lesions may occur after surgery

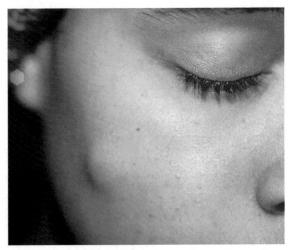

Figure 7-1 Epidermoid cyst. (Used with permission from Goodheart HP. *Goodheart's photoguide of common skin disorders.* Philadelphia: Lippincott Williams & Wilkins; 2003:4.)

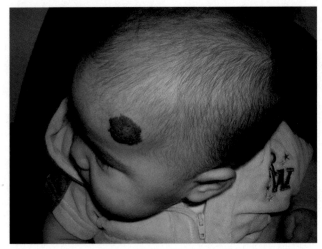

Figure 7-2 Hemangioma. (Courtesy of Scott Van Duzer, MD.)

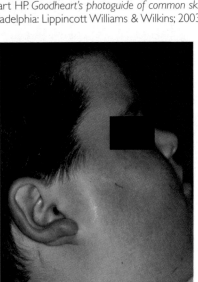

Figure 7-3 Parotitis. (Courtesy of Kathleen Cronan, MD.)

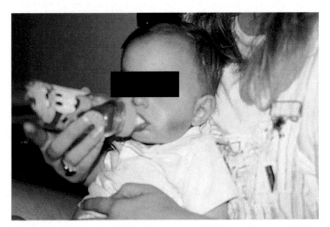

Figure 7-4 Buccal cellulitis. (Courtesy of Kathleen Cronan, MD.)

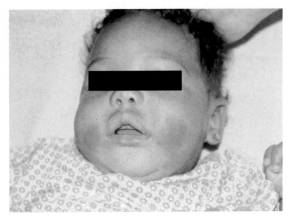

Figure 7-5 Popsicle panniculitis. (Courtesy of Kathleen Cronan, MD.)

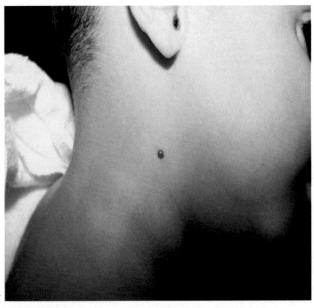

Figure 7-6 Pyogenic granuloma. (Courtesy of Kathleen Cronan, MD.)

OTHER
DIAGNOSES TO
CONSIDER

- Trichoepithelioma

- Pilomatrixoma

- Idiopathic neuroma

- Multiple mucosal neuromas (MEN IIB)

- Lymphocytoma cutis

SUGGESTED READINGS

Fisher RG, Benjamin DK Jr. Facial cellulitis in childhood: a changing spectrum. *South Med J.* 2002;95(7):672–674.

Goodheart HP. *Goodheart's photoguide of common skin disorders.* Philadelphia: Lippincott Williams & Wilkins; 2003:4.

Lin RL, Janniger CK. Pyogenic granuloma. *Cutis.* 2004;74(4):229–233.

McKinzie JP. Clinical pearls: fever and facial swelling—buccal cellulitis. *Acad Emerg Med.* 1998;5(4):347, 368–370.

Miller T, Frieden IJ. Hemangiomas: new insights and classification. *Pediatr Ann.* 2005;34(3):179–190.

Nahlieli O, Shachem R, Shlesinger M, et al. Juvenile recurrent parotitis: a new method of diagnosis and treatment. *Pediatrics.* 2004;114(1):9–12.

Pagliai KA, Cohen BA. Pyogenic granuloma in children. *Pediatr Dermatol.* 2004;21(1):10–13.

Section
THREE

Eyes

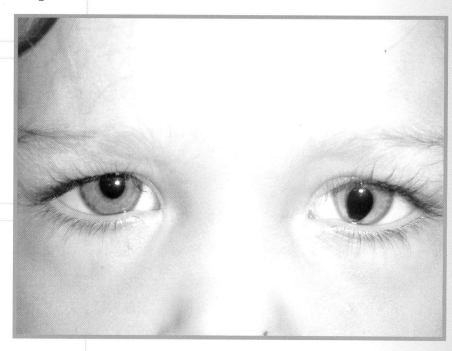

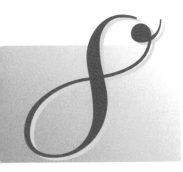

PARUL B. PATEL AND STEVEN M. SELBST

Red Eye

APPROACH TO THE PROBLEM

The red eye is an eye with vascular congestion of the conjunctiva resulting from inflammation, trauma, conjunctivitis, glaucoma, or secondary to eyelid pathology. Conjunctivitis is the most common cause of a red eye, while glaucoma is rare in pediatrics. Conjunctivitis, commonly referred to as "pink eye," may have a viral, bacterial, or allergic etiology. Trauma to the eye can cause eye redness in association with corneal abrasions, iritis, and subconjunctival hemorrhage. The red eye may be related to eyelid pathology such as blepharitis and preseptal (periorbital) or postseptal (orbital) cellulitis. Red eyes also may be seen in some systemic diseases such as Kawasaki disease.

KEY POINTS IN THE HISTORY

- A history of atopy, allergen exposure, or seasonality will often help distinguish viral from allergic conjunctivitis.

- Pruritus is a common complaint with allergic conjunctivitis.

- While both viral and bacterial conjunctivitis sometimes may have a purulent discharge, early morning lid crusting or gluey eyes usually points to a bacterial etiology.

- Time at presentation is very important in a neonate with conjunctivitis; chemical conjunctivitis usually occurs in the first 24 hours, conjunctivitis secondary to gonococcal infection usually appears within 1 week after birth, and conjunctivitis secondary to chlamydia infection usually appears 1 to 2 weeks after birth.

- Pain after trauma suggests corneal abrasion or iritis, while subconjunctival hemorrhages are usually painless.

- Decreased vision and marked photophobia suggest a more serious diagnosis, such as glaucoma.

- Ocular pain with eye movement distinguishes orbital cellulitis from preseptal cellulitis.

- Consider Kawasaki disease when an irritable child with fever has red eyes but no eye discharge.

**KEY POINTS IN
THE PHYSICAL
EXAMINATION**

- Unilateral conjunctivitis with surrounding vesicular lesions is highly suspicious for keratoconjunctivitis resulting from herpes simplex virus.

- Visual acuity, because it may be impaired, should be tested whenever orbital cellulitis is suspected.

- Fluorescein examination is extremely helpful in diagnosing a corneal abrasion. Holding the fluorescein strip near the outer canthus, while having the patient blink, allows the dye to taint the tears. To further limit discomfort, fluorescein dye may be applied to the conjunctiva following the application of an ocular anesthetic.

- Signs of orbital cellulitis, such as limited eye movement and decreased vision, may mimic those of orbital pseudotumor and neoplasm.

- A preauricular node in association with conjunctivitis is suspicious for viral conjunctivitis.

- Forty percent to fifty percent of those who have conjunctivitis in association with acute otitis media (formerly described as the otitis media-conjunctivitis syndrome) suggests nontypeable *Haemophilus influenzae*.

- Consider other diagnoses, such as keratitis, iritis, or uveitis, when the limbus (the sclerocorneal junction) is involved.

- Conjunctivitis associated with pharyngitis is often caused by adenovirus.

PHOTOGRAPHS OF SELECTED DIAGNOSES

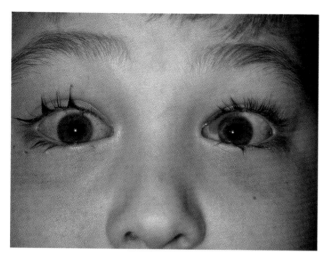

Figure 8-1 Conjunctivitis with a subconjunctival hemorrhage. Note the subconjunctival hemorrhage on the left. (Courtesy of Steven M. Selbst, MD.)

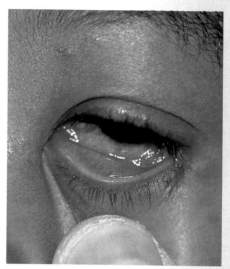

Figure 8-2 Allergic conjunctivitis with lid edema and conjunctival injection. (Used with permission from Fleisher GR, Ludwig S, Baskin MN. *Atlas of pediatric emergency medicine.* Philadelphia: Lippincott Williams & Wilkins; 2004:271.)

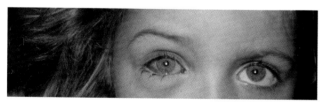

Figure 8-3 Viral conjunctivitis. (Courtesy of Steven M. Selbst, MD.)

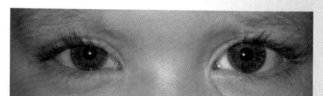

Figure 8-4 Bacterial conjunctivitis. (Courtesy of Steven M. Selbst, MD.)

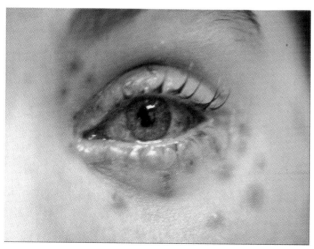

Figure 8-5 Herpes keratoconjunctivitis. (Courtesy of Steven M. Selbst, MD.)

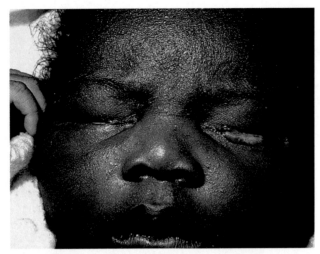

Figure 8-6 Gonococcal ophthalmia neonatorum. (Used with permission from Ostler HB, Maibach HI, Hoke AW, et al. *Diseases of the eye and skin: a color atlas.* Philadelphia: Lippincott Williams & Wilkins; 2004:269.)

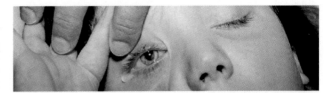

Figure 8-7 Corneal abrasion. (Courtesy of Steven M. Selbst, MD.)

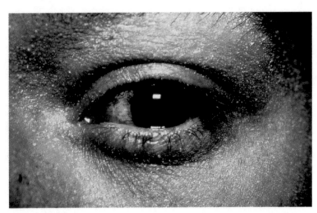

Figure 8-8 Conjunctivitis seen with Kawasaki disease. (Used with permission from Goodheart HP. *Goodheart's photoguide to common skin disorders.* 2nd ed. Philadelphia: Lippincott Williams & Wilkins; 2003:198.)

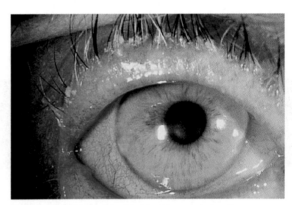

Figure 8-9 Blepharitis. (Used with permission from Weber J, Kelley J. *Health assessment in nursing.* 2nd ed. Philadelphia: Lippincott Williams & Wilkins; 2003:196.)

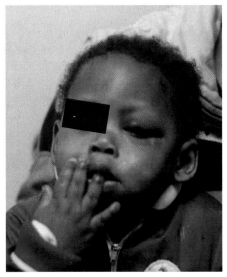

Figure 8-10 Periorbital cellulitis. (Courtesy of Steven M. Selbst, MD.)

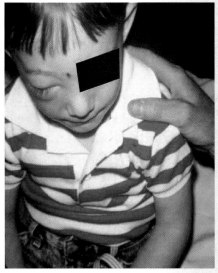

Figure 8-11 Orbital cellulitis. Note erythema, swelling, and proptosis on right. (Courtesy of Steven M. Selbst, MD.)

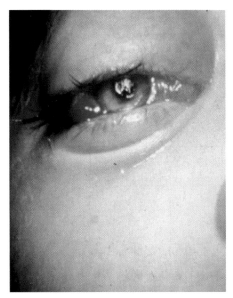

Figure 8-12 Chemosis. (Courtesy of Steven M. Selbst, MD.)

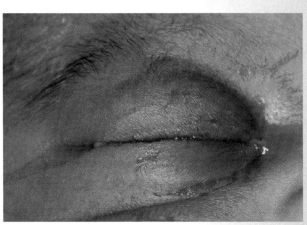

Figure 8-13 Chlamydia conjunctivitis. (Courtesy of Steven M. Selbst, MD.)

DIFFERENTIAL DIAGNOSIS

DIAGNOSIS	ICD-9	DISTINGUISHING CHARACTERISTICS	DISTRIBUTION
Subconjunctival Hemorrhage	372.72	Painless Benign Spontaneous resolution	Localized rupture of small subconjunctival vessels
Allergic Conjunctivitis	372.14	Seasonal Pruritic Conjunctival edema (chemosis) Usually watery discharge Bilateral	Diffuse (involves whole conjunctiva and sclera)
Viral Conjunctivitis	077.99	History of exposure Ocular discomfort Watery discharge Tender preauricular node Follicular aggregates	Diffuse (involves whole conjunctiva and sclera)
Bacterial Conjunctivitis	372.30	Usually mucopurulent discharge Early morning crusty or "gluey" eye	Diffuse marked erythema

	098.4	Gonococcal conjunctivitis
		    Profuse purulent discharge
		    Lids often swollen
		    High risk in neonates usually less than 2 weeks old
		    and sexually active adolescents
			Diffuse hyperacute conjunctival injection

Herpes Keratoconjunctivitis	370.40	Lid often swollen Watery discharge Painful Unilateral Photophobia Foreign body sensation Periorbital vesicles Dendritic pattern with fluorescent stain	Diffuse
Corneal Abrasion	918.1	Intense pain Tearing (+ / −) photophobia	Localized
Conjunctivitis with Kawasaki Disease (KD)	446.1	Nonpurulent Nonulcerative Bilateral	Bulbar conjunctivitis (spares limbus)
Blepharitis	373.00	Redness and swelling of eyelid margins Scaly, flaky debris on lid margins Gritty, burning sensation Matting upon awakening	Eyelid margins
Preseptal (Periorbital) Cellulitis	373.13	Infection of space anterior to orbital septum Lid warmth, edema, erythema, and tenderness More common in children <5 yrs	Eyelids, upper and lower
Postseptal (Orbital) Cellulitis	376.01	Infection involving the orbital structures posterior to the orbital septum Lid warmth, edema, erythema, and tenderness Chemosis Proptosis Decreased ocular movement Periocular pain Usually unilateral	Eyelids, upper and lower Mild, diffuse conjunctival injection
Glaucoma	365.9	Cloudy or hazy cornea (because of corneal edema) Tearing but discharge is unusual Photophobia, blurred vision Irregular corneal reflex Rare in children except congenital variety Eye may appear large	Circumcorneal injection (ciliary flush)

DURATION/ CHRONICITY	ASSOCIATED FINDINGS	COMPLICATIONS	PREDISPOSING FACTORS
Resolves in 2–3 weeks	Periorbital trauma	None	Direct trauma Spontaneous Childbirth Increased intrathoracic pressure (from coughing, vomiting)
Resolves with allergen removal and/or treatment Recurs every season	Atopy Teary eyes Photophobia	Usually none	Allergens including pollen, ragweed, dust, animal dander (usually airborne)
3–7 days Self-limited	Viral syndrome (fever, pharyngitis, adenopathy) Ocular discomfort Eyelid swelling	Infectious to others	Exposure from direct contact or from fomites
7–10 days Generally self-limited in infants and older children	Sometimes occurs with otitis media (usually because of nontypable *H. influenzae*) Ocular discomfort	Infectious to others	Exposure from direct contact with other infected individuals
Variable, depends on treatment	Sepsis-like picture in neonates May be associated with disseminated gonococcal disease (arthritis, rash) or urethral discharge in adolescents	Loss of eye from abscess, corneal ulceration, and perforation when untreated Infectious to others	Vertical transmission (mother to baby) Sexually active adolescents Victims of sexual abuse Exposure to (direct contact) infected person
Variable, depends on treatment May be recurrent	Mucocutaneous or predominantly periorbital vesicles Corneal ulceration Systemic involvement Sepsis-like picture or seizures in neonates	Systemic infection in neonates Infectious to others	Neonates of infected mothers are at risk Sexually active adolescents
Improved in 24–48 hours	Facial trauma Other eye injury	Infection Ulceration (contact lens wearers)	Direct trauma Rubbing eyes Foreign body Insertion/removal of contact lenses
1–2 weeks if untreated	Signs and symptoms of acute phase of KD (fever, irritability, rash, lymphadenopathy, mucous membrane and extremities changes) Transient anterior uveitis or acute iridocyclitis in 83%	Coronary artery aneurysms, myocardial infarction, and/or death when KD is left untreated	Uncertain
Chronic/recurrent	Rosacea or seborrheic dermatitis	Hordeolum	Usually none
7–10 days with oral antibiotic treatment	Fever and pain	Orbital cellulitis Bacteremia/sepsis Meningitis	Minor trauma or insect bite Localized lid infections Bacteremia because of *H. influenza* type B
10–14 days with IV+ oral antibiotic treatment	Fever Associated URI (upper respiratory infection) symptoms Decreased visual acuity Malaise	Blindness Brain abscess Meningitis Death secondary to cavernous sinus thrombosis	Minor trauma Sinusitis Dental abscess Preseptal cellulitis
Variable	Increased intraocular pressure Acute periocular pain Nausea and vomiting with acute angle glaucoma	Blindness	Trauma Congenital Other ocular diseases

OTHER DIAGNOSES TO CONSIDER	• Keratitis

- • Keratitis

- • Episcleritis/scleritis

- • Chemical or toxic conjunctivitis

- • Iritis (anterior uveitis or iridocyclitis)

- • Dacrocystitis

SUGGESTED READINGS

Alessandrini EA. The case of the red eye. *Pediatr Ann.* 2000;29(2):112–116.

Coote MA. Sticky eye, tricky diagnosis. *Aust Fam Physician.* 2002;31(3):225–231.

Fleisher GR, Ludwig S, Baskin MN. *Atlas of pediatric emergency medicine.* Philadelphia: Lippincott Williams & Wilkins; 2004:271.

Gigliotti F. Acute conjunctivitis. *Pediatr Rev.* 1993;16:203–208.

Goodheart HP. *Goodheart's photoguide to common skin disorders.* 2nd ed. Philadelphia: Lippincott Williams & Wilkins; 2003:198.

Ostler HB, Maibach HI, Hoke AW, et al. *Diseases of the eye and skin: a color atlas.* Philadelphia: Lippincott Williams & Wilkins; 2004:269.

Pasternak A, Irish B. Ophthalmologic infection in primary care. *Clin Fam Pract.* 2004;6(1):19–25.

Rietveld RP, van Weert HCPM, ter Riet G, et al. Predicting bacterial cause in infectious conjunctivitis: cohort study on informativeness of combinations of signs and symptoms. *BMJ.* 2004;329:206–210.

Teoh DL, Reynolds S. Diagnosis and management of pediatric conjunctivitis. *Pediatr Emerg Care.* 2003;19(1):48–55.

Weber J, Kelley J. *Health assessment in nursing.* 2nd ed. Philadelphia: Lippincott Williams & Wilkins; 2003:196.

ENGLISH D. WILLIS AND TERRI L. YOUNG

Swelling of/Around the Eye

APPROACH TO THE PROBLEM

Several disorders exist that may cause swelling of or around the eye. Most can be distinguished by the age of onset, clinical appearance, and pattern of enlargement. The two most common eyelid lesions are caused by chalazia and hordeola (stye). The most concerning cause of swelling for which an etiology must be determined is an expanding orbital process causing proptosis.

KEY POINTS IN THE HISTORY

- Patients with hordeola complain of pain; those with chalazia generally have no discomfort.

- Dermoid cysts are among the most common orbital tumors of childhood. Most of these cysts form near the frontal zygomatic or frontonasal suture, rather than on the eyelid. If cystic rupture occurs, extruded keratin can cause an acute inflammatory reaction with periocular erythema, tenderness, and swelling, which mimics orbital cellulitis.

- Congenital dacryocystocele (also a mucocele, amniotocele, or lacrimal sac cyst) is a result of nasolacrimal duct obstruction with distention of the lacrimal sac. This bluish colored mass is present at birth or shortly thereafter and usually is filled with tear fluid or mucopurulent material.

- Nephrotic syndrome commonly presents with bilateral periorbital edema that may be most notable upon awakening, and improves throughout the day.

- Angioedema causes diffuse swelling of the eyes and a burning sensation of the skin.

- A capillary hemangioma of the eyelid presents within the first few weeks of life as a small red patch that slowly progresses during the first years of life to a soft, strawberry red or bluish colored, round mass.

- Proptosis generally refers to a forward displacement of the orbit or a bulging of the eye. Proptosis may be the result of many causes including infectious or inflammatory lesions, tumors, neurogenic lesions, cystic lesions, and vascular lesions.

- Cystic lesions, such as a dermoid cyst, are generally nontender and nonprogressive.

- Vascular lesions, such as hemangiomas and lymphangiomas, are generally nontender and are associated with dilated conjunctival vessels that manifest as a red eye.

- Pingueculae are degenerative collagenous collections of the conjunctiva that can occur spontaneously or from chronic exposure to sunlight or wind.

KEY POINTS IN
THE PHYSICAL
EXAMINATION

- Consider the diagnosis of a chalazion when a warm, tender, erythematous, and indurated nodule is present on the conjunctival side of the eyelid.

- Juvenile xanthogranulomas are rubbery, red to yellow-orange papules most commonly affecting the eye area. Overlying telangiectatic blood vessels occasionally may be seen.

- In childhood, most dermoid cysts are superficial, and they present as firm, painless, round, smooth, mobile, subcutaneous masses commonly located in the superotemporal and anterior orbit.

- Palpation of a congenital dacryocystocele may force the mucopurulent contents of the distended lacrimal sac to extrude retrograde onto the ocular surface appearing as a white-yellow discharge. This is both diagnostic and therapeutic, mainly because extrusion decreases the likelihood of developing periorbital cellulitis.

- An insect bite or sting of the eyelid presents as a unilateral, diffuse, nontender, and nonpurulent swelling of the eyelid. The presence of a central entry mark may be helpful in distinguishing a bite from a cellulitis because both entities may present with mild erythema, warmth, and induration. In addition, cellulitis is tender, but insect bites are not.

- Children with periorbital swelling caused by idiopathic nephrotic syndrome are distinguished from those with an allergic reaction by the presence of generalized edema or edema in dependent areas such as the scrotum, vulva, and lower extremities.

- Capillary hemangiomas of the dermal layer have a strawberry red pigmentation, while lesions within the subcutaneous tissue may appear bluish in color.

- Children with proptosis should have a complete visual examination that includes visual acuity testing, assessment of ocular duction and versions, and testing of the cranial nerves III, IV, and VI.

- Increasing proptosis with crying or straining is suggestive of a capillary hemangioma or lymphangioma.

PHOTOGRAPHS OF SELECTED DIAGNOSES

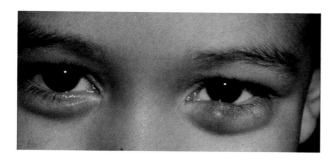

Figure 9-1 Chalazion. (Courtesy of Terri Young, MD.)

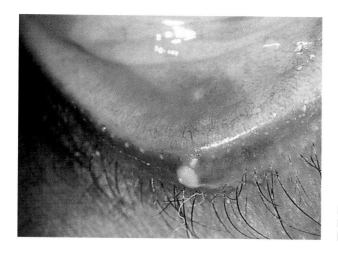

Figure 9-2 Hordeolum. (Used with permission from Weber J, Kelley J. *Health assessment in nursing.* 2nd ed. Philadelphia: Lippincott Williams & Wilkins; 2003:196.)

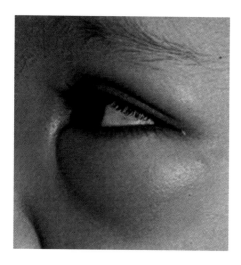

Figure 9-3 Insect bite. (Courtesy of George A. Datto, III, MD.)

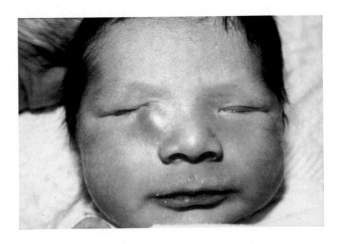

Figure 9-4 Congenital dacryocystocele. (Courtesy of Terri Young, MD.)

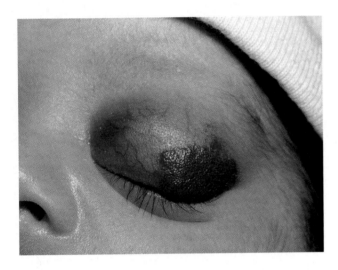

Figure 9-5 Capillary hemangioma of the eyelid. (Courtesy of Dean John Bonsall, MD.)

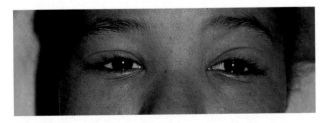

Figure 9-6 Eyelid edema in child with nephrotic syndrome. (Courtesy of George A. Datto, III, MD.)

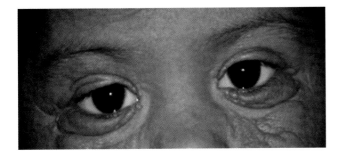

Figure 9-7 Xanthogranuloma. (Courtesy of Terri Young, MD.)

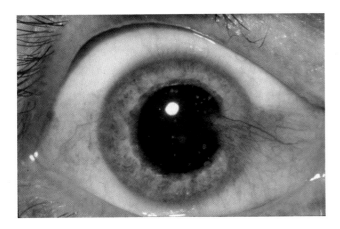

Figure 9-8 Pterygium. (Courtesy of Terri Young, MD.)

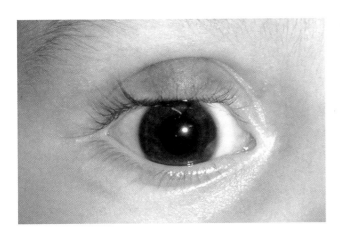

Figure 9-9 Lymphangioma of eyelid. (Courtesy of Brian Forbes, MD.)

DIFFERENTIAL DIAGNOSIS

DIAGNOSIS	ICD-9	DISTINGUISHING CHARACTERISTICS	DISTRIBUTION
Chalazion	373.2	Erythematous rubbery nodule Painless Sometimes, foreign body sensation with blinking	Develops around a Meibomian gland located just under the conjunctival side of the eyelid
Hordeolum	373.11 (external) 373.12 (internal)	Erythematous purulent nodule Painful Usually caused by *Staphylococcus aureus* May be associated with some drainage	External hordeola involve the anterior eyelid in the Zeis glands or lash follicles (stye) Internal hordeola involve the Meibomian glands located on the conjunctival side of the eyelid and may be infectious or sterile
Insect Bite	E906.4 918.0	Acute Nontender, slightly erythematous, nonpurulent edema of the eyelid A central punctate mark may be visible	Unilateral, diffuse swelling of the eyelid
Dermoid Cyst	238.2 239.2	Present in infancy and childhood Firm, smooth, painless, slightly mobile oval masses Enlarges slowly	Orbital and periorbital Lateral brow adjacent to the frontozygomatic suture or medial upper eyelid adjacent to the frontoethmoidal suture
Congenital Dacryocystocele	375.30	10–12 mm diameter, fluctuant bluish-appearing mass	Nasolacrimal sac region
Capillary Hemangioma of the Eyelid	228.01	Presents within the first 2 weeks of life, enlarges during the next 1 to 2 years and involutes by age 5 years if untreated	Periorbital region in the dermal or subcutaneous tissue
Nephrotic Syndrome	581.9	Bilateral periorbital edema Pitting edema in the lower extremities, increase in abdominal girth, anorexia, abdominal pain	Nephrotic syndrome secondary to minimal change disease occurs primarily between ages 2 and 6 years and more often in males
Plane Xanthoma of the Eyelid (Xanthelasma)	272.2 374.51	Lipid-filled soft yellow plagues and nodules of the upper eyelids	Medial aspects of the upper eyelids, bilaterally along with face, truck, and proximal extremities; rare in children
Pterygium	372.40	Conjunctival growth Erythema Irritation	Medially on the ocular surface, extending horizontally from the nasal conjunctiva onto the cornea Wing or triangular wedged shaped

ASSOCIATED FINDINGS	COMPLICATIONS	PREDISPOSING FACTORS
Seen in some patients with blepharitis	Blurred vision as a result of astigmatism secondary to corneal compression	May result from an internal hordeolum or blepharitis
None	Cellulitis of the eyelid	May result in patients with blepharitis
Possible presence of insect bites or stings on other areas	Secondary infection with excessive scratching	Allergic reactions to specific insects
If the cyst is posterior and in the temporal fossa, must evaluate for a "dumbbell" expansion into the orbit If medial, must distinguish from a congenital encephalocele	Proptosis with mastication from pressure on the cyst caused by temporalis contraction Astigmatism caused by pressure on the globe	None
None	Dacryocystitis Respiratory compromise if bilateral and extending onto the lateral nasal wall Cellulitis	None
None	Amblyopia Stigmatism Ptosis	None
Proteinuria, hypoalbuminemia, and hypercholesterolemia	Complications related to the severity of the renal disease	Minor infections or allergic reactions to insect bites, bee stings, or poison ivy
Hyperlipidemia, familial hypercholesterolemia, lipoprotein abnormalities, diabetes, and biliary cirrhosis; also seen with Hand-Schüller-Christian disease, myeloma, and liver disease	Complications related to abnormal lipid metabolism	None
None	Extension onto the cornea may cause irregular astigmatism and decrease in vision Decrease in visual acuity with impingement of the visual axis	Excessive exposure to ultraviolet light and wind Common in tropical regions

- Immune-mediated diseases

- Rhabdomyosarcoma

- Orbital cyst

SUGGESTED READINGS

The Foundation of the American Academy of Ophthalmology. Course faculty: Wilhelmus KR, Huang AJW, Hwang DG, Parrish CM, Sutphin JE, and Whitsett JC. *External disease and cornea. Basic and clinical science course.* Section 8; 2000–2001.

The Foundation of the American Academy of Ophthalmology. Course faculty: Kersten R, Bartley GB, Nerad JA, Neuhaus RW, Nowinski TS, Popham, JK, and Beardsley, TL. *Orbit, eyelids, and lacrimal system. Basic and clinical science course.* Section 7; 2000–2001.

Hertle RW, Schaffer DB, Foster JA. *Pediatric eye disease color atlas and synopsis.* New York: McGraw-Hill; 2002.

Katowitz J. *Pediatric oculoplastic surgery.* New York: Springer-Verlag; 2002.

Lederman C, Miller M. Hordeola and chalazia. *Pediatr Rev.* 1999;20:283–284.

Robb RM. Congenital nasolacrimal duct obstruction. *Ophthalmol Clin North Am.* 2001;14:443.

Taylor D. *Paediatric ophthalmology.* 2nd ed. Oxford: Blackwell Science; 1997.

Weber J, Kelley J. *Health assessment in nursing.* 2nd ed. Philadelphia: Lippincott Williams & Wilkins; 2003:196.

MARYELLEN E. GUSIC AND
DEAN JOHN BONSALL

Discoloration of/Around the Eye

APPROACH TO THE PROBLEM

Visual inspection of the eye may reveal discoloration of the lids and tissues around the eye or a change in color of the bulbar conjunctivae. Blunt trauma to the eye or forehead may lead to extravasation of blood into the surrounding tissues. Neuroblastoma, a tumor of embryonic sympathetic neuroblasts, may metastasize to involve the orbit. The unilateral or bilateral discoloration associated with spread of the tumor to the eye, and subsequent obstruction of palpebral blood vessels, appears similar to the ecchymosis following trauma. Allergic shiners result from venous congestion because of nasal and paranasal sinus mucosal edema; and the sclerae are usually white in appearance. Children and adults with increased skin pigmentation may have increased pigmentation in the basal layer of the bulbar conjunctivae. This normal discoloration is usually bilateral and is most evident in the intrapalpebral area. Icterus is a yellow discoloration of the sclerae that is more uniform in distribution and occurs as a result of bilirubin binding to the bulbar conjunctivae. In disorders such as Ehler Danlos syndrome, Marfan syndrome, and osteogenesis imperfecta, the sclerae appear blue because the underlying brown uvea showing through thinned sclerae. Bluish sclerae are also noted in congenital glaucoma and aniridia.

KEY POINTS IN THE HISTORY

- In traumatic injuries, the timing of the injury determines the discoloration observed—initially purple or deep blue that changes later to a yellowish color as the bruising resolves.

- Visual complaints may occur with concomitant trauma to the eye and its surrounding tissues.

- Poor visual acuity or double vision may also occur with infiltrative disease of the orbit and extraocular muscles.

- A family history of atopic disease including rhinitis, dermatitis, and asthma may be present in patients with allergic shiners. Patients with allergic rhinitis often report nasal itching, sneezing, congestion, and rhinorrhea; and may have other atopic diseases.

- Scleral epithelial melanosis, seen as a result of pigmentation of the conjunctivae, does not change in appearance or location. It is more common in African American, Hispanic, and Asian children. The amount of pigment may increase after sun exposure or when conjunctivae are inflamed.

- Nevus of Ota is a congenital hyperpigmentation of the tissues of the eye (melanosis oculi) in association with pigmentation of the surrounding skin.

KEY POINTS IN THE PHYSICAL EXAMINATION

- Jaundice in an otherwise healthy child should raise suspicion for hemolytic or hepatic disease.

- Proptosis seen in association with eye discoloration is consistent with infiltrative disease of the orbit.

- The lesions of scleral epithelial melanosis are stationary and flat and are not inflamed or vascularized. They are usually brown in appearance.

- The increased pigmentation of a nevus of Ota is usually unilateral and located below the conjunctiva. The eye is gray or blue in appearance.

- Blue sclerae and joint hyperextensibility are associated with Ehlers Danlos and Marfan syndromes.

- The ecchymotic discoloration seen with metastatic neuroblastoma may precede diagnosis of the primary tumor, which is typically the abdomen or thorax.

PHOTOGRAPHS OF SELECTED DIAGNOSES

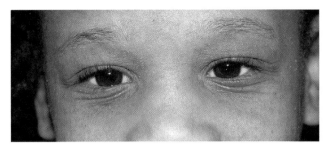

Figure 10-1 Allergic shiners. Note the darkening of the periorbital areas, the lichenification, and the characteristic double-fold (Dennie-Morgan line) that extends from the inner to the outer canthus of the lower eyelid. (Used with permission from Goodheart HP. *Goodheart's photoguide of common skin disorders.* 2nd ed. Philadelphia: Lippincott Williams & Wilkins; 2003:48.)

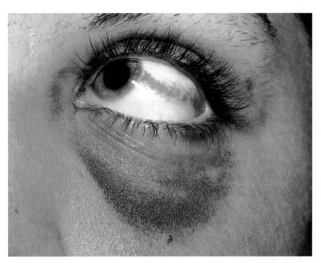

Figure 10-2 Black eye from trauma. (Courtesy of Dean John Bonsall, MD, FACS.)

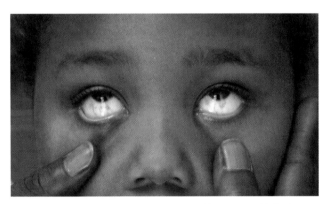

Figure 10-3 Scleral epithelial melanosis. (Courtesy of Julie A. Boom, MD.)

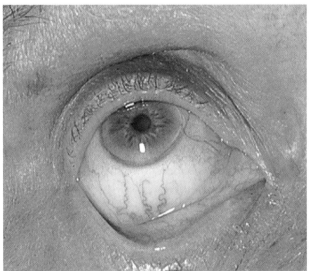

Figure 10-4 Scleral icterus. (Used with permission from Bickley LS, Szilagyi P. *Bates' guide to physical examination and history taking.* 8th ed. Philadelphia: Lippincott Williams & Wilkins; 2003:147.)

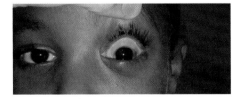

Figure 10-5 Nevus of Ota. (Courtesy of Brian Forbes, MD.)

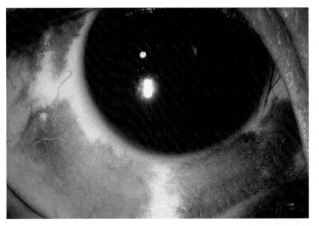

Figure 10-6 Nevus of Ota. (Courtesy of Dean John Bonsall, MD, FACS.)

DIFFERENTIAL DIAGNOSIS

DIAGNOSIS	ICD-9	DISTINGUISHING CHARACTERISTICS	DISTRIBUTION
Allergic Shiners	477.9 (allergic rhinitis)	Bilateral darkening of skin below orbits Symptoms and signs of allergic rhinitis	Skin below eyelids
Scleral Epithelial Melanosis	743.49	Flat, patchy pigmentation of conjunctivae Moves with conjunctivae	Bilateral, although not necessarily symmetric Limbal area
Scleral Icterus	782.4	Yellow discoloration of scleral conjunctivae Jaundice of skin	Sclera Conjunctivae
Raccoon Eyes seen with Basilar Skull Fracture	Basilar skull Fracture 801.00	History of trauma Bilateral periorbital ecchymoses (Raccoon eyes) Bruising behind auricle (Battle's sign)	Periorbital
Metastatic Neuroblastoma	198.4	Unilateral or bilateral ecchymoses Proptosis Periorbital swelling Palpable abdominal mass	Periorbital

DURATION/ CHRONICITY	ASSOCIATED FINDINGS	COMPLICATIONS	PREDISPOSING FACTORS
Concurrent with symptoms of rhinitis	Dennie-Morgan lines Allergic salute Deepened nasolabial folds Mouth breathing	Of rhinitis: • Epistaxis • Infection • Change in bony structure of face and palate • Malocclusion	Inhaled allergens
Congenital	Pigmentation of skin	*Not* risk factor for ocular melanoma	More common in African American, Hispanic, and Asian children May be induced by UV light exposure or inflammation of conjunctivae
Associated with serum hyperbilirubinemia May persist after normalization of serum bilirubin level	Yellow discoloration of skin and mucous membranes May be associated with hepatomegaly May be associated with signs of anemia	Of hyperbilirubinemia in neonates: • Kernicterus	Increased bilirubin production Impaired uptake or conjugation of bilirubin Biliary obstruction Hepatocellular injury
Raccoon eyes resolve with time	CSF otorrhea and/or rhinorrhea	Of basilar skull fracture: • Intracranial infection • Intracranial air collections • Cerebral injury/bleed • Increased intracranial pressure • Seizures	Trauma
Precedes, follows, or is concurrent with primary tumor	Proptosis Palpable abdominal mass Fever Opsoclonus myoclonus Ataxia Bone pain Anemia	Flushing Hypertension Tachycardia Urinary obstruction Airway obstruction Superior vena cava syndrome	Unknown

OTHER
DIAGNOSES TO
CONSIDER

- Orbital tumors

- Conjunctival nevus

- Phlyctenule—a vesicle or ulcer on the cornea or conjunctivae

- Ruptured globe

- Episcleritis/scleritis

- Uveitis

SUGGESTED READINGS

Bickley LS, Szilagyi P. *Bates' guide to physical examination and history taking.* 8th ed. Philadelphia: Lippincott Williams & Wilkins; 2003:147.
Goodheart HP. *Goodheart's photoguide of common skin disorders.* 2nd ed. Philadelphia: Lippincott Williams & Wilkins; 2003:48.
Kanski JJ. *Clinical ophthalmology: a systemic approach.* 5th ed. Edinburgh: Butterworth-Heinemann; 2003.
Liesegang TJ. Pigmented conjunctival and scleral lesions. *Mayo Clin Proc.* 1994;69:151–161.
Oski FA, DeAngelis CD, Feigin RD, et al. Metastatic neuroblastoma. In: *Principles and practice of pediatrics.* 2nd ed. Philadelphia: JB Lippincott Co; 1994:892.
Oski FA, DeAngelis CD, Feigin RD, et al. Allergy. In: *Principles and practice of pediatrics.* 2nd ed. Philadelphia: JB Lippincott Co; 1994:213, 237.
Wright KW. Eyelid, orbital masses, and ocular pigmentation abnormalities. In: *Pediatric ophthalmology for pediatricians.* Baltimore: Williams & Wilkins; 1999:229–247, 283–286.

RENEE M. TURCHI AND ESTHER K. CHUNG
Pupil, Iris, and Lens Abnormalities

APPROACH TO THE PROBLEM

There are various abnormalities of the pupils, iris, and lens in children. In most cases, timely diagnosis and management are critical. Assessment of visual acuity is the most integral facet of the ophthalmologic examination. More than half of the visual abnormalities in children are first discerned by their primary care physician. Many diagnoses, such as leukocoria, require prompt referral to an ophthalmologist. When in doubt, referral is a prudent approach in managing many of these diagnoses.

KEY POINTS IN THE HISTORY

- Congenital cataracts are associated with intrauterine infections (such as congenital rubella and congenital varicella syndrome) and metabolic disorders, and they may be associated with Down, Edward, and Turner syndromes.

- One third of cataracts are hereditary, and nearly one third of cataracts in children have no identifiable etiology.

- Brushfield spots occur in up to 85% of children with Down syndrome, but they may be seen in normal children as well.

- Colobomas may occur in normal children or as part of genetic syndromes (such as CHARGE syndrome).

- Hyphemas are often the result of blunt trauma to the globe.

KEY POINTS IN THE PHYSICAL EXAMINATION

- Small, centrally located cataracts are often clinically stable without an impact on vision.

- Leukocoria, or a white pupillary reflex, is an important clinical sign of intraocular tumors, such as retinoblastoma.

- Leukocoria is bilateral in 30% to 40% of cases.

- It is important to rule out scleral rupture or the presence of a foreign body when chemosis is present.

- Kaiser-Fleischer rings are rims of brown-green pigment in the cornea. Although occasionally visible to the naked eye, slit lamp examination is sometimes necessary to visualize these rings.

- Iritis is characterized by pain, tearing, photophobia, and decreased visual acuity. It may be asymptomatic in children with rheumatologic disease such as juvenile rheumatoid arthritis.

- Blunt traumatic injuries to the eye warrant an inspection of the anterior chamber (space between cornea and iris) for hyphemas.

- Small hyphemas require slit lamp examination, while larger ones may be visible to the naked eye.

- When blood pools in the inferior portion of the eye from a hyphema, it often causes elevated intraocular pressure and decreased visual acuity.

PHOTOGRAPHS OF SELECTED DIAGNOSES

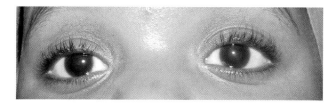

Figure 11-1 Aniridia. This photograph shows a child with bilateral aniridia. (Courtesy of Brian Forbes, MD.)

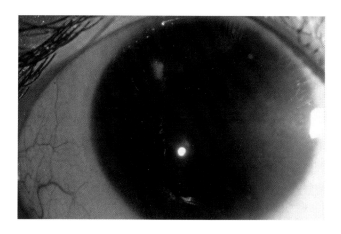

Figure 11-2 Aniridia. (Courtesy of Sophia M. Chung, MD.)

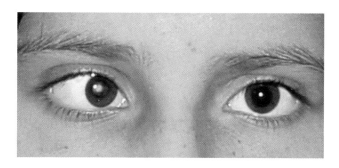

Figure 11-3 Cataract. Note the central haze in the right eye of this patient. (Courtesy of Brian Forbes, MD.)

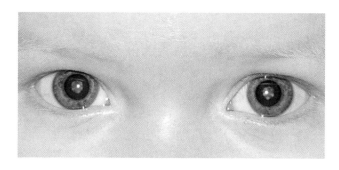

Figure 11-4 Bilateral central cataracts. (Courtesy of Brian Forbes, MD.)

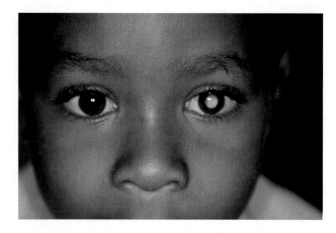

Figure 11-5 Leukocoria. (Used with permission from Rubin E, Farber JL. *Pathology*. 3rd ed. Philadelphia: Lippincott Williams & Wilkins; 1999:765.)

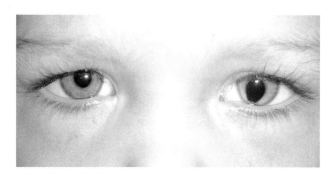

Figure 11-6 Coloboma in the left eye. (Courtesy of Brian Forbes, MD.)

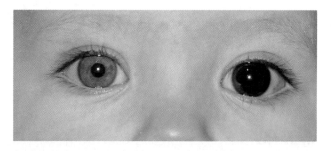

Figure 11-7 Heterochromia iridium. (Courtesy of Brian Forbes, MD.)

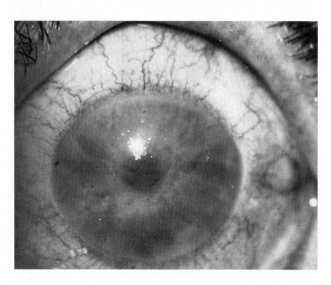

Figure 11-8 Iritis. (Used with permission from Harwood-Nuss A, Wolfson, et al. *The clinical practice of emergency medicine*. 3rd ed. Philadelphia: Lippincott Williams & Wilkins; 2001:66.)

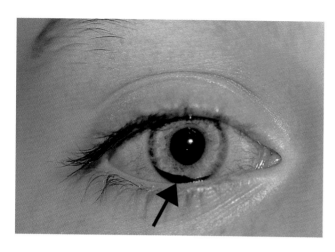

Figure 11-9 Hyphema. This 7-year-old girl was struck by a hard rubber ball and presented with blurred vision. The 1-mm hyphema was only visible when she was upright. (Used with permission from Fleisher GR, Ludwig S, Baskin MN. *Atlas of pediatric emergency medicine*. Philadelphia: Lippincott Williams & Wilkins; 2004:403.)

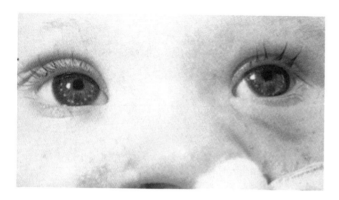

Figure 11-10 Brushfield spots. (Used with permission from Bickley LS, Szilagyi P. *Bates' guide to physical examination and history taking*. 8th ed. Philadelphia: Lippincott Williams & Wilkins; 2003:771.)

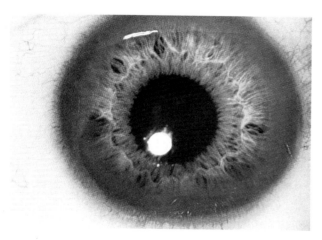

Figure 11-11 Kaiser-Fleischer ring. (Used with permission from Tasman W, Jaeger E. *The Wills Eye Hospital atlas of clinical ophthalmology*. 2nd ed. Philadelphia: Lippincott Williams & Wilkins; 2001:466.)

DIFFERENTIAL DIAGNOSIS

DIAGNOSIS	ICD-9	DISTINGUISHING CHARACTERISTICS	DISTRIBUTION
Aniridia	743.45	Iris hypoplasia Pupil is same size as cornea Edge of lens visible Incidence 1:64,000–1:96,000	Usually bilateral Some cases asymmetrical
Anisocoria	379.41 (pupil) 743.46 (cong)	Unequal pupil size Change in light reactivity	N/A
Cataract	366.9	Haze over eyes Apparent with red reflex testing	Location and density of cataract determines visual effects
Leukocoria	360.44	White pupillary reflex	May be unilateral or bilateral, depending on etiology (up to 40% of time bilateral in retinoblastoma)
Coloboma	743.49	Notch, hole, or defect in iris or choroids	Defect often located inferior and nasal May be unilateral or bilateral
Heterochromia Iridium	364.53 Acquired heterochromia of the iris	Rare May be isolated finding	Iridium–different colors between irises Iridis–different colors within one iris
Iritis	364.3	Pain, redness, and photophobia In severe cases, may have vision disturbances and hypotonia of the eye	Inflammation of the iris
Hyphema	364.41 Traumatic-921.3	Collection of blood in anterior chamber of the eye	Superior located meniscus in anterior chamber
Brushfield Spots	743.800	White and yellow spots evenly arranged around pupil in iris Iris looks speckled	Often bilateral
Kaiser-Fleischer Rings	275.1	Corneal staining from copper that is brown to orange-green in color	Staining more common at upper pole or cornea

DURATION/ CHRONICITY	ASSOCIATED FINDINGS	COMPLICATIONS	PREDISPOSING FACTORS
May employ pigmented contact lens to ameliorate symptoms	Photophobia Nystagmus Cataracts Glaucoma Part of WAGR and Gillespie syndromes	Poor vision	May be genetically inherited (usually autosomal dominant—sporadic in one-third)
Related to etiology	Horner syndrome Drugs Lesion of parasympathetic system (including CN III)	Changes in vision with severe cases:	Horner syndrome Drugs Lesion of parasympathetic system (including CN III)
Dense bilateral cataracts require urgent surgery Partial cataracts removed after visual assessment	Decrease in visual acuity	Blindness Amblyopia Glaucoma Strabismus	Intrauterine infections Metabolic disorders (i.e., hypoglycemia, hypocalcemia) Genetic disorders (Trisomy 21)
Related to diagnosis and ability to treat	Orbital tumors also may find: proptosis, pain, diplopia, conjunctival edema	Blindness Myopia Cataracts	Retinoblastoma is most serious etiology Other etiologies: • Congenital cataracts • Retinopathy of prematurity • Retinal detachment • Persistent hyperplastic primary vitreous • Coat disease • Toxocariasis
Visual loss related to affected area	Small eye Glaucoma Retinal detachment Disc degeneration	Poor vision	Dominant inheritance when present without systemic manifestations Syndromes associated: • Trisomy 13 and 18 • Cat eye syndrome • Wolf-Hirschhorn • Rieger syndrome • CHARGE association
N/A	N/A	N/A	Trauma Congenital pigmented nevi Waardenburg syndrome Piebald trait Horner syndrome
Pain, redness, and photophobia may last weeks in acute cases Chronic cases may have milder symptoms for months/years Blurred vision Poor pupillary light response	Cataract Glaucoma	Amblyopia Corneal changes and blurry vision Band keratopathy Macular edema	JRA (most common) Trauma Kawasaki disease Infections (measles, mumps, varicella, EBV, leprosy, Lyme) Spondyloarthropathies Sarcoidosis
Clot often gone in 3–5 days Rebleeding can occur if there is inadequate rest, unstable intraocular pressure; is more prevalent in sickle-cell disease	Occasional blood staining of the cornea	Glaucoma (10%) Increased intraocular pressure Rebleeding	Trauma (most common) Herpes zoster Iritis Orbital tumors Juvenile xanthogranulomatosis
N/A	Most often seen in children with Trisomy 21	N/A	Trisomy 21 (most often)
Often present after systemic disease treated	Liver disease, neurological impairment, and cognitive deficits in Wilson disease	No visual impairment Often fade with treatment	Wilson disease (defect in copper metabolism) Liver failure Carotenemia Multiple myeloma

OTHER
DIAGNOSES TO
CONSIDER

Pupil Abnormalities:

- Horner's syndrome

- Adie syndrome

- Third cranial nerve palsy

- Persistent pupillary membrane

Lens Abnormalities:

- Lens subluxation

- Dystrophy

- Cystinosis

- Lenticular myopia

Iris Abnormalities:

- Ocular albinism

- Iridodialysis

- Cyclodialysis

SUGGESTED READINGS

Bickley LS, Szilagyi P. *Bates' guide to physical examination and history taking.* 8th ed. Philadelphia: Lippincott Williams & Wilkins; 2003:771.

Fleisher GR, Ludwig S, Baskin MN. *Atlas of pediatric emergency medicine.* Philadelphia: Lippincott Williams & Wilkins; 2004:403.

Harwood-Nuss A, Wolfson, et al. *The clinical practice of emergency medicine.* 3rd ed. Philadelphia: Lippincott Williams & Wilkins; 2001:66.

Holland GN, Stiehm ER. Special considerations in the evaluation and management of uveitis in children. *Am J Ophthalmol.* 2003;135(6):867–878.

Khaw PT. Aniridia. *J Glaucoma.* 2002;11(2):164–168.

Lai JC, Ferkat S, Barron Y, et al. Traumatic hyphema in children: risk factors for complications. *Arch Ophthalmol.* 2001;119(1):64–70.

Nelson LB. *Harley's pediatric ophthalmology.* 4th ed. Philadelphia: WB Saunders; 1998.

Patel H. Pediatric uveitis. *Pediatr Clin North Am.* 2003;50:125–136.

Rubin E, Farber JL. *Pathology.* 3rd ed. Philadelphia: Lippincott Williams & Wilkins; 1999:765.

Tasman W, Jaeger E. *The Wills Eye Hospital atlas of clinical ophthalmology.* 2nd ed. Philadelphia: Lippincott Williams & Wilkins; 2001:466.

Terraciano AJ, Sidoti PA. Management of refractory glaucoma in childhood. *Curr Opin Ophthalmol.* 2002;13:97–102.

12

MARYELLEN E. GUSIC AND
DEAN JOHN BONSALL

Misalignment of the Eyes

APPROACH TO THE PROBLEM

Strabismus or ocular misalignment is a common disorder in pediatrics, with esotropia (medial deviation) being more common than exotropia (lateral deviation). Esotropia or exotropia may be a normal occurrence for infants fewer than 3 months old. Fixed and intermittent eye misalignment in older infants and children interferes with visual development and, if not detected and corrected, may lead to amblyopia or vision loss in the affected eye. It is important to examine the movement of the eyes in all visual fields to assess for differences in the degree of deviation or to determine whether there is limited movement of the extraocular muscles because these findings may be associated with neurologic conditions such as increased intracranial pressure. Children may also have vertical deviation in the alignment of their eyes.

KEY POINTS IN THE HISTORY

- Parents are often the first to notice ocular misalignment.

- Intermittent esotropia or exotropia may occur with greater frequency when the child is fatigued.

- Preterm birth and prenatal alcohol and drug exposure are factors that increase a child's risk for misalignment of the eyes. The mechanism by which this occurs is unknown. Other risk factors include a family history of strabismus and having cerebral palsy, genetic disorders, and a history of structural abnormalities of the eyes or of significant head injury.

- The onset of esotropia after 6 months of age may be associated with farsightedness.

- Complaints of double vision (diplopia) in an older child are worrisome because they may be a result of acquired esotropia (onset after infancy), exotropia, or extraocular muscle paresis. Limited movement of one of the extraocular muscles may be associated with neurologic disease and intracranial pathology. Children with double vision may squint or close an eye to avoid seeing two images.

- Children with myasthenia gravis may complain of difficulty opening their eyes fully, of double vision, and of extremity weakness.

KEY POINTS IN THE PHYSICAL EXAMINATION

- Family photos may be helpful supplements to the physical exam, particularly when pseudostrabismus is suspected.

- A child with pseudostrabismus often has a broad nasal bridge or wide epicanthal folds that partially cover the medial portion of the sclerae.

- The corneal light reflex, as detected by the Hirschberg test, should be in a symmetric, central position on both eyes in a child with pseudostrabismus. The Hirschberg test involves asking the child to look directly toward a light source. The examiner then determines the position of the light reflex on each eye. If the location of the reflex is asymmetric, ocular misalignment is present.

- The Bruckner test, or red reflex test, is used to detect symmetry of the size, color, and brightness of the red reflex in each eye. This test is performed using the ophthalmoscope to view both red reflexes simultaneously. If the child has a strabismus, the red reflex will be brighter in the deviated eye.

- If the child has an esotropia, the corneal light reflex will be displaced laterally. If the child has an exotropia, the corneal light reflex will be displaced medially. In both cases, the red reflex will appear brighter in the affected eye.

- The cover test may be a useful additional test in the evaluation of strabismus. The observer covers one of the child's eyes while having him or her focus on an object approximately two feet away and watches for movement of that eye after the cover is removed. An esophoria or exophoria is latent and may be revealed only when an eye is uncovered during this test.

- An upward deviation (hypertropia) or a downward deviation (hypotropia) may also be detected by looking for symmetry of the light reflex and movement during the cover test.

- A child with a sixth nerve palsy will not be able to abduct the affected eye when asked to look to that side. A full neurologic exam should be performed to rule out intracranial pathology.

- A child with a congenital or acquired third cranial nerve palsy will not be able to move the affected eye up or down and will not be able to adduct that eye (move medially). Ptosis may be present, and the pupil may be large and nonreactive to light. A third nerve palsy may be congenital or may occur in association with migraines, trauma, or increased intraocular pressure.

- Brown's syndrome, congenital or secondary to trauma or inflammation, describes a disorder in which a child cannot elevate the affected eye when in full lateral gaze. This condition is caused by limited movement (tightness) of the superior oblique muscle, tendon, or both.

- A child may have a head tilt or turn to compensate for ocular misalignment.

PHOTOGRAPHS OF SELECTED DIAGNOSES

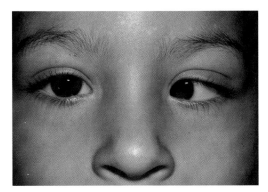

Figure 12-1 Esotropia. (Courtesy of Dean John Bonsall, MD, FACS.)

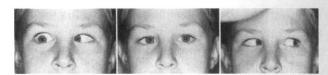

Figure 12-4 Right sixth nerve palsy. (Used with permission from Wright KW. *Pediatric ophthalmology for pediatricians*. Baltimore: Williams and Wilkins; 1999:59.)

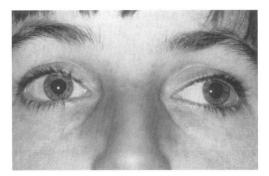

Figure 12-2 Exotropia. (Used with permission from Wright KW. *Pediatric ophthalmology for pediatricians*. Baltimore: Williams and Wilkins; 1999:41.)

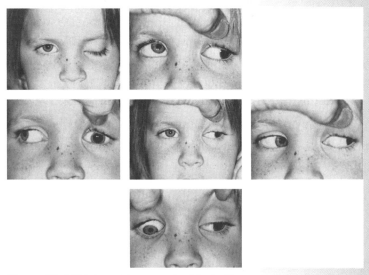

Figure 12-5 Third cranial nerve palsy. (Used with permission from Wright KW. *Pediatric ophthalmology for pediatricians*. Baltimore: Williams and Wilkins; 1999:63.)

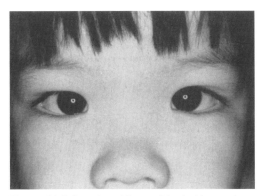

Figure 12-3 Pseudostrabismus. (Used with permission from Wright KW. *Pediatric ophthalmology for pediatricians*. Baltimore: Williams and Wilkins; 1999:49.)

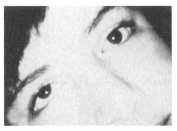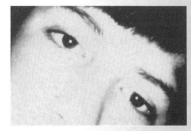

Figure 12-6 Fourth cranial nerve palsy. (Used with permission from Wright KW. *Pediatric ophthalmology for pediatricians*. Baltimore: Williams and Wilkins; 1999:57,58.)

DIAGNOSIS	ICD-9	DISTINGUISHING CHARACTERISTICS	DURATION/CHRONICITY
Esotropia	378.00	Lateral displacement of corneal light reflex Increased brightness of red reflex in involved eye Lateral movement of involved eye when other eye is covered	May resolve spontaneously in an infant under age 3 months
Exotropia	378.10	Medial displacement of corneal light reflex Increased brightness of red reflex in affected eye Medial movement of involved eye when other eye is covered	May resolve spontaneously in an infant under age 3 months
Pseudostrabismus	743.63	Symmetric corneal light and red reflex No movement on alternate cover, cover/uncover testing Visual acuity equal in each eye	N/A
Sixth nerve palsy	378.54	Inability to move affected eye laterally	Post viral palsy resolves in weeks to months
Third nerve palsy	378.52	Inability to move affected eye medially; eye also unable to move up or down	Palsy may persist after resolution of headache when associated with migraine
Fourth nerve palsy	378.53	Affected eye deviated upward and turned toward the temple Often presents as a head tilt	Variable

ASSOCIATED FINDINGS	COMPLICATIONS	PREDISPOSING FACTORS
Fixation preference in uninvolved eye Decreased visual acuity in involved eye Head may be turned to side of affected eye	Amblyopia	Idiopathic May be more common in children born prematurely and in children who were exposed to drugs and alcohol during gestation More common in children with: • Cerebral palsy • Genetic syndromes • Structural abnormalities of the eyes • History of significant head trauma • Decreased visual acuity or vision loss in one eye • Paralysis of a cranial nerve • Restriction of movement of extraocular muscle • Head trauma • Neurologic disease including disorders associated with increased intracranial pressure (tumors, hydrocephalus, Arnold-Chiari malformation) • Muscular disorders such as myasthenia gravis
Fixation preference in uninvolved eye Decreased visual acuity in involved eye Head may be turned to side of unaffected eye	Amblyopia	Idiopathic More common in children with: • Decreased visual acuity in one eye • Paralysis of a cranial nerve • Restriction of movement of extraocular muscle • Neurologic disease including disorders associated with increased intracranial pressure
Wide epicanthal folds Broad nasal bridge	N/A	Wide nasal bridge Epicanthal folds
Diplopia Head turned to side of palsy to prevent diplopia	Neurologic complications of associated systemic diseases	Idiopathic Preceding viral infection CNS infection Increased intracranial pressure Ocular or intracranial masses
Ptosis Pupil is dilated and does not react to light	Neurologic complications of conditions causing increased intracranial pressure	Congenital Trauma Viral infection Increased intracranial pressure Migraine headaches
Diplopia Head tilted to side opposite the palsy to maintain alignment of the eyes. Side of face opposite to affected eye may have some degree of atrophy and appear smaller in comparison to other side of face.	The upward deviation of the eye is worse when the head is tilted toward the affected side.	Congenital Head trauma Viral infection Rarely, may be caused by intracranial tumor

OTHER
DIAGNOSES TO
CONSIDER

- Duane syndrome—medial and lateral rectus innervated by same nerve; both contract with adduction of the involved eye

- Möbius syndrome—palsy of the sixth and seventh cranial nerve; associated limb and craniofacial anomalies

- Hydrocephalus

- Myasthenia gravis

SUGGESTED READINGS

American Academy of Pediatrics, Committee on Practice and Ambulatory Medicine and Section of Ophthalmology. *Policy statement on eye examination in infants, children, and young adults by pediatricians.* Pediatrics. 2003;111(4):902–907.

Curnyn KM, Kaufman LM. The eye examination in the pediatrician's office. Pediatr Clin North Am. 2003;50:25–40.

Mittelman D. Amblyopia. Pediatr Clin North Am. 2003;50:189–196.

Oski FA, DeAngelis CD, Feigin RD, et al. Eye problems. In: *Principles and practice of pediatrics.* 2nd ed. Philadelphia: JB Lippincott Co; 1994:888–890.

Ticho BH. Strabismus. Pediatr Clin North Am. 2003;50:173–188.

Wright KW. *Pediatric ophthalmology for pediatricians.* Baltimore: Williams & Wilkins; 1999:21–29, 31–44, 45–69.

Ears

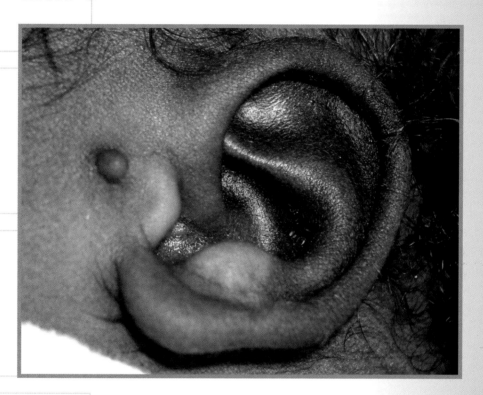

CHARLES A. POHL

Abnormalities in Ear Shape and Position

APPROACH TO THE PROBLEM

Normally, there is a wide variation of shapes, sizes, and positions of ears in children. Most auricular growth (85%) is completed by 3 years of age, cartilaginous formation by 5 to 6 years, and ear width and its distance from the scalp by 10 years. Abnormalities in ear shape or position may occur as isolated findings or as part of a complex of congenital anomalies. Congenital malformations of the external ear, which occur in 1:10,000 to 1:20,000 live births, include problems with ear size (e.g., micro-ear), position (e.g., posteriorly rotated, low-set ears), maldevelopment (e.g., anotia, microtia, cleft earlobe, lobular attachment), and protrusion (e.g., prominent, lopped, cupped).

Malformed or underdeveloped auricles are frequently seen with genetic problems such as Beckwith-Wiedemann syndrome (creased lobes), CHARGE association (lopped or cupped ears), facio-auriculo-vertebral spectrum (Goldenhar syndrome; microtia), Levy-Hollister (cupped ears), or Trisomy 21 (small ears). Low-set ears commonly occur in syndromes such as Noonan, Smith-Lemli-Opitz, Treacher Collins, and Trisomy 18. Several studies have found an association between renal anomalies and various ear abnormalities. Although the underlying etiology is unclear, the anomalies usually are not found as isolated findings, but rather as components of more complex congenital syndromes, such as Beckwith-Wiedemann or Trisomy 18.

When inspecting the external ear, it is important to evaluate its position, size, shape, and symmetry compared with the other ear. The protrusion angle of the ear should not exceed 15 degrees in children. Fifteen percent of the auricle (the superior attachment of the pinna) should be above the horizontal line (an imaginary line drawn from the inner canthus through the outer canthus). The angle between the vertical axis (the line perpendicular to the horizontal line) and the longitudinal axis of the ear (superior aspect of the outer helix to the inferior border of the earlobe) is normally between 10 degrees and 30 degrees. In addition, the length of an ear can be roughly estimated by measuring the distance between the arch of the eyebrow and the base of the ala nasi.

KEY POINTS IN THE HISTORY

- Because hearing impairment is associated with microtia, lopped, or cupped ears, and with meatal atresia, it is essential to ask about hearing and language development.

- Underlying renal anomalies should be considered when children with ear abnormalities have a history of deafness or a maternal history of gestational diabetes.

- Children with microtia often have hearing loss on the side of their normal-appearing auricle.

- Familial inheritance patterns are seen with abnormal earlobe attachments and cupped ears; therefore, asking about a family history of ear abnormalities may be helpful.

KEY POINTS IN THE PHYSICAL EXAMINATION

- Children with posteriorly rotated, low-set ears should be inspected carefully for other congenital abnormalities.

- When a child has protruding ears, normal auricular architecture distinguishes prominent ears from lopped or cupped ears.

- Micro-ears, unlike maldeveloped auricles such as microtia, are small but normally formed.

- Marked skull molding can make normal auricles appear protruded.

- Abnormal facial features including small chin, midfacial or nose hypoplasia, and highly arched eyebrows, can give the false impression of low-set, posteriorly rotated ears.

- Normally developed helices distinguish intrauterine compression abnormalities from the array of helix deformities. Also, intrauterine positioning effects do not generally result in symmetric abnormalities.

- Evaluation for renal anomalies should be considered when a patient with an auricular abnormality has other dysmorphic features, including facial asymmetry, choanal atresia, micrognathia, colobomas of the eye, branchial cysts, cardiac abnormalities, imperforate anus, and/or distal limb abnormalities.

DIFFERENTIAL DIAGNOSIS

CATEGORY	DIAGNOSIS	ICD-9	DISTINGUISHING CHARACTERISTICS	ASSOCIATED FINDINGS	OTHER FEATURES
Ear Size	Micro-ear	872.11	Normal auricular architecture, but smaller size	Usually none	N/A
Ear Position	Posteriorly rotated, low-set ears	744.2	External ear located inferior to normal location and rotated posteriorly	Isolated or component of complex syndrome, often involving the renal system	N/A
Maldeveloped Auricles	Microtia	744.23	Dysplastic or disorganized external ear Variable presentation—from a small deformed auricular appendage to gross hypoplasia with a blind or absent external canal	Hearing loss (even in normal appearing ear) Other auditory malformations common (e.g., external auditory meatus, middle ear abnormality, ossicular abnormality)	1.7/10,000 live births 2:1 male to female ratio Autosomal dominant or recessive
	Helix deformity	744.29	Partial abnormality of auricle	Usually isolated	N/A
	Cleft ear (bifid lobule)	744.2	Isolated maldevelopment of earlobe	N/A	N/A
	Adherent lobule/ lobular attachment	744.21	Earlobe attached anteriorly	Usually isolated	Familial
Protrusion	Prominent	744.29	Helix of ear is normally shaped and attached to the skull, but protrudes forward	N/A	N/A
	Lopped ear	744.29	Ear's helix and scapula fold downward because of inadequate development of antihelix; absence of antihelical fold	Hearing loss Similar to microtia Associated with anencephaly, microencephaly, severe congenital neuromotor deficiency; ossicular malformation	N/A
	Cupped ear	744.29	Ear malformation causes anterior protrusion of pinna and an exaggerated concave concha	Similar to lopped ear	Familial or sporadic
Maldevelopment of Ear Canal	Meatal atresia (aural atresia)	872	Atresia of auditory canal with or without pinna abnormality	Microtia Hearing impairment Craniofacial abnormality	1.5/20,000 live births Sporadic, autosomal dominant or recessive, chromosomal syndrome (e.g., Goldenhar syndrome)

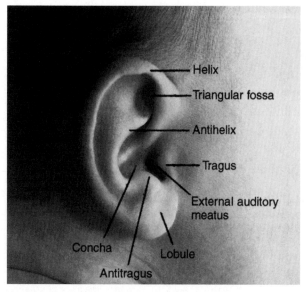

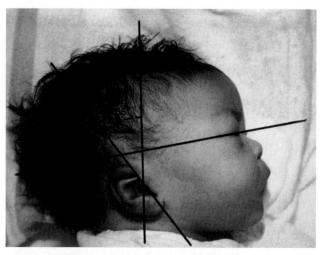

Figure 13-1 Normal anatomy of external ear. (Used with permission from Fletcher MA, ed. *Physical diagnosis in neonatology.* Philadelphia: Lippincott–Raven Publishers; 1998:285.)

Figure 13-2 Posteriorly rotated, low-set ears. (Used with permission from Fletcher MA, ed. *Physical diagnosis in neonatology.* Philadelphia: Lippincott–Raven Publishers; 1998:287.)

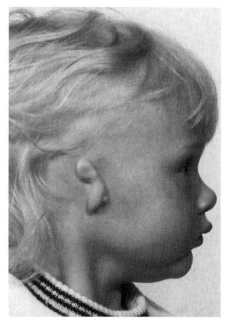

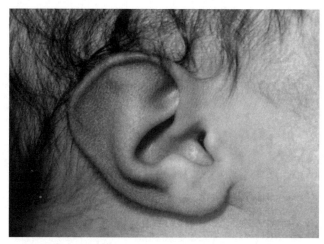

Figure 13-4 Helix deformity. (Used with permission from Fletcher MA, ed. *Physical diagnosis in neonatology.* Philadelphia: Lippincott–Raven Publishers; 1998:288.)

Figure 13-3 Microtia. (Used with permission from Cotton RT, Myer CM III, eds. *Practical pediatric otolaryngology.* Philadelphia: Lippincott–Raven Publishers; 1999:345.)

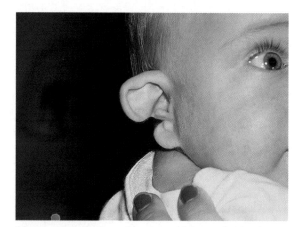

Figure 13-5 Cleft ear. (Courtesy of Steven D. Handler, MD, MBE.)

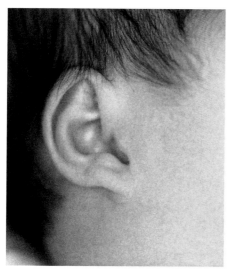

Figure 13-6 Adherent lobule/lobular attachment. (Used with permission from Fletcher MA, ed. *Physical diagnosis in neonatology.* Philadelphia: Lippincott–Raven Publishers; 1998:289.)

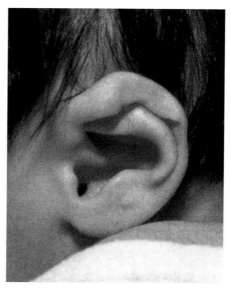

Figure 13-7 Lopped ear. (Used with permission from Fletcher MA, ed. *Physical diagnosis in neonatology.* Philadelphia: Lippincott–Raven Publishers; 1998:297.)

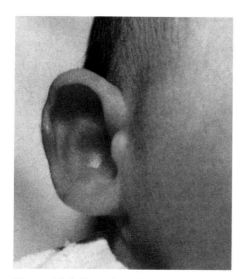

Figure 13-8 Cupped ear. (Used with permission from Fletcher MA, ed. *Physical diagnosis in neonatology.* Philadelphia: Lippincott–Raven Publishers; 1998:298.)

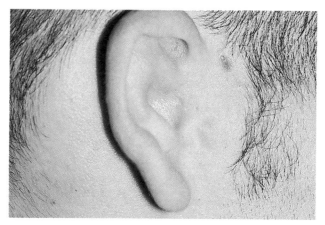

Figure 13-9 Meatal atresia. (Courtesy of Steven D. Handler, MD, MBE.)

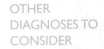

OTHER
DIAGNOSES TO
CONSIDER

- Intrauterine compression, such as folded helix

- Marked skull molding (appears "protruded")

- Craniofacial disproportion forms such as severe microcephaly (ear appears large)

- Appearance of "low-set" or "posteriorly rotated" ears when abnormal facial features are present, such as a small chin, midface hypoplasia, or highly arched eyebrows

- Epidermal nevus on ear

- Arteriovenous malformation

SUGGESTED READINGS
Bellucci RJ. Congenital aural malformation: diagnosis and treatment. *Otolaryngol Clin North Am.* 1981;14:95–124.
Bordley JE, Brookhouser PE, Tucker GK (eds.). *Ear, nose & throat disorders in children.* New York: Raven Press; 1986.
Cotton RT, Myer CM III, eds. *Practical pediatric otolaryngology.* Philadelphia: Lippincott–Raven Publishers; 1999:345.
Fletcher MA, ed. *Physical diagnosis in neonatology.* Philadelphia: Lippincott–Raven Publishers; 1998:285, 287, 288, 289, 297, 298.
Jones KL. *Smith's recognizable patterns of human malformation.* 5th ed. Philadelphia: WB Saunders; 1997.
Wang RY, Earl DL, Ruder RO, et al. Syndromic ear anomalies and renal ultrasounds. *Pediatrics.* 2001;108(2):E32.

Ear Swelling

KATHLEEN CRONAN

APPROACH TO THE PROBLEM

Swelling of the external ear may be a concerning symptom to parents. Most causes of ear swelling are benign. Insect bites, for example, are a common cause of ear swelling in pediatric patients. However, the swelling seen with insect bites and other benign entities may mimic other diseases, such as cellulitis, bacterial chondritis, and mastoiditis, that require immediate attention. Blunt trauma to the ear results in swelling and discoloration of the auricle, pinna, or both. Mastoiditis, an uncommon bacterial infection, causes swelling and erythema of the pinna in addition to posterior auricular swelling and tenderness.

KEY POINTS IN THE HISTORY

- Pruritus, associated with swelling and erythema, is the typical presentation of an insect bite to the ear.

- A previous history of ear piercing or laceration to the ear lobe should raise the suspicion for a keloid. Patients with keloids will often have a history of keloids on other parts of their body.

- Recent ear pain with or without drainage in conjunction with posterior auricular swelling, fever, or both may indicate mastoiditis.

- Duration of symptoms often helps to distinguish an insect bite from cellulitis. Swelling and erythema resulting from an insect bite occur suddenly, whereas the swelling, tenderness, and redness of cellulitis gradually develop.

- A history of recent otitis externa may precede cellulitis of the auricle.

**KEY POINTS IN
THE PHYSICAL
EXAMINATION**

- Trauma, which may present as an auricular hematoma, and cellulitis typically present as swelling of the pinna and auricle, whereas mastoiditis presents as swelling and redness of the posterior auricular (for example, in the area of the mastoid) and auricular areas.

- Forward displacement of the pinna usually indicates mastoiditis, although a posterior auricular insect bite can cause ear displacement when significant associated swelling is present.

- A rubbery, fleshy mass that extends beyond the wound margins indicates keloid formation.

- Erythema, swelling, warmth, and tenderness of the auricle usually indicate cellulitis. If there is no tenderness in association with the swelling and redness, an insect bite is more likely than cellulitis.

- Pain elicited with traction on the pinna and/or pressure on the tragus is associated with otitis externa.

- A bluish discoloration of the auricle accompanied by swelling suggests trauma. Petechial lesions on top of or inside the pinna are highly suspicious for an intentional injury that may be the result of pinching and pulling the pinna as seen with boxing or child physical abuse.

- Erythema and tenderness of the overlying skin and perichondrium suggests perichondritis.

DIFFERENTIAL DIAGNOSIS

DIAGNOSIS	ICD-9	DISTINGUISHING CHARACTERISTICS	DISTRIBUTION	ASSOCIATED FINDINGS	PREDISPOSING FACTORS
Cellulitis	380.10	Erythema Warmth Tenderness Originating from a wound Edema	Pinna Earlobe	Fever Red streaking Wound	Insect bites Laceration Earring related Ear piercing
Insect Bite	910.8	Erythema Swelling Nontender Papule or punctum at site of bite Pruritus	Pinna Posterior auricular space	Other papules on skin surface	Insect bite Sting
Mastoiditis	383.00	Edema of pinna and skin overlying mastoid Erythema of pinna/skin over mastoid process Tenderness of mastoid process Displacement of pinna inferiorly and anteriorly	Postauricular area Mastoid periosteum Pinna	Otitis media Purulent otorrhea Fever Toxicity	Otitis media
Trauma	959.09	Discoloration with ecchymoses Hematoma between the perichondrium and the cartilage Pallor of area	Pinna Earlobe Auricle	Hemotympanum Perforated tympanic membrane	Direct blow to the ear Frost bite
Keloid	701.4	Flesh colored mass May be tender and pruritic initially Rubbery Extends beyond margins of wound	Ear lobe Site of wound	Other sites of keloid formation	Pierced ear Ear laceration Insect bites
Perichondritis	380.00 (pinna, auricle) 380.01 (acute, of pinna) 380.02 (chronic, of pinna)	Erythema Tenderness Swelling	Pinna Site of wound	Puncture from earring Laceration Nodule Fever	Ear piercing through the cartilage Laceration through cartilage

PHOTOGRAPHS OF SELECTED DIAGNOSES

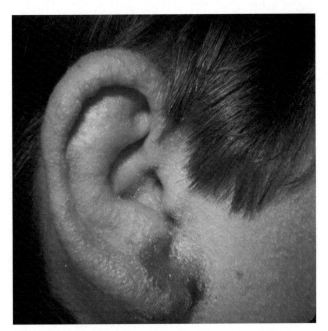

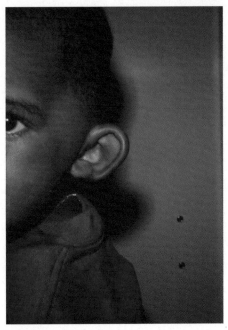

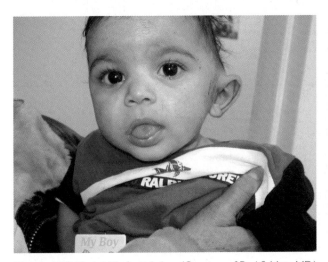

Figure 14-1 Cellulitis. (Courtesy of Kathleen Cronan, MD.)

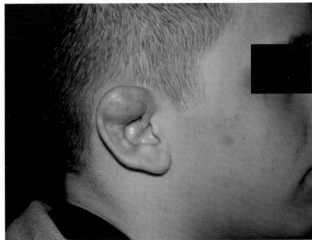

Figure 14-2 Insect bite to ear. (Courtesy of Kathleen Cronan, MD.)

Figure 14-3 Mastoiditis, frontal view. (Courtesy of Paul S. Matz, MD.)

Figure 14-4 Auricular hematoma from trauma to the ear. (Courtesy of Kathleen Cronan, MD.)

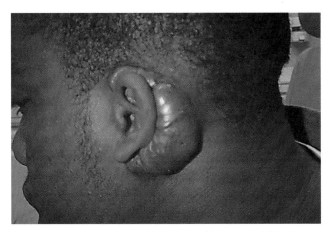

Figure 14-5 Keloid at ear piercing site. (Courtesy of Steven Cook, MD.)

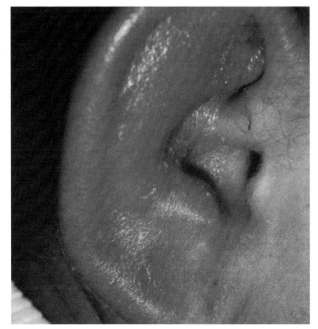

Figure 14-6 Perichondritis. (Used with permission from Handler SD, Myer CM. *Atlas of ear, nose and throat disorders in children.* Ontario, Canada: BC Decker; 1998:12.)

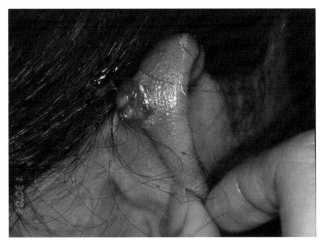

Figure 14-7 Infected ear piercing site. (Courtesy of Ellen Deutsch, MD.)

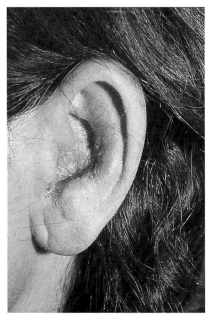

Figure 14-8 Ramsay Hunt syndrome. (Courtesy of Steven D. Handler, MD, MBE.)

OTHER DIAGNOSES TO CONSIDER

- Malignant otitis externa

- Xanthomatosis

- Relapsing polychondritis

- Henoch-Schönlein purpura involving the ear lobe and pinna

- Ramsay Hunt syndrome or herpes zoster oticus

SUGGESTED READINGS

Arnett AM. Pain-earache. In: Fleisher GR, Ludwig S, eds. *Textbook of pediatric emergency medicine.* 4th ed. Philadelphia: Lippincott Williams & Wilkins; 2000:454–455.

Feigin RD, Alexander JJ. Otitis externa. In: Feigin RD, Cherry JD, Demmler GJ, Kaplan SL, eds. *Textbook of pediatric infectious diseases.* 5th ed. Philadelphia: WB Saunders; 2004:212–213.

Handler SD, Myer CM. *Atlas of ear, nose and throat disorders in children.* Ontario, Canada: B.C. Decker, Inc.; 1998:12.

Lewis K, Shapiro NL, Cherry JD. Mastoiditis. In: Feigin RD, Cherry JD, Demmler GJ, Kaplan SL, eds. *Textbook of pediatric infectious diseases.* 5th ed. Philadelphia: WB Saunders; 2004:235–240.

Maffei FA, Davis HW. Minor lesions and injuries. In: Feigin RD, Cherry JD, Demmler GJ, Kaplan SL, eds. *Textbook of pediatric infectious diseases.* 4th ed. Philadelphia: WB Saunders; 2000:1509.

RENEE M. TURCHI AND DAVID E. TUNKEL
Ear Pits and Tags

APPROACH TO THE PROBLEM

Preauricular pits (ear pits or sinuses) and tags (ear tags) have a prevalence rate of approximately 0.5% to 1.0% in newborns. Preauricular sinuses are reportedly more common in Asian and African American children. These congenital anomalies may be unsightly and also may be associated with abnormalities in other organ systems as part of a syndrome (e.g., Goldenhar syndrome). While some pits are shallow, others are deeper and associated with a sinus tract (preauricular sinuses) or a cystic dilatation (preauricular cysts) that may contain sebaceous material. Preauricular cysts and sinuses are embryologically distinct from first branchial cysts as preauricular cysts are the result of faulty resorption or fusion of the auricular hillocks. When infected, prompt antimicrobial therapy and even surgical treatment may be necessary to treat preauricular sinuses and cysts. Symptomatic or unsightly external ear pits and tags can be removed by surgeons under general or local anesthesia, with few complications. Recurrence rates are nominal when complete excision is performed.

Recent literature has documented the low yield of routine renal ultrasonography in the evaluation of infants with preauricular sinuses and tags in the absence of other anomalies. The yield of routine renal ultrasonography in children with preauricular pits or tags is 0% to 9%. In general, renal ultrasonography should be obtained when preauricular pits and tags are found in children with other congenital anomalies or dysmorphisms. Routine audiological screening of children with ear sinuses and tags is generally accepted—early diagnosis of hearing loss facilitates favorable outcomes.

KEY POINTS IN THE HISTORY

- Ear pits and tags are usually asymptomatic.

- Ear pits and tags typically are isolated entities, but they occur more frequently in children with craniofacial abnormalities.

- Ear pits and tags can be unilateral or bilateral.

- Multiple ear tags have been described in the literature, but multiple ear pits have rarely been reported.

- Ear tags do not grow rapidly.

- Approximately 50% of children with preauricular sinuses have positive family histories. Having families identify other affected members may help to allay fears or address concerns they may have.

- Signs and symptoms of preauricular pit, sinus, or cyst infection are: swelling, erythema, pain, and purulent drainage. Infection of ear pits is usually the result of self-manipulation, and the causative agents include staphylococcus and streptococcus.

- Ear pits associated with recurrent infections and/or drainage require surgical removal.

- First branchial cleft cysts and sinuses are usually present at birth and may go unnoticed until they become infected. They may present with preauricular or postauricular swelling, or with drainage from a sinus tract.

KEY POINTS IN THE PHYSICAL EXAMINATION

- Ear tags are usually nontender, flesh-colored, nondraining mounds of epithelial tissue located anterior to the tragus or the crus of the helix and attached to the surface of the cheek. They may have cartilaginous tissue in the center.

- Ear pits or sinus tracts are usually located in the front of the ear, above the tragus, proximal to the anterior helix border. Preauricular sinus tracts may extend and tunnel under the skin.

- Infected pits are often erythematous, edematous, and tender, and they may have purulent drainage or granulation tissue present. Swelling or fluctuance from infection may occur at a site 1 cm to 2 cm away from the sinus tract opening, as the infected sac may be remote from the tract opening.

- First branchial cleft cysts are usually preauricular at the angle of the mandible, along the anterior border of the sternocleidomastoid. They are nontender unless infected. The sinus tracts associated with first branchial clefts are usually more anterior and inferior than preauricular sinus tracts.

DIAGNOSIS	ICD-9	DISTINGUISHING CHARACTERISTICS	DISTRIBUTION	ASSOCIATED FINDINGS	COMPLICATIONS
Preauricular Tags	744.1	Painless Flesh-colored No or minimal growth	Located anterior to tragus or crus of the helix Attached to cheek, pinna, tragus, or lobe	Found in patients with "oculoauriculovertebral" syndromes, chromosome 11q duplications and 4p deletions	Rarely infected Hearing loss and renal anomalies are uncommon associated findings
Preauricular Pits, Sinuses/ Cysts	744.46 744.47	Small, pin-sized hole most commonly found at junction of pinna and temporal skin Nonerythematous May have scanty drainage No swelling	Usually in front of ear; anterior and superior to the tragus	Found in patients with branchio-otorenal syndrome, Beckwith-Wiedemann syndrome, and chromosome 11q duplication	Can become infected May have associated sinus tract or cystic mass below skin Hearing loss and renal anomalies are uncommon associated findings
Infected Preauricular Pits	682.9 (cellulitis)	Erythema, edema Tenderness Draining purulent fluid	(See Preauricular Pits in Diagnosis)	Edema may obscure the opening of the ear pit	Require antibiotics and surgical drainage by specialists Subsequent removal recommended after infection clears
First Branchial Cleft Sinus/ Cyst	744.41 (sinus tract) 744.42 (cyst)	Slowly enlarging (cyst) sinus—pitlike opening in front and below ear canal Often fluctuant and unattached	Preauricular to upper neck region	Associated ear pit may be found close to cyst	May become infected Surgical removal usually necessary Tract often intimately involved with facial nerve, making surgical removal challenging

PHOTOGRAPHS OF SELECTED DIAGNOSES

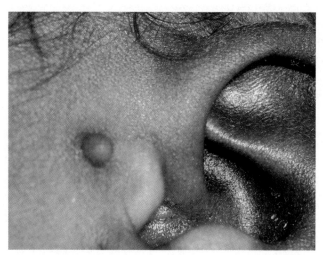

Figure 15-1 Simple preauricular tag. (Courtesy of Esther K. Chung, MD, MPH.)

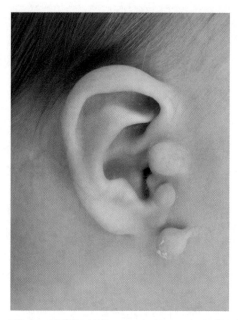

Figure 15-2 Multiple preauricular tags in a child with oculoauriculovertebral spectrum disorder. (Courtesy of David Tunkel, MD.)

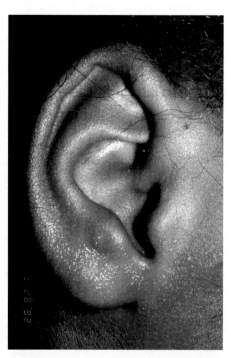

Figure 15-3 Preauricular pit. Note how visualization can be obscured by hairline. (Courtesy of David Tunkel, MD.)

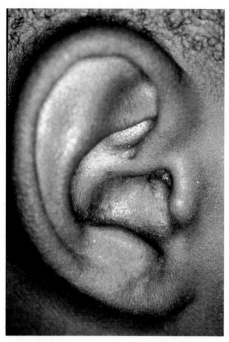

Figure 15-4 Auricular sinus on the inferior crus area of the pinna. (Courtesy of David Tunkel, MD.)

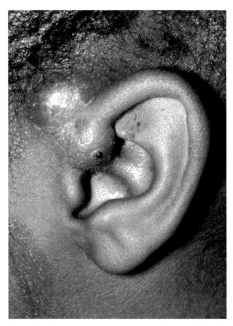

Figure 15-5 Infected preauricular sinus. The swelling nearly obscures identification of the offending sinus tract opening. (Courtesy of David Tunkel, MD.)

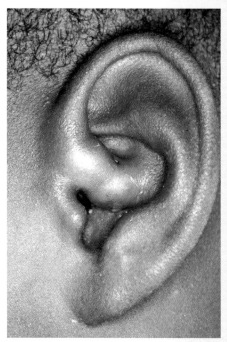

Figure 15-6 Infected auricular pit on the inferior crus. Note erythema and edema. (Courtesy of David Tunkel, MD.)

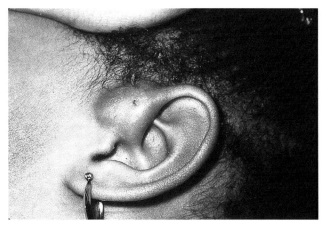

Figure 15-7 Preauricular abscess. (Courtesy of Steven D. Handler, MD, MBE.)

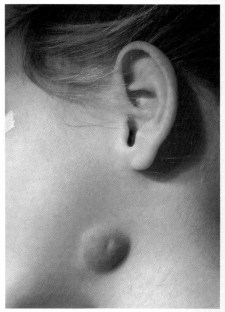

Figure 15-8 First branchial cleft sinus. While not a true a preauricular sinus, this lesion must be considered in the differential diagnosis. (Courtesy of David Tunkel, MD.)

OTHER
DIAGNOSES TO
CONSIDER

- Duplication of ear canal

- Cellulitis from otitis externa

- Reaction to body piercing

- Association with craniofacial or chromosomal syndromes, such as:

    - Oculoauriculovertebral malformation (hemifacial microsomia or Goldenhar syndrome)

    - Chromosome 11q duplication

    - Chromosome 4p deletions

    - Branchio-otorenal (Melnick Fraser) syndrome

    - Beckwith-Wiedemann syndrome

SUGGESTED READINGS
Bianca S, Ingegnosi C, Ettore G. Preauricular tags and associated anomalies: considerations for genetic counseling. *Genet Couns*. 2003;14(3):321–324.
Handler SD, Myer CM. *Atlas of ear, nose and throat disorders in children*. Ontario, Canada: B.C. Decker, Inc.; 1998:6–8.
Kohelet D, Arbel E. A prospective search for urinary tract abnormalities in infants with isolated preauricular tags. *Pediatrics*. 2000;105(5):E61.
Kugelman A, Tubi A, Bader D, et al. Preauricular tags and pits in the newborn: the role of renal ultrasonography. *J Pediatr*. 2002;141(3):388–391.
Prasad S, Grundfast K, Milmoe G. Management of congenital preauricular pit and sinus tract in children. *Laryngoscope*. 1990;100(3):320–321.
Wang RY, Earl DL, Ruder RO, et al. Syndromic ear anomalies and renal ultrasounds. *Pediatrics*. 2001;108(2):E32.

16

LEE R. ATKINSON-MCEVOY AND
ESTHER K. CHUNG

Ear Canal Findings

APPROACH TO THE PROBLEM

Physicians caring for children frequently see patients who have complaints about the ear, including pain, itching, drainage, and decreased hearing. Often, the initial concern is focused on middle ear abnormalities, but external auditory canal (EAC) abnormalities may cause complaints that are similar to those caused by middle ear pathology. Common diseases of the EAC include otitis externa (affecting up to 10% of the population), impacted cerumen, trauma, and foreign bodies in the ear.

There are many variations in cerumen in the canal and canal size and shape. In some cases, as in Down syndrome, the canals may be narrowed, making it difficult for the examiner to evaluate the tympanic membrane on routine otoscopy.

KEY POINTS IN THE HISTORY

- School-aged children may be exceptionally precise in their description of pain. Therefore, it is important to ask them to describe what they are feeling. Often, when parents report pain, the child instead reports ringing or fullness. For example, one child with water in his ear reported, "It sounds like I am under water."

- Use of cotton swabs or other objects to clean the ear may result in trauma to the EAC and tympanic membrane. Retained pieces of cotton may cause subsequent inflammation.

- Placement of a foreign body in the ear may lead to trauma and most often presents with pain. If the foreign body is not promptly removed, the EAC may become infected.

- Tinnitus and bleeding, in addition to pain, may be symptoms that occur from trauma to the external ear canal.

- Decreased hearing often occurs with cerumen impaction, fluid in the external canal, or otitis externa, but it may also be seen in trauma, particularly when perforation of the tympanic membrane exists.

- Drainage from the EAC may occur in acute otitis media with perforation, otitis externa, and external fluid in the canal (residual from swimming or baths).

- The drainage seen with acute otitis media with perforation is often described as brownish and sticky.

- Pseudomonas and fungal infections should be considered in children with chronic symptoms of otitis externa.

- History of frequent swimming or submersion of ears while in the bathtub is suggestive of otitis externa (also known as *swimmer's ear*). Water from the pool or tub is believed to cause alterations in the normal flora of the EAC.

- Patients with eczema, seborrhea, or psoriasis may have involvement of the epidermis of the EAC and may complain of pruritus.

- Use of medication or topical substances to the ear may result in an eczematous dermatitis.

- Earrings, particularly those made of alloy metals, may cause inflammation at the earring site and an eczematous dermatitis of the surrounding tissues.

KEY POINTS IN THE PHYSICAL EXAMINATION

- It is important to note that there may be variations in the amount, color, and consistency of cerumen.

- If blood is present, suspect trauma and carefully inspect the tympanic membrane for perforation or other injury.

- Pain elicited from pressure on the tragus and/or outward traction on the pinna is suggestive of otitis externa.

- Edema and inflammation of the ear canal is typically seen with otitis externa.

- When a significant amount of discharge is present, it may be difficult to differentiate acute otitis media with perforation and otitis externa.

- Greasy scales, dry or flaky skin, excoriation, and crusting of the external ear canal and pinna may be seen with eczematous or psoriatic dermatitis and seborrhea.

- Pustules on the outer portion of the EAC suggest furunculosis.

DIFFERENTIAL DIAGNOSIS

DIAGNOSIS	ICD-9	DISTINGUISHING CHARACTERISTICS	ASSOCIATED FINDINGS	COMPLICATIONS	PREDISPOSING FACTORS
Foreign Body in EAC	385.83	Foreign bodies—most commonly seen in younger children	Acute setting—possibly pain or decreased hearing Chronic setting—foul odor or discharge	Hearing loss	Cleaning ears with cotton swabs Toddler-aged children frequently place foreign bodies in their ears
Trauma/ Superficial Injury to EAC	910.8	Bleeding or pain of the ear	Bloody discharge—may be decreased hearing whenever the tympanic membrane is affected	Hearing loss	Foreign body in ear Aggressive cleaning with an object
Acute Otitis Media with Perforation	382.01	Mucoid, whitish to grayish discharge in canal Canal walls, when visualized, are not irritated or red	May be associated with systemic symptoms, such as fever.	Hearing loss Speech delays if recurrent	Associated with preceding upper respiratory infection
Otitis Externa	380.10	Tenderness with pressure on the tragus and outward traction on the pinna	Edema of the external ear canal with seropurulent discharge or whitish to grayish exudate Generally no fever	Rarely, otitis media from invasion through the tympanic membrane Cellulitis	Trauma to external ear canal or exposure to water
Seborrheic Otitis Externa	690.10	Greasy appearing scales that may involve the auricle	Patient may have seborrheic dermatitis in other areas, especially the scalp	Scarring and narrowing of external ear canal	Family history of seborrheic dermatitis
Eczematous Otitis Externa	380.22	Dry, flaky skin that may be pruritic	History of diffuse eczema	Scarring and narrowing of external ear canal	Use of topical medications or exposure to metals (earrings) or cosmetics
Psoriatic Otitis Externa	696.1	Dry scaly plaques with a silvery quality	History of psoriasis	Scarring and narrowing of external ear canal	History of psoriasis
Chronic Mycotic Otitis Externa	380.15	Intense itching, but usually painless	May form an exudate that may have a musty odor	Untreated infections can lead to bacterial superinfection	Recurrent or chronic otitis externa
Furunculosis	680.0	Erythematous pustules in the anterior portion of the external ear canal	Point tenderness at the site of the furuncle	Scarring and narrowing of external ear canal	Infection of hair follicle

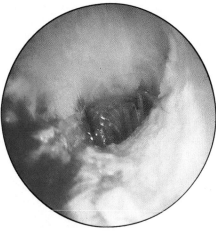

Figure 16-1 Cockroach in external canal. (Courtesy of Ellen Deutsch, MD.)

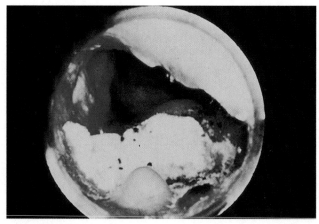

Figure 16-2 Otitis externa. (Courtesy of Steven D. Handler, MD, MBE.)

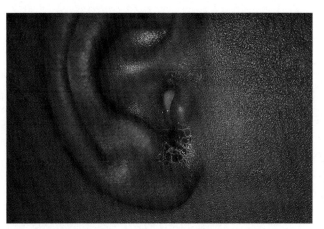

Figure 16-3 Otorrhea associated with a cholesteatoma. (Courtesy of Ellen Deutsch, MD.)

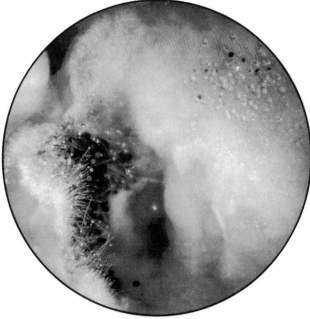

Figure 16-4 Mycotic otitis externa. (Used with permission from Mycotic Handler SD, Myer CM. *Atlas of ear, nose and throat disorders in children.* Hamilton: BC Decker; 1998:24.)

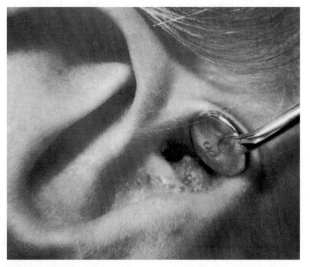

Figure 16-5 Furuncle of the external auditory canal. (Used with permission from Handler SD, Myer CM. *Atlas of ear, nose and throat disorders in children.* Hamilton: BC Decker; 1998:24.)

OTHER
DIAGNOSES TO
CONSIDER

- Osteomyelitis

- Acne

- Cholesteatoma

- External auditory canal exostosis

- Malignant otitis externa

SUGGESTED READINGS

Beers SL, Abramo TJ. Otitis externa review. *Pediatr Emerg Care*. 2004;20(4):250–253.

Dohar JE. Evolution of management approaches for otitis externa. *Pediatr Infect Dis J*. 2003;22(4):299–308.

Handler SD, Myer CM. *Atlas of ear, nose, and throat disorders in children*. Hamilton: B.C. Decker; 1998:22–27.

McCoy SI, Zell ER, Besser RE. Antimicrobial prescribing for otitis externa in children. *Pediatr Infect Dis J*. 2004;23(2):181–183.

Roland PS, Stroman DW. Microbiology of acute otitis externa. *Laryngoscope*. 2002;112:1166–1177.

van Balen FA, Smit WM, Zuithoff NP, et al. Clinical efficacy of three common treatments in acute otitis externa in primary care: randomized controlled trial. *BMJ*. 2003;327:1201–1205.

Tympanic Membrane Abnormalities

APPROACH TO THE PROBLEM

Acute otitis media (AOM) is one of the most common diagnoses and reasons for antibiotic prescriptions in children. With more than five million cases diagnosed annually, it is associated with individual discomfort, family disruption, financial costs, serious sequelae, and antimicrobial resistance. For these reasons, it is important to make the correct diagnosis when evaluating the tympanic membrane (TM).

Pneumatic otoscopy allows visualization of TM characteristics: color, contour, position (normal, retracted, full, bulging), and mobility. A normal TM is described as translucent, pearly gray, and mobile. A light reflex and bony landmarks, such as the arm of the malleus, are generally easily viewed. The examination, though, requires the child to be restrained or held still and to have a clean ear canal. Also, a pneumatic otoscope with a good seal and light source must be available.

KEY POINTS IN THE HISTORY

- Acute onset, hyperpyrexia, and otalgia are features of AOM and not otitis media with effusion (OME).

- Concomitant or recent upper respiratory infections or allergies are commonly seen with AOM and OME.

- Hearing loss is a nonspecific finding that may be caused by middle ear fluid (AOM, OME), as well as by structural damage of the TM or ossicles (severe tympanosclerosis, TM perforation, or cholesteotoma).

- Refer children to a pediatric otolaryngologist whenever TM perforation is accompanied by either hearing loss or vertigo, or when middle ear fluid is chronic and associated with hearing loss and/or speech delay.

- Suspect cholesteatoma if persistent middle ear effusion (MEE) or hearing impairment, greasy and/or whitish mass, or no clinical response is present when treating another suspected TM problem.

- When a cholesteatoma is associated with ataxia or headaches, neuroimaging should be considered to evaluate for the presence of a brain abscess.

KEY POINTS IN THE PHYSICAL EXAMINATION

- Must immobilize head carefully and firmly when evaluating the TM and ear canal, while using a snug-fitting ear speculum. The small (2.5 mm diameter) ear speculum should be used in infants and preschool children, while the large (4 mm diameter) ear speculum should be used in school-aged children and adolescents.

- The light reflex may be absent in some normal children.

- Mobility, assessed by pneumatic otoscopy, should be measured especially when the history and/or physical examination suggest a problem. Poor TM mobility is associated with AOM, middle ear effusion (MEE), TM perforation, or TM structural damage (e.g., tympanosclerosis).

- Mild TM erythema can occur in association with fever, crying, upper respiratory viral infections, or irritation from cerumen or foreign objects.

- AOM should have evidence of MEE *and* acute inflammation (TM bulging or fullness, marked erythema, otorrhea, or yellow or cloudy fluid).

- Air bubbles and amber TM discoloration are associated with serous middle ear fluid or OME.

- Blood in the ME causes a bluish, deep red, or brown ("chocolate") appearance of the TM.

- Chalky white plaques on TM (tympanosclerosis) are seen with healed inflammation.

- TM mobility is absent or decreased with TM perforation.

- Manipulation of the ear pinna to ensure proper visualization of TM varies with age. As in adults, the pinna should be lifted posteriosuperiorly in older children. Pinna should be pulled horizontally backward in infants and younger children.

- Localized TM atelectasis, especially in the posteriosuperior quadrant of pars tensa, is seen with retraction pockets.

- Excessive localized mobility reflects a healed perforation or TM thinning.

- OME is evidenced by fluid bubbles and air-fluid levels or by at least two of the following TM changes: abnormal color including white, yellow, amber, or blue; opacification; decreased mobility.

DIAGNOSIS	ICD-9	DISTINGUISHING CHARACTERISTICS	ASSOCIATED FINDINGS	PREDISPOSING FACTORS	COMPLICATIONS
Acute Otitis Media (AOM)	382.0	Usually under age 6 years MEE and features of acute inflammation: otalgia, fullness or bulging TM, marked TM erythema, otorrhea, yellow or cloudy fluid Malleus may be obscured; TM will have poor mobility Acute onset	Fever Otalgia Dizziness Unsteady gait	Upper respiratory infection Allergies Environmental tobacco smoke	Structural damage of TM or ear bones (ossicles) Hearing impairment Mastoiditis Facial paralysis Persistent perforation Intracranial infection (rare) Cholesteatoma formation
Otitis Media with Effusion (OME)	381.4	Absence of pain or fever Nonerythemeatous, nonmobile TM with serous or mucuid fluid Bubbles or air-fluid interface noted on otoscopy TM discolorations(white, yellow, or amber) TM atelectasis common (prominence of the short process of the malleus) Usually indolent course	Ear popping Feeling of fullness or pressure Hearing loss Vertigo	Concomitant resolving AOM Allergies Upper respiratory viral infection	Hearing loss Speech/language delay TM atelectasis Developmental/learning impairment Cholesteatoma Usually spontaneously resolves (50% to 60% resolve 2 weeks after AOM treated, 80% 4 weeks after treatment, 90% after 8 weeks)
Tympanosclerosis (Myringosclerosis)	385.0	"Chalky white plaque" in fibrous layer of TM Reddish or yellowish localized deposit early Poor mobility when severe	Conductive hearing loss when AOM is present Asymptomatic if small patch	Ear infections (severe AOM) Ventilation tube insertion	Conductive hearing loss
TM Perforation	384.2 382.01	Hole in TM Everted, ragged edges resulting from sudden pressure changes; bloody when resulting from direct TM trauma Anteroinferior quadrant when resulting from sudden pressure changes; posteriorly when resulting from direct trauma	Refer if vertigo, persistent hearing loss, or when perforation does not heal Hearing loss Bleeding Pain Tinnitus	Direct TM trauma (e.g., cotton swab, hairpins) Ear trauma Sudden ear pressure changes in ear canal (e.g., gunfire or violent slap) AOM Chronic OME	Usually heals spontaneously Marginal perforation less likely to heal than central ones and more likely to lead to cholesteatoma or intracranial infection Residual perforation Water entering middle ear Ear infections Ossicular damage (more likely when resulting from direct TM trauma)
Cholesteatoma	385.32	Greasy, whitish mass of keratin debris	Dizziness Ataxia and headaches (suggests brain abscess) Hearing loss Chronic otorrhea	Congenital Recurrent AOM Persistent MEE	Bony structure erosion Hearing loss Facial nerve paralysis Intracranial process (e.g., brain abscess, meningitis)
Hemotympanum	385.89	Extravasated blood or blood stained fluid in ME space Bright red or dark red, blue, or brown ("chocolate" ear drum) TM	Hearing loss Pain Feeling of pressure or fullness	Head injury Barotrauma (e.g., flying, diving) Temporal bone fracture Severe AOM Middle ear surgery	Usually resolves spontaneously Hearing loss TM perforation
Atelectasis	384.9	Retracted and atrophic TM Golden-yellow serous effusion TM thinning and transparent over time (may resemble perforation)	Often asymptomatic Muffled sounds; feeling of pressure or fullness	Untreated OME (prolonged negative pressure)	Fluctuating conductive hearing loss
Retraction Pockets	384.9	Localized atelectasis Usually on posteriosuperior quadrants of pars tensa	Usually asymptomatic	Atrophic TM from recurrent OM, atelectasis, chronic eustachian tube dysfunction Trauma	Cholesteatoma Hearing loss

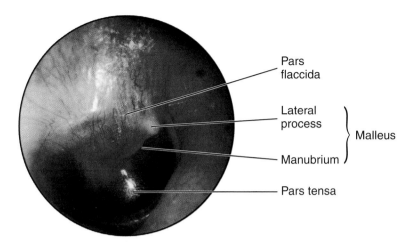

Pars
flaccida

Lateral
process

Manubrium

} Malleus

Pars tensa

Figure 17-1 Normal tympanic membrane. (Photo used with permission from Handler SD, Myer CM. *Atlas of ear, nose and throat disorders in children.* Ontario, Canada: BC Decker; 1998:28.)

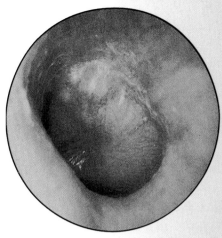

Figure 17-2 Acute otitis media. (Courtesy of Steven D. Handler, MD, MBE.)

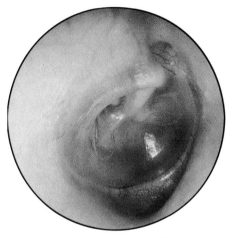

Figure 17-3 Otitis media with effusion. (Courtesy of Glenn Isaacson, MD.)

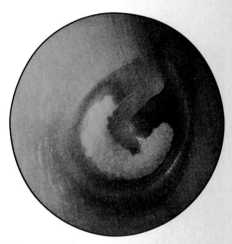

Figure 17-4 Tympanosclerosis. (Courtesy of Steven D. Handler, MD, MBE.)

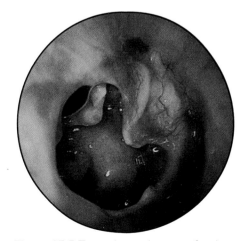

Figure 17-5 Tympanic membrane perforation. (Courtesy of Steven D. Handler, MD, MBE.)

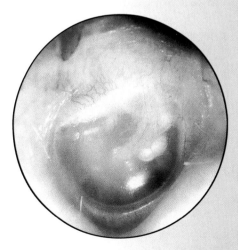

Figure 17-6 Cholesteatoma. (Used with permission from Handler SD, Myer CM. *Atlas of ear, nose and throat disorders in children.* Ontario, Canada: BC Decker; 1998:30.)

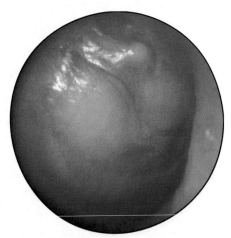

Figure 17-7 Cholesteatoma. Note the white, pearly lesion seen behind the tympanic membrane in the anterior and posterior superior quadrants. (Courtesy of John A. Germiller, MD, PhD.)

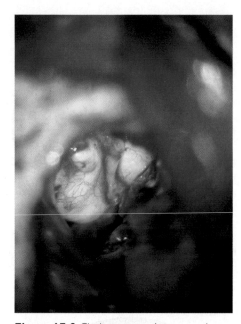

Figure 17-8 Cholesteatoma. Intraoperative view of the lesion that corresponds with the previous figure. (Courtesy of John A. Germiller, MD, PhD.)

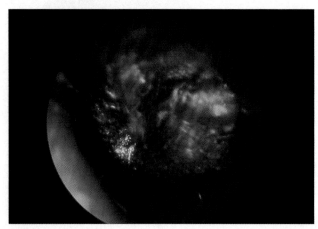

Figure 17-9 Hemotympanum. This hemotympanum was seen in association with a left temporal bone fracture. (Courtesy of Ellen Deutsch, MD.)

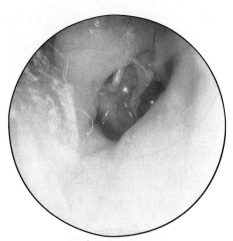

Figure 17-10 Atelectasis, severe. (Courtesy of Ellen Deutsch, MD.)

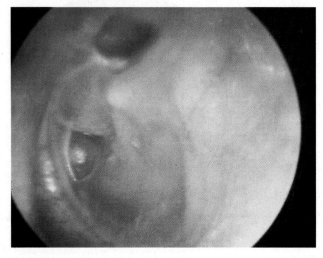

Figure 17-11 Retraction pocket. (Courtesy of Steven D. Handler, MD, MBE.)

OTHER
DIAGNOSES TO
CONSIDER

- Bullous myringitis

- Improper technique (e.g., inadequate light resource, poor speculum seal)

- Cerumen

- Mastoiditis

- Trauma to temporal bone

- Foreign body in ear canal

- Bleeding disorder

- Glomus tympanicum or glomus jugulare tumor

- Otosclerosis (Schwartze's sign)

SUGGESTED READINGS

American Academy of Family Physicians, American Academy of Otolaryngology—Head and Neck Surgery, American Academy of Pediatrics Subcommittee on Otitis Media With Effusion. Otitis media with effusion. *Pediatrics.* 2004;113:1412–1429.

Handler SD, Myer CM. *Atlas of ear, nose and throat disorders in children.* Ontario, Canada: B.C. Decker, Inc.; 1998:28,30.

Kaeida PH. The COMPLETES exam for otitis. *Contemp Pediatr.* 1997;14:93–101.

Paradise JL. Otitis media in infants and children. *Pediatrics.* 1980;65:917–943.

Paradise JL. Managing otitis media: a time for change. *Pediatrics.* 1995;96:712–715.

Paradise JL. On classifying otitis media as suppurative or nonsuppurative, with a suggested clinical schema. *J Pediatr.* 1987;111:948–951.

Pichichero ME. Acute otitis media: improving diagnostic accuracy—Part I. *AFP.* 2000;61:2051–2056.

Stool SE, Berg AO, Berman S, et al. Otitis media with effusion in young children. Clinical Practice Guideline, No. 12. AHCPR Publication No. 94-0622. Rockville, MD: Agency for Health Care Policy and Research, Public Health Service, US Department of Health and Human Services; July 1994.

Subcommittee on Management of Acute Otitis Media. American Academy of Pediatrics. Diagnosis and management of acute otitis media. *Pediatrics.* 2004;113:1451–1465.

FIVE

Nose

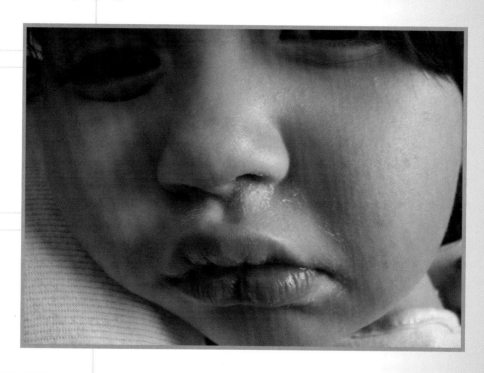

SHOSHANA MELMAN

Nasal Bridge Swelling

APPROACH TO THE PROBLEM

Nasal bridge swelling may be the result of masses, including dermoid cysts, encephaloceles, or hemangiomas; infectious processes; inflammatory conditions; and trauma. Nasal bridge lesions may cause airway obstruction, impairment of vision, bleeding, and central nervous system infections. Additionally, patients and their families often fear the facial disfigurement that may result from these lesions.

KEY POINTS IN THE HISTORY

- Nasal dermoid sinus cysts are the most common of congenital midline nasal masses. They may be present at birth or discovered years later when symptomatic.

- Patients with nasal bridge encephaloceles may also have chromosomal anomalies, other congenital malformations, and cerebrospinal fluid rhinorrhea.

- Nasal fractures are most commonly a result of blunt trauma.

- A history of high-energy impact accompanied by an immediate nasal deformity and subsequent nasal obstruction suggests a diagnosis of nasal fracture.

- Hemangiomas typically undergo a proliferative phase averaging 6 to 12 months, followed by a slower involutional phase averaging 2 to 10 years.

| KEY POINTS IN THE PHYSICAL EXAMINATION | • In contrast to nasal dermoid cysts, encephaloceles expand with Valsalva maneuvers and will transilluminate. |

• A positive Furstenberg test, characterized by enlargement of a mass upon bilateral compression of the internal jugular veins, favors the diagnosis of an encephalocele over a dermoid cyst or nasal glioma.

• Nasal fractures may present with deformity of the nose, swelling, lacerations, ecchymoses, mucosal tears, and cerebrospinal fluid rhinorrhea.

• Hemangiomas may occur in isolation or may be associated with other external and/or internal hemangiomas as seen in diffuse neonatal hemangiomatosis. Therefore, a complete physical examination should be performed in these patients. Depending on the location of the hemangiomas, complications of diffuse hemangiomatosis may include congestive heart failure, hepatomegaly, anemia, and tethered cord.

• Nasal bridge hemangiomas may be superficial (often bright red, with clear margins), deep (often bluish, with indistinct margins), or mixed.

• A nasal bridge hemangioma should be distinguished from a nasal tip hemangioma, which is sometimes described as a "Cyrano de Bergerac nose" or "Pinocchio nose."

DIFFERENTIAL DIAGNOSIS

DIAGNOSIS	ICD-9	DISTINGUISHING CHARACTERISTICS	ASSOCIATED FINDINGS	COMPLICATIONS
Dermoid Cyst	216.9	Midline nasal mass, pit, or fistula	Sinus tract to skin with secretion of pus or sebum	Localized abscess Osteomyelitis Orbital cellulitis Meningitis Brain abscess
Nasal Bridge Encephalocele	742.0	Soft, compressible mass May have a translucent appearance and/or a blue hue Postive Furstenberg test	Chromosomal abnormalities	Meningitis
Nasal Glioma	748.1	Firm nonpulsatile mass Nasal dorsum and/or the lateral nasal wall May have telangiectasias of the overlying skin Negative Furstenberg test	CSF rhinorrhea Epiphora (watery eyes)	Nasal obstruction Meningitis Epistaxis
Nasal Bridge Trauma	959.09	Epistaxis Skin lacerations Hematomas Ecchymosis	Septal hematoma CSF rhinorrhea (consider cribriform plate fracture)	Nasolacrimal duct injury Septal necrosis Facial deformity Impaired vision Intracranial infection
Nasal Hemangioma	228.00	Soft, raised, compressible red or bluish masses	Posterior fossa abnormalities Ocular abnormalities Malformations of the great arteries	Ulceration Bleeding Obscured vision Amblyopia Breathing difficulties Facial deformity

PHOTOGRAPHS OF SELECTED DIAGNOSES

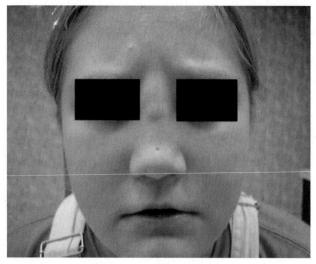

Figure 18-1 Dermoid cyst. (Courtesy of Kathleen Cronan, MD.)

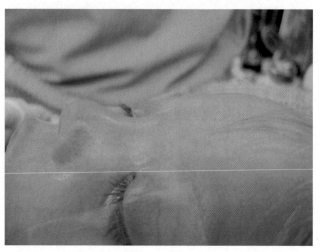

Figure 18-2 Dermoid cyst. (Courtesy of John A. Germiller, MD, PhD.)

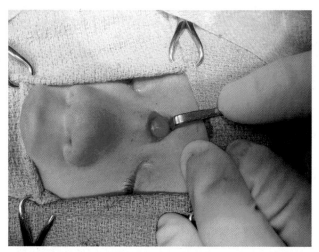

Figure 18-3 Dermoid cyst. Intraoperative view of a well-circumscribed dermoid cyst that corresponds with the previous figure. (Courtesy of John A. Germiller, MD, PhD.)

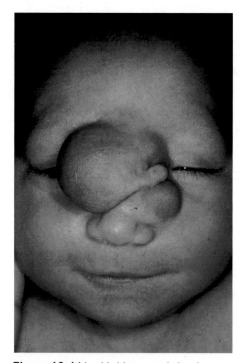

Figure 18-4 Nasal bridge encephalocele. (Courtesy of Joseph Piatt, MD.)

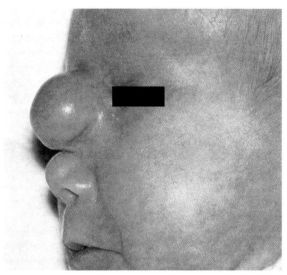

Figure 18-5 Large frontal encephalocele. (Used with permission from Handler SD, Myer CM. *Atlas of ear, nose and throat disorders in children.* Ontario, Canada: BC Decker; 1998:48.)

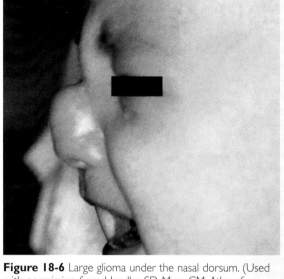

Figure 18-6 Large glioma under the nasal dorsum. (Used with permission from Handler SD, Myer CM. *Atlas of ear, nose and throat disorders in children.* Ontario, Canada: BC Decker; 1998:48.)

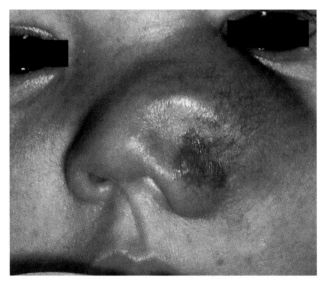

Figure 18-7 Nasal hemangioma in a child 6 months of age. (Used with permission from Handler SD, Myer CM. *Atlas of ear, nose and throat disorders in children.* Ontario, Canada: BC Decker; 1998:55.)

OTHER
DIAGNOSES TO
CONSIDER

- Epignathus

- Nasopharyngeal teratoma

- Proboscis lateralis

SUGGESTED READINGS

Carroll CM, Gaffney R, McShane D. Congenital nasal dermoids in children. *Ir J Med Sci*. 1997:149–151.

East CA, O'Donaghue G. Acute nasal trauma in children. *J Pediatr Surg*. 1987;22(4):308–310.

Handler SD, Myer CM. *Atlas of ear, nose and throat disorders in children*. Ontario, Canada: B.C. Decker, Inc.; 1998:48, 55.

Metry DW. Hemangiomas of infancy. *Postgrad Medicine Online*. 2003;114(1). Available at: http://www.postgradmed.com/issues/2003/07_03/metry.htm.

Paller AS, Pensler JM, Tomita T. Nasal midline masses in infants and children: dermoids, encephaloceles, and gliomas. *Arch Dermatol*. 1991;127:362–366.

SHAREEN F. KELLY

19 Nasal Swelling, Discharge, and Crusting

APPROACH TO THE PROBLEM

Investigating the causes of nasal swelling and discharge involves acquiring a careful history that includes the duration and timing of symptoms, the environment in which the symptoms occurred, whether anything has relieved the symptoms, and to what extent the problem has disrupted the child's daily functioning. Radiological studies may be useful in select cases. Noting the age of the patient is important because the sinus and nasopharyngeal complex changes with age. Asking about sick contacts will help to identify infectious causes of rhinorrhea that may vary with age.

KEY POINTS IN THE HISTORY

- Most rhinorrhea from viral upper respiratory tract infections resolves in 6 to 10 days.

- Rhinorrhea accompanying viral infections may be associated with fever, cough, and/or lymphadenopathy.

- Seasonal allergic rhinitis is generally accompanied by intense nasal itching (and is often associated with eye itching).

- Children with allergic rhinitis often have family members with atopic diseases.

- Fits of sneezing soon after rising from sleep and nasal symptoms in the presence of specific allergens, such as dust and animals, are characteristic of seasonal allergic rhinitis.

- Nasal drainage resulting from a foreign body, typically occurring in young children, is usually acute and unilateral, and often associated with a foul odor.

- Children with impetigo generally do not complain of pain at the affected site.

- Prolonged purulent rhinorrhea (>10 days) associated with headache and/or fever is suggestive of bacterial rhinosinusitis.

- Recurrent nasal infections or persistent inflammation may contribute to the development of nasal polyps.

KEY POINTS IN THE PHYSICAL EXAMINATION

- Viral rhinorrhea may be of varied color and thickness.

- Difficulty with nasal breathing in the absence of swollen turbinates is usually indicative of enlarged adenoids.

- Rhinorrhea from allergic rhinitis is generally thin, profuse, and clear.

- Children with allergic rhinitis often have associated Dennie-Morgan lines and allergic shiners.

- Nasal drainage from a foreign body is unilateral, thick, purulent, sometimes, bloody and foul smelling.

- Impetigo may occur as a single "honey-crusted" lesion of the nares. Because of auto-innoculation, it often presents with multiple lesions in close proximity to the original lesion.

- Nasal polyps are painless, lucent-gray nasal masses that are most often solitary.

- Tenderness over the facial bones and increased headache and/or facial pain on forward bending of the neck are signs of sinusitis.

- Following nasal trauma, children should be examined carefully for septal hematomas.

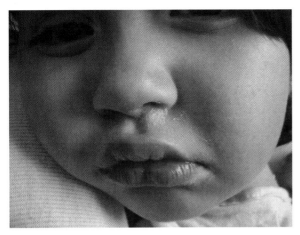

Figure 19-1 Viral rhinorrhea. (Courtesy of Paul S. Matz, MD.)

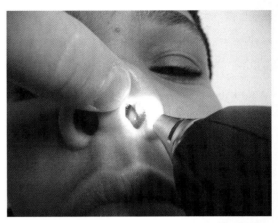

Figure 19-2 Boggy inferior turbinates seen with allergic rhinitis. (Courtesy of Paul S. Matz, MD.)

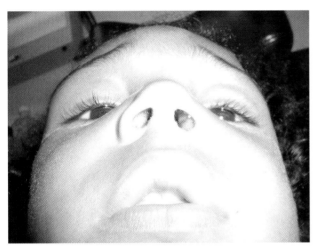

Figure 19-3 Nasal discharge/crusting because of a foreign body. This child had persistent unilateral, foul-smelling discharge until paper was removed from the left side by an otolaryngologist. (Courtesy of Paul S. Matz, MD.)

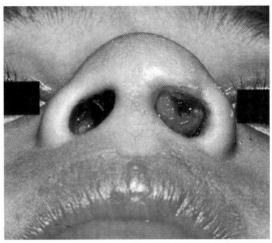

Figure 19-4 Nasal polyp. (Used with permission from Handler SD, Myer CM. *Atlas of ear, nose and throat disorders in children.* Ontario, Canada: BC Decker; 1998:59.)

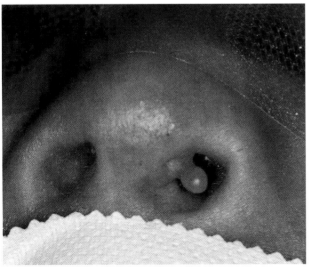

Figure 19-5 Skin tag at nasal vestibule. (Used with permission from Handler SD, Myer CM. *Atlas of ear, nose and throat disorders in children.* Ontario, Canada: BC Decker; 1998:49.)

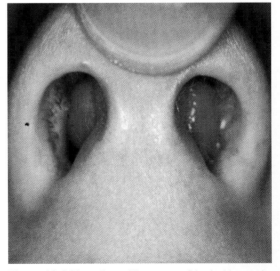

Figure 19-6 Bilateral septal hematoma. (Used with permission from Handler SD, Myer CM. *Atlas of ear, nose and throat disorders in children.* Ontario, Canada: BC Decker; 1998:52.)

DIFFERENTIAL DIAGNOSIS

DIAGNOSIS	ICD-9	DISTINGUISHING CHARACTERISTICS	DISTRIBUTION
Viral Rhinorrhea	478.1	Thin and clear or thick white or yellow rhinorrhea	Any age; more frequent in daycare attendees
Allergic Rhinitis	477.9	Thin, profuse, watery rhinorrhea	Unusual in children less than 3 years of age; peak incidence in adolescence
Impetigo	684	Golden "honey-crusted" erythematous area	Any age but may be associated with children who pick their noses Usually near the nares but may be seen anywhere on the body
Nasal Foreign Body	932	Unilateral purulent nasal discharge	Most common in preschoolers
Nasal Polyp	471.9	Glistening gray mass in nares	Usually solitary Unusual in children less than 10 years old

DURATION/ CHRONICITY	ASSOCIATED FINDINGS	COMPLICATIONS	PREDISPOSING FACTORS
Lasts 5–10 days. Occurs most often in winter	Sore throat, cough, fever, enlarged cervical lymph nodes	Bacterial rhinosinusitis	Exposure to others with upper respiratory tract infections
Occurs more seasonally or upon exposure to allergens or irritants, such as smoke, animals, and dust	Associated with ocular symptoms of tearing and itchiness; often associated with atopic dermatitis	Headaches from sinus pressure Postnasal drip with or without halitosis	Allergens Familial predisposition with other allergic symptoms
Easy to treat but contagious in young children. May recur if child is colonized with *Staphylecoccus aureus*	May have skin lesions in other areas	Rarely, invasive infection with *Staphylecoccus aureus* Generally does not result in scarring	Nasal colonization with *Staphylecoccus aureus* Nose picking
N/A	Malodorous nasal discharge, sometimes bloody	Nasal septum erosion whenever foreign body not removed.	Behavior of child Follows foreign body placement in nare
Long-lasting unless removed	May be associated with epistaxis	Persistent nasal congestion and decreased ability to breathe through affected side	Recurrent infections and persistent inflammation Associated with cystic fibrosis

- Cerebrospinal fluid leak

- Rhinitis medicamentosa

- Nasal glioma or encephalocele

- Nasopharyngitis from gastroesophageal reflux

- Choanal atresia

- Anterior nasal stenosis

SUGGESTED READINGS
Handler SD, Myer CM. *Atlas of ear, nose and throat disorders in children.* Ontario, Canada: B.C. Decker, Inc.; 1998:49, 52, 59.
Nash DR. Allergic rhinitis. *Pediatr Ann.* 1998;27:799–808.
Schoem SR, Josephson GD, Mendelson LM, et al. Why won't this child's nose stop running? *Contemp Pediatr.* 2002;19:48–63.
Turner RB. The common cold. *Pediatr Ann.* 1998;27:790–795.
Yellon RF, McBride TB, Davis HW. Otolaryngology. In: *Atlas of pediatric physical diagnosis.* 4th ed. Philadelphia: Mosby, 2002:832–838.

SIX

Mouth

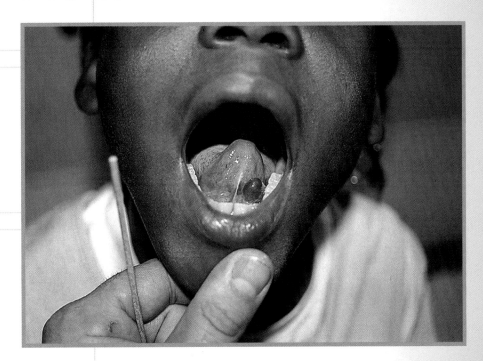

20 Mouth Sores and Patches

APPROACH TO THE PROBLEM

In the pediatric patient, lesions of the oral cavity may range from those that are asymptomatic to those that are extremely painful and uncomfortable. Oral lesions may arise from birth to adolescence and are often self-limited. An oral lesion may occur in isolation or may be part of a systemic infection or disorder. An accurate diagnosis is essential for treatment. Managing pain is particularly important to prevent dehydration because children will often refuse to eat or drink when painful oral lesions are present.

KEY POINTS IN THE HISTORY

- The most common types of ulcers are aphthous ulcers.

- The presence of aphthous ulcers and systemic symptoms such as fever may be an indication of an inflammatory, autoimmune, or connective tissue disease.

- Fever, headaches, and erythematous oral vesicles in the posterior pharynx during the summer months are suggestive of herpangina resulting from coxsackie virus infection.

- Viral etiologies of oral ulcerations usually present as vesicles before becoming ulcerated.

- Herpes gingivostomatitis most commonly presents in children younger than 4 years of age.

- White nodules on the palate of a neonate are consistent with Epstein pearls. These self-limited benign nests of sebaceous and keratin material are extremely common.

- Thrush will have an insidious onset, and parents may report decreased oral intake.

- Palatal burns will have an acute onset with localization to the palate.

- Lip-licking dermatitis can be an isolated lesion but is often seen in conjunction with atopic dermatitis.

**KEY POINTS IN
THE PHYSICAL
EXAMINATION**

- HSV gingivostomatitis causes ulcer formation predominately at the anterior and posterior oropharynx, while herpangina causes ulcers in the posterior pharynx.

- The ulcers of herpangina have erythematous borders with a white to gray base whereas the ulcers of HSV gingivostomatitis are erythematous and associated with gingival erythema and edema.

- Aphthous ulcers present on nonkeratinized mucosa of the mouth, which includes the buccal and labial mucosae as well as the floor of the mouth.

- Ulcerative lesions may be so painful that drooling may be apparent on examination.

- Epstein pearls are seen in the first few weeks of life as white, nodular lesions of the mucosa.

- Koplik spots are often missed because these lesions arise only during the prodrome of measles.

- Thrush is typically seen throughout the oropharynx on the buccal and labial mucosae. Scraping of the white plaque-like lesion of thrush will reveal an erythematous superficial ulceration of the mucosae.

DIFFERENTIAL DIAGNOSIS

DIAGNOSIS	ICD-9	DISTINGUISHING CHARACTERISTICS	DISTRIBUTION	ASSOCIATED FINDINGS	COMPLICATIONS
HSV Gingivostomatitis	054.2	Clusters of erythematous, painful vesicles Edematous gingiva Yellow exudative ulcers with an erythematous halo	Anterior oral pharynx: • Lips • Gingival • Tongue • Buccal mucosa • Palate	High fever Irritability Odynophagia	Dehydration
Herpangina	074.0	Discrete erythematous vesicles Painful gray ulcers on an erythematous base	Posterior pharynx: • Soft palate • Tonsillar pillars • Uvula	Fever Headache Malaise	Dehydration
Aphthous Ulcers	528.2	Ulcers with pseudomembrane and erythematous halo	Buccal and labial mucosa, floor of mouth and ventral surface of tongue	Fever and may manifest systemic symptoms	None
Palatal Erosion (Burn, Sucking Blister)	947.0	Erythematous ulcerated lesions	Palate	Pain Decreased intake	Dysphagia
Thrush	771.7	White plaques on an erythematous base	Throughout anterior and posterior oral pharynx, including buccal and labial mucosae	Often concurrent with candidal diaper dermatitis	Poor feeding
Koplik Spots	055.9	Bluish-white papules on an erythematous base	Buccal mucosa opposite the first molar and soft palate	Fever Cough Coryza Conjunctivitis Morbilliform rash	None from lesions
Lip-Licking Dermatitis	528.5	Perioral dryness Scaly and lichenified Hyperpigmentation	Perioral	May have eczematous changes to skin elsewhere	None
Epstein Pearls	528.4	Small, white pearly cysts	Midline of palate Gums (may have similar lesions that are referred to as Bohn nodules)	None	None

PHOTOGRAPHS OF SELECTED DIAGNOSES

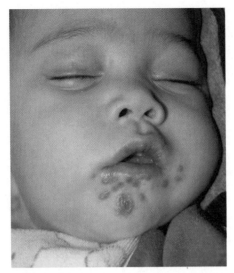

Figure 20-1 Herpes simplex viral stomatitis. (Courtesy of George A. Datto, III, MD.)

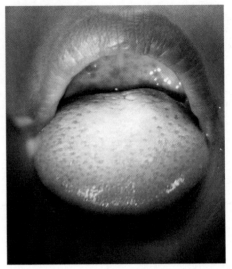

Figure 20-2 Herpangina. (Courtesy of Paul S. Matz, MD.)

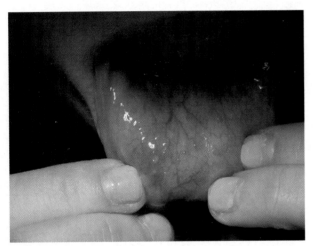

Figure 20-3 Aphthous ulcers. (Courtesy of Michael Lemper, DDS.)

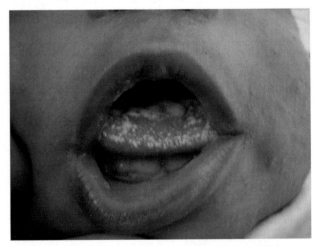

Figure 20-4 Oral thrush. (Courtesy of Paul S. Matz, MD.)

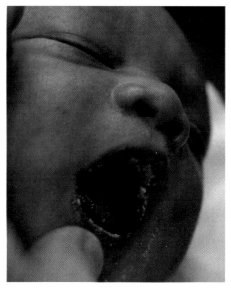

Figure 20-5 Oral thrush. (Courtesy of George A. Datto, III, MD.)

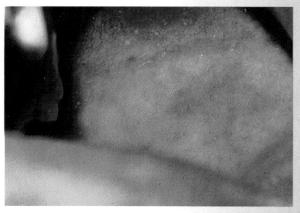

Figure 20-6 Koplik spots. (Used with permission from The Wellcome Trust, National Medical Slide Bank, London, UK.)

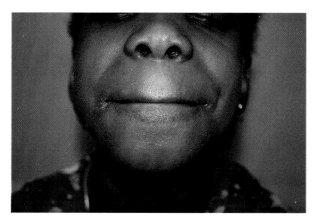

Figure 20-7 Lip-licking dermatitis. (Courtesy of George Datto, III, MD.)

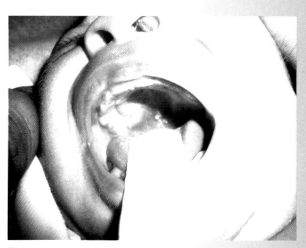

Figure 20-8 Epstein pearls. (Courtesy of Paul S. Matz, MD.)

OTHER
DIAGNOSES TO
CONSIDER

- Mucoceles or ranulas

- Hemangiomas

- Leukoplakia

- White sponge nevus

SUGGESTED READINGS

Milano M. Oral electrical and thermal burns in children: review and report of case. *ASDC J Dent Child.* 1999;March–April:116–119.

Patel NJ, Sciubba J. Oral lesions in young children. *Pediatr Clin North Am.* 2003;50:469–486.

Perry RT, Halsey NA. The clinical significance of measles: a review. *J Infect Dis.* 2004;189(Suppl 1):S4–S16.

Peter JR, Haney HM. Infections of the oral cavity. *Pediatr Ann.* 1996;25:10:572–576.

Witman PM, Rogers RS. Pediatric oral medicine. *Dermatol Clin.* 2003;21:157–170.

21 Focal Gum Lesions

APPROACH TO THE PROBLEM

Oral lesions are very common in newborns, infants, and young children. Parents may be particularly concerned when there is a focal swelling on their child's gum. Fortunately, most of these lesions are benign. The prevalence and incidence of the most commonly noted gum lesions, Bohn nodules and eruption cysts, are unknown. Both typically resolve without intervention, and their presence does not have adverse effects. Some lesions, however, represent infections that are the result of untreated dental caries and poor oral hygiene. Dental abscesses, if left untreated, may extend to involve the adjacent tissue, resulting in formation of a fistula to the gum surface, facial cellulitis, and even osteomyelitis involving the facial bones.

KEY POINTS IN THE HISTORY

- Eruption cysts are common in infants and children during the mixed-dentition stage, when primary and permanent teeth are present in the mouth.

- Eruption cysts tend to rupture spontaneously.

- Bohn nodules and alveolar cysts, often present at the time of birth, generally do not interfere with feeding.

- Parents may confuse Bohn nodules with oral thrush.

- Poor dental hygiene and dental caries are risk factors for dental abscesses.

- Children with dental abscesses may have a history of fever or mouth pain.

- Some children with a fistula between a dental abscess and the gum may note drainage, a funny taste in their mouth, or both.

KEY POINTS IN THE PHYSICAL EXAMINATION

- Bohn nodules are smooth, translucent, pearly white, and approximately 1- to 3-mm cysts.

- Alveolar cysts are visible along the alveolar ridges.

- Eruption cysts are usually found in the region of the incisors on the edge of the alveolar ridge where a tooth is erupting.

- Eruption cysts may feel rubbery and have a bluish hue.

- Natal teeth are erupted teeth that are present at the time of birth.

- The presence of fever in association with a focal gum lesion should raise suspicion for a dental abscess.

- Dental abscesses may appear as a swelling of the gum, often in the region of a dental carie.

- Dental abscesses may cause swelling of the overlying cheek.

- Dental abscesses may develop a fistula between the tooth apex and the oral cavity.

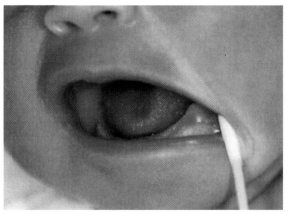

Figure 21-1 Bohn nodule. (Used with permission from Fletcher MA. *Physical diagnosis in neonatology.* Philadelphia: Lippincott–Raven Publishers; 1998:216.)

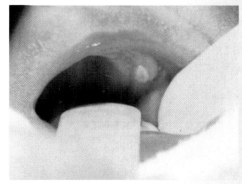

Figure 21-2 Alveolar cyst. (Used with permission from Fletcher MA. *Physical diagnosis in neonatology.* Philadelphia: Lippincott–Raven Publishers; 1998:216.)

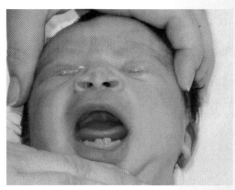

Figure 21-4 Natal teeth. (Courtesy of Denise. Salerno, MD.)

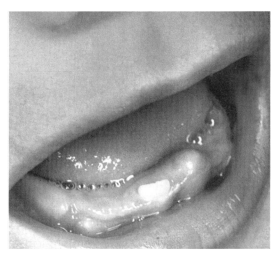

Figure 21-3 Eruption cyst. (Used with permission from Fleisher GR, Ludwig S, Baskin MN, eds. *Atlas of pediatric emergency medicine.* Philadelphia: Lippincott Williams & Wilkins; 2004:78.)

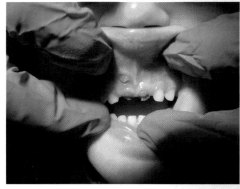

Figure 21-6 Dental abscess and fistula associated with severe dental caries. (Courtesy of Michael Lemper, DDS.)

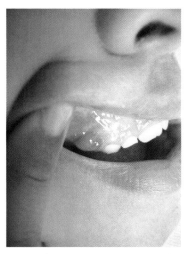

Figure 21-5 Dental abscess with fistula to the gum. (Courtesy of Paul S. Matz, MD.)

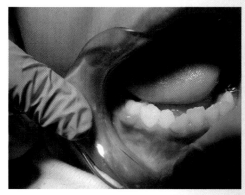

Figure 21-7 Gingival abscess. (Courtesy of Michael Lemper, DDS.)

DIFFERENTIAL DIAGNOSIS

DIAGNOSIS	ICD-9	DISTINGUISHING CHARACTERISTICS	DISTRIBUTION
Bohn Nodules	528.4 (oral cyst)	Occur in 85% of newborns Smooth, translucent, pearly white, keratin-filled, 1- to 3-mm cysts	Buccal or alveolar surface of the gums
Eruption Cyst	526.0	Common in infants and children during the mixed-dentition phase Dome-shaped, fluid filled, rubbery cysts Bluish hue Rupture spontaneously	On the edge of the alveolar ridge where the tooth is erupting Usually, in the region of the incisors Less often in the region of the permanent molars
Alveolar Cyst	525.5	Gingival cysts that appear in up to 50% of newborns Smooth, translucent, pearly white, keratin filled, 1- to 3-mm cysts Single or multiple Discrete or clustered	Alveolar mucosa, most commonly on the maxillary mucosa
Dental Abscess with Fistula to the Gum	522.7	Dental caries progress to involve the tooth pulp, causing an abscess, which may progress to development of a fistula to the gum Tooth and gum pain	Fistula between the tooth apex and the oral cavity

DURATION/ CHRONICITY	ASSOCIATED FINDINGS	COMPLICATIONS	PREDISPOSING FACTORS
Rupture spontaneously in the first month of life	None	None	None
Related to tooth eruption	Mixed dentition Eruption hematoma	May precede neonatal teeth	Tooth eruption
Rupture spontaneously in first 3 months of life	None	None	None
Takes months to develop Will not resolve without intervention	Pain Discharge from the gum	Facial space infection Sepsis Primary tooth infection may disrupt normal development of the secondary tooth Destruction of underlying bone	Dental caries

OTHER
DIAGNOSES TO
CONSIDER

- Congenital epulis

- Teratomas and dermoid cysts

- Peripheral giant cell granuloma

- Alveolar lymphangioma

- Rhabdomyosarcoma

- Osteogenic sarcoma

- Fibrosarcoma

- Mucoepidermoid carcinoma

- Oral lymphoepithelialized cyst

SUGGESTED READINGS

Caufield PW, Griffen AL. Dental caries: an infectious and transmissible disease. *Pediatr Clin North Am.* 2000;47(5):1001–1019.

Fleisher GR, Ludwig S, Baskin MN. *Atlas of pediatric emergency medicine.* Philadelphia: Lippincott Williams & Wilkins; 2004:78.

Fletcher MA. *Physical diagnosis in neonatology.* Philadelphia: Lippincott–Raven Publishers; 1998:216.

Pinkham JR, Casamassimo PS, McTigue DJ, et al., eds. *Pediatric dentistry: infancy through adolescence.* 4th ed. St. Louis: Elsevier Science; 2005:9–60.

Wright JT. Normal formation and development defects of the human dentition. *Pediatr Clin North Am.* 2000;47(5):975–1000.

HAROLD V. SALVATI
Discoloration of the Teeth

APPROACH TO THE PROBLEM

Staining of the teeth may result from certain medications, congenital defects, food and beverage ingestion, systemic disease, and infection. The discoloration may be intrinsic or extrinsic. *Intrinsic* discoloration follows a change in the structural composition or thickness of the dental hard tissues. *Extrinsic* discoloration occurs outside the tooth on the surface or in the acquired pellicle. Tooth staining depends on the timing and the duration of exposure to various agents. Proper dental hygiene and the avoidance of specific products at sensitive periods of dental development may prevent many of the more common causes of tooth discoloration.

KEY POINTS IN THE HISTORY

- Deciduous incisors and canines (cosmetically important) are most susceptible to tetracycline staining between 4 months gestation and 5 months postnatally, while permanent dentition is most susceptible from 4 months to approximately 7 years of age.

- Fluoride from supplemented water, vitamins, toothpaste, and topical cleansing agents may stain teeth (fluorosis) if ingested in higher than recommended quantities.

- The permanent central upper incisors are most susceptible to fluoride staining between 15 to 24 months of age in boys and 21 to 30 months of age in girls.

- The younger a child begins brushing with fluoride-containing toothpaste, the higher the risk of accidental ingestion and subsequent fluorosis.

- Vitamins containing iron may extrinsically stain teeth.

- Ingestion of large quantities of juice or soft drinks without good dental hygiene following meals (or through a bottle at bedtime) puts a child at higher risk for caries.

- Cigarette smoking and ingestion of coffee, tea, and wine are other risk factors for dental staining.

**KEY POINTS IN
THE PHYSICAL
EXAMINATION**

- Teeth stained by tetracycline may fluoresce under ultraviolet light.

- Tetracycline imparts a brown/yellow appearance to the teeth that cannot be removed by scraping.

- Fluoride stains may range from mild white markings to dark brown staining with pitting of the teeth.

- Iron causes a characteristic black discoloration of the teeth that may be removed by scraping or professional cleaning.

- Staining and damage limited to maxillary teeth suggest bottle caries. The mandibular dentition is believed to be spared because of the protective barrier formed by the presence of the lower lip and tongue.

- Dental changes associated with other abnormalities on examination, such as scleral changes or lax joints, suggest a systemic illness.

DIFFERENTIAL DIAGNOSIS

DIAGNOSIS	ICD-9	DISTINGUISHING CHARACTERISTICS	DISTRIBUTION	PREDISPOSING FACTORS
Bottle Caries	521.0	Brown, eroded teeth Halitosis	Primarily maxillary central and lateral incisors with sparing of mandibular teeth	Sleeping with bottles Prolonged or frequent bottle use Lack of good dental hygiene
Iron Staining	521.7	Black, removable stain	Lingual surfaces of anterior and posterior teeth	Ingestion of iron-containing products
Tetracycline Staining	520.8	Yellow and brown staining that cannot be scraped off	Depends on timing of exposure	Tetracycline exposure during critical time of tooth development
Fluorosis	520.3	White to brown staining that cannot be scraped off	Permanent central incisors, but may affect others as well	Ingestion of excess fluoride Early use of fluoride-containing toothpaste

PHOTOGRAPHS OF SELECTED DIAGNOSES

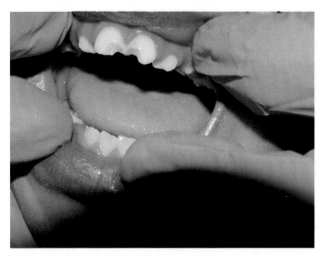

Figure 22-1 Bottle caries. (Courtesy of Michael Lemper, DDS.)

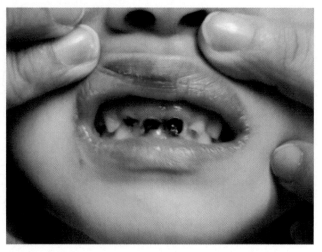

Figure 22-2 Bottle caries. (Courtesy of Philip Siu, MD.)

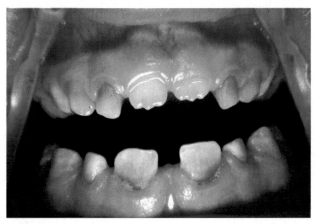

Figure 22-3 Tetracycline staining. (Courtesy of the Department of Pediatric Dental Medicine at St. Christopher's Hospital for Children.)

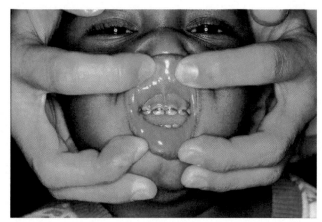

Figure 22-4 Tetracycline staining. (Courtesy of Jan E. Drutz, MD.)

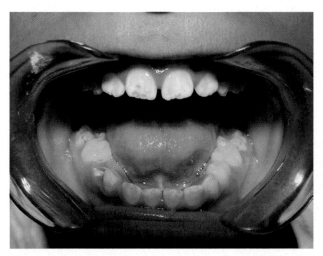

Figure 22-5 Fluorosis. (Courtesy of Michael Lemper, DDS.)

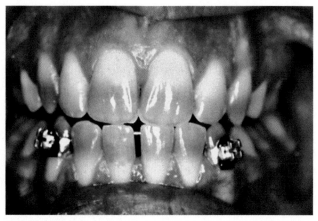

Figure 22-6 Dental erosion. (Courtesy of American Academy of Pediatrics.)

OTHER
DIAGNOSES TO
CONSIDER

- Enamel hypoplasia

- Erythroblastosis fetalis

- Dentinogenesis imperfecta

- Alkaptonuria

- Congenital porphyria

- Trauma

SUGGESTED READINGS

Lewis CS, Milgrom P. Fluoride. *Pediatr Rev.* 2003;24:327–336.

Martof A. Consultation with the specialist: dental care. *Pediatr Rev.* 2001;22:13–15.

Nazif M, McKibben D, Davis H, et al. Oral disorders. In: Zitelli B, Davis H, eds. *Atlas of pediatric physical diagnosis.* 3rd ed. St Louis, Missouri: Mosby-Wolfe; 1997:603–624.

Watts A, Addy M. Tooth discolouration and staining: a review of the literature. *Br Dent J.* 2001;190:309–316.

Weiss PA, Czerepak CS, Hale KJ, et al. American Academy of Pediatrics Policy Statement. Oral health risk assessment timing and establishment of the dental home. *Pediatrics.* 2003;111:1113–1116.

CYNTHIA COLLIER WARREN
AND PAUL S. MATZ

23

Oral Clefts and Other Variants

APPROACH TO THE PROBLEM

A cleft is a gap or separation resulting from a failure of the soft tissue or skeleton to fuse normally. Although cleft lip and palate occur in all races, the highest incidence is among Asians and the lowest is among African Americans. Rates of bifid uvula and ankyloglossia (tongue tie) are approximately 2% to 5%. The male-to-female ratio for cleft lip and palate is approximately 2:1. In unilateral clefts, the ratio of left-sided to right-sided is approximately 2:1. As many as 30% of cases of combined cleft lip and palate—and 50% of isolated cleft palate—are associated with genetic syndromes. Isolated cleft palate may involve the soft palate only or may extend to the hard palate as well.

KEY POINTS IN THE HISTORY

- Some patients with cleft lip or palate may have a positive family history for clefts or other congenital abnormalities.

- Maternal exposure to teratogens may cause cleft lip or palate.

- A cleft lip or palate may interfere with the infant's ability to create the oral vacuum necessary for the extraction of liquid during bottle feeding or breastfeeding, which may lead to poor oral intake and failure to thrive.

- Children with clefts have higher rates of dental abnormalities and caries.

- Excessive air intake, nasal regurgitation, fatigue, coughing, choking, gagging on fluids, and prolonged feeds are sequelae of the oral-nasal coupling seen with cleft palate.

- Recurrent otitis media and hearing loss are common among children with cleft palate.

- Some infants with ankyloglossia may have difficulty with breastfeeding.

- Ankyloglossia in older children may be associated with speech articulation problems; however, ankyloglossia does not cause speech delay.

- Older children with ankyloglossia may have difficulty with intraoral hygiene (cleaning the teeth with the tongue), playing musical instruments, and kissing.

KEY POINTS IN THE PHYSICAL EXAMINATION

- Cleft lip may vary from a small notch on the vermillion border to a complete separation that extends to the floor of the nose.

- Patients with an isolated cleft palate, cleft lip and palate, submucosal cleft palate, or a bifid uvula may demonstrate impaired articulation, nasal speech, and poor enunciation of certain consonant sounds.

- In some cases, a bifid uvula may be associated with a submucosal cleft palate, often only diagnosed by direct palpation.

- Failure to thrive in a patient with cleft lip and palate or isolated cleft palate suggests inadequate caloric intake.

- A cleft palate may also involve the teeth, maxilla, and labial musculature.

- Primary palatal clefting occurs most commonly between the primary and secondary palate at the incisive fissure dividing the lateral incisors and the canine teeth.

- Ankyloglossia leads to decreased tongue movement in all directions, most notably with tongue protrusion, and may be associated with a notched or heart-shaped appearance.

- The presence of other abnormalities may suggest a specific genetic syndrome.

DIFFERENTIAL DIAGNOSIS

DIAGNOSIS	ICD-9	DISTINGUISHING CHARACTERISTICS
Cleft Lip	749.10	Fissure in the upper lip May be unilateral or bilateral Variation in presentation from a notch on the vermillion border to a large separation extending to the floor of the nose
Cleft Palate	749.00	Unilateral or bilateral clefting of the hard and/or soft palate May involve just the uvula and soft palate (incomplete clefts) or the entire palate (complete clefts)
Bifid Uvula	749.02	Notched or cleft uvula
Ankyloglossia (Tongue Tie)	750.0	Very short frenulum; may be fibrous or thin, membranous tissue Limited tongue protrusion Tongue with notched appearance on tongue protrusion

DISTRIBUTION	ASSOCIATED FINDINGS	COMPLICATIONS	PREDISPOSING FACTORS
Orofacial region, specifically the lip. May involve the maxilla May involve the gums	Deformed, absent, or supernumery teeth Orofacial clefts	Abnormal speech Difficulty feeding	Intrauterine drug exposure (teratogens): phenytoin, valproic acid, thalidomide, alcohol, cigarettes, isotretinoin, digoxin Genetic syndromes
Hard palate Soft palate Uvula	Velopharyngeal insufficiency Cleft lip Dental agenesis Dental displacement Orofacial clefts	Abnormal speech Difficulty feeding	Teratogenic exposures Genetic syndromes
Uvula	Submucosal cleft palate	None	Genetic syndromes
Tongue	Cleft lip or palate	Abnormal speech Difficulty feeding Poor oral hygiene	Genetic syndromes

PHOTOGRAPHS OF SELECTED DIAGNOSES

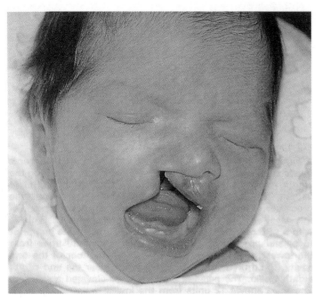

Figure 23-1 Cleft lip. (Used with permission from Moore KL, Dalley AF. *Clinical oriented anatomy.* 4th ed. Baltimore: Lippincott Williams & Wilkins; 1999:929.)

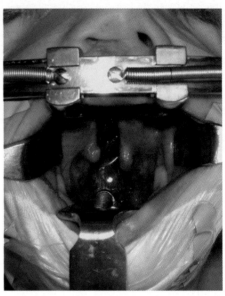

Figure 23-2 Cleft palate. (Courtesy of Scott T. VanDuzer, MD.)

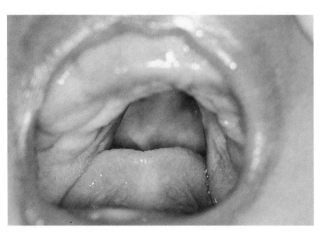

Figure 23-3 Cleft palate in a child with Robin sequence. (Courtesy of Ellen Deutsch, MD.)

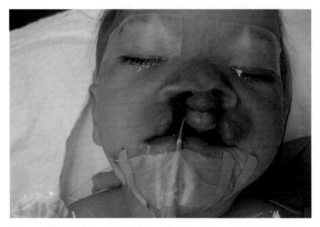

Figure 23-4 Bilateral cleft lip and palate. (Courtesy of Scott T. VanDuzer, MD.)

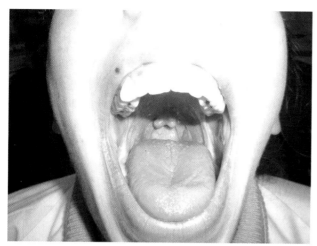

Figure 23-5 Bifid uvula. (Courtesy of Paul S. Matz, MD.)

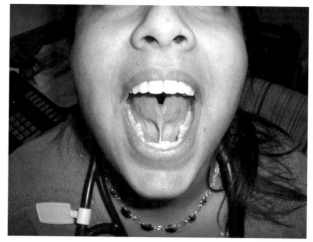

Figure 23-6 Ankyloglossia. (Courtesy of Paul S. Matz, MD.)

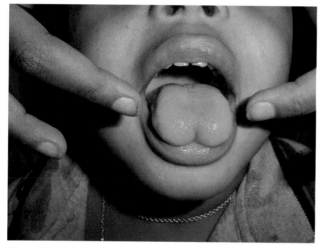

Figure 23-7 Ankyloglossia—notched or heart-shaped tongue visible on protrusion of the tongue. (Courtesy of Michael Lemper, DDS.)

OTHER
DIAGNOSES TO
CONSIDER

- Pierre-Robin syndrome

- Robinow syndrome

- Kallmann syndrome

- Orofacial digital syndrome

- Mucopolysachharidosis, Type IX

- Fetal alcohol syndrome

SUGGESTED READINGS

Behrman RE. Nelson. *Textbook of pediatrics.* 17th ed. Philadelphia: WB Saunders; 2004:1207–1208.

Lalakea ML, Messner AH. Ankyloglossia: does it matter? *Pediatr Clin North Am.* 2003;50(2):381–397.

Moore KL, Dalley AF. *Clinical oriented anatomy.* 4th ed. Baltimore: Lippincott Williams & Wilkins; 1999:929.

Morris H, Ozanne A. Phonetic, phonological, and language skills of children with a cleft palate. *Cleft Palate Craniofac J.* 2003;40(5):460–469.

Murray JC. Gene/environment causes of cleft lip and/or palate. *Clin Genet.* 2002;61:248–256.

Redford-Badwal DA, Mabry K, Frassinelli JD. Impact of cleft lip and/or palate on nutritional health and oral-motor development. *Dent Clin North Am.* 2003;47:305–317.

Shprintzen RJ, Schwartz RH, Daniller, et al. Morphologic significance of bifid uvula. *Pediatrics.* 1985;75(3):553–561.

Wharton P, Mowrer DE. Prevalence of cleft uvula among school children in kindergarten through grade five. *Cleft Palate Craniofac J.* 1992;29(1):10–12.

CHRISTOPHER O'HARA

24 Tongue Discoloration and Surface Changes

APPROACH TO THE PROBLEM

The surface of the tongue may develop changes in color or texture because of intrinsic and extrinsic factors. Discolorations may be related to chewed (betel, for example), ingested (coffee), or topical products (mouthwash); and certain infections. It is important to be familiar with some of the more common tongue abnormalities that may present in pediatrics so that appropriate guidance and reassurance may be given to families.

KEY POINTS IN THE HISTORY

- Medications such as antibiotics, antimalarial drugs, psychotropic agents—including selective serotonin reuptake inhibitors (SSRIs), phenothiazines, and benzodiazepines and phenytoin—may cause tongue discoloration.

- Hairy tongue, elongated filiform papillae in the midline tongue, is associated with the use of tobacco, tea, coffee, antibiotics, griseofulvin, or certain mouthwashes containing an oxidizing agent (such as sodium perborate, sodium peroxide, or hydrogen peroxide).

- The presence of an immunodeficiency or a history of recent radiation or cytotoxic therapy may predispose patients to oral thrush or oral hairy leukoplakia. Hairy leukoplakia, seen more commonly in adults affected by human immunodeficiency virus (HIV), is rare in children affected by HIV.

- Syphilis and lichen planus may be associated with white plaques on the tongue.

- The use of broad-spectrum antibiotics or systemic or inhaled corticosteroids may predispose patients to oral thrush.

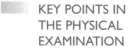 **KEY POINTS IN THE PHYSICAL EXAMINATION**

- A white plaque that wipes off easily with gauze may be because of milk or food. If it can be scraped off with a tongue blade and it bleeds or leaves a denuded surface, it is generally the result of a fungal infection.

- Oral hairy leukoplakia generally cannot be scraped off and often is located on the lateral surface of the tongue.

- A red tongue that is smooth indicates glossitis, while a red tongue with enlarged papillae is more consistent with strawberry tongue.

- Patches of hyperpigmentation on the tongue may be a normal variant in darkly pigmented individuals.

- A tongue with denuded areas of papillae surrounded by annular loops of normal papillae is geographic tongue. Median rhomboid glossitis is a reddish smooth rhomboid-shaped area of papillary atrophy just anterior to the circumvallate papillae.

- Hairy tongue discoloration may be brown, black, green, or yellow.

DIFFERENTIAL DIAGNOSIS

DIAGNOSIS	ICD-9	DISTINGUISHING CHARACTERISTICS	DISTRIBUTION	ASSOCIATED CONDITIONS	COMPLICATIONS
Blackening from Medication	E980.9	Black discoloration of dorsal surface without changes in size or distribution of papillae	Affects dorsal tongue surface; may affect lateral edges, especially in Addison's disease	Discoloration resulting from penicllins, tetracyclines, lansoprazole, Aldomet, heavy metals (Pb, Ag), chlorpromazine, Addison's disease	Salicylate found in bismuth products made in the United States
White Plaques from Thrush	112.0 771.7 (newborn)	When scraped off the tongue, bleeds or reveals a denuded surface Mostly in infants—peak prevalence is fourth week of life	Localized; may be widespread especially in immunodeficient states May be on buccal mucosa as well	Erythema multiforme Fifth disease Viral stomatitis Antimalarial side effect Lichen planus (rare) Secondary syphilis (rare) Oral hairy leukoplakia Stevens-Johnson syndrome	Breastfed infants with oral thrush may spread the infection to the mother's nipple Recurrent thrush should raise suspicion for immunodeficiency, particularly if seen beyond infancy
Strawberry Tongue	529.3	Reddened dorsal surface with enlarged fungiform papillae White or yellow papillae resembling seeds on a strawberry's surface	Usually generalized and found on the anterior two thirds of the dorsal and lateral tongue surfaces	Strep pharyngitis Kawasaki disease Staph toxic shock Strep toxic shock Adenoviral infection Ehrlichiosis Mediterranean spotted fever Yersinia pseudotuberculosis Candy tongue Glossitis Pernicious anemia AED hypersensitivity*	Rheumatic fever from strep infection Kawasaki-related coronary artery aneurysms Depends on the underlying cause
Geographic Tongue	529.1	Whitish bands of normal papillae surrounding reddish areas of atrophic papillae	Dorsal surface Widespread Migrates across tongue over time	Associated with fissured tongue and possibly psoriasis Case report of association with lithium treatment	Benign condition but alarming to parents and patients
Hairy Tongue	529.3	Elongated filiform papillae in the midline dorsally with a plaque of discoloration over this (the color depends on the offending agent) Color resulting from chromogenic bacteria or trapped particles underneath hyperplastic layers of keratin on the filiform papillae	Medial aspect of dorsal surface just anterior to circumvallate papillae	Hyperkeratosis Hyperplastic candidiasis Sometimes related to poor oral hygiene Seen with use of tetracyclines	Undesirable cosmetic appearance

*A reaction to one of the aromatic anti-epileptic drugs—phenytoin, carbamazepine, phenobarbital, and primidone.

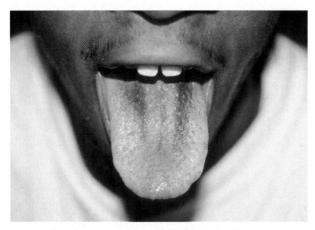

Figure 24-1 Black tongue from bismuth. (Courtesy of Kathleen Cronan, MD.)

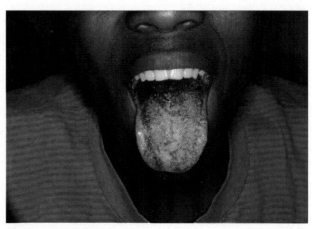

Figure 24-2 Black tongue from bismuth exposure. (Courtesy of Jan E. Drutz, MD.)

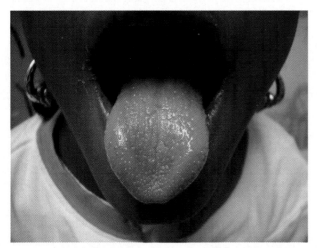

Figure 24-3 Strawberry tongue. (Courtesy of Paul S. Matz, MD.)

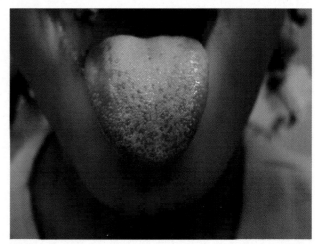

Figure 24-4 Strawberry tongue. (Courtesy of Esther K. Chung, MD.)

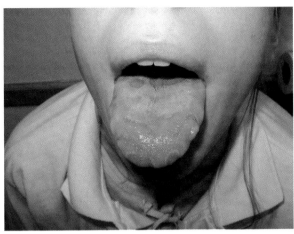

Figure 24-5 Geographic tongue. (Courtesy of Paul S. Matz, MD.)

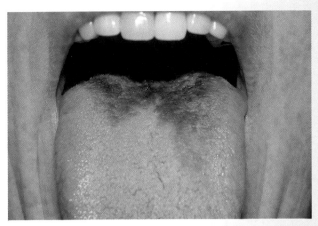

Figure 24-6 Black hairy tongue. (Used with permission from Goodheart HP. *Goodheart's photoguide of common skin disorders.* 2nd ed. Philadelphia: Lippincott Williams & Wilkins; 2003:228.)

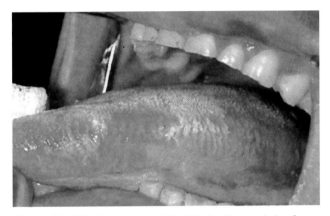

Figure 24-7 Oral hairy leukoplakia. (Used with permission from Weber J, Kelley J. *Health assessment in nursing.* 2nd ed. Philadelphia: Lippincott Williams & Wilkins; 2003:244.)

SUGGESTED READINGS

Cleveland DB, Rinaggio J. Oral and maxillofacial manifestations of systemic and generalized disease. *Endodont Topics.* 2003;4:69–90.

Goodheart HP. *Goodheart's photoguide of common skin disorders.* 2nd ed. Philadelphia: Lippincott Williams & Wilkins; 2003:228.

Hoppe J. Treatment of oropharyngeal candidiasis and candidal diaper dermatitis in neonates and infants: review and reappraisal. *Pediatr Infect Dis J.* 1997;16:885–894.

Mirowski GW, Waibel JS. Pigmented lesions of the oral cavity. *Dermatol Ther.* 2002;15:218–228.

Rogers RS III, Bruce AJ. The tongue in clinical diagnosis. *J. Eur Acad Dermatol Venereol.* 2004;18:254–259.

Sarti GM, Haddy RI, Schaffer D, et al. Black hairy tongue. *Am Fam Physician.* 1990;41:1751–1755.

Tack DA, Rogers RS III. Oral drug reactions. *Dermatol Ther.* 2002;15:236–250.

Weber J, Kelley J. *Health assessment in nursing.* 2nd ed. Philadelphia: Lippincott Williams & Wilkins; 2003:244.

NANCY D. SPECTOR

Swellings Within the Mouth

APPROACH TO THE PROBLEM

A variety of swellings exist that may occur in the mouths of children and adolescents. These swellings range from benign lesions to very serious infections. The incidence and prevalence of many of the benign lesions are unknown. The more serious swellings of the mouth are secondary to bacterial infections of the deep soft tissues of the mouth and pharynx. These more serious entities can be distinguished from the benign lesions by the presence of systemic signs of illness. Peritonsillar abscess and Ludwig's angina have potentially life-threatening complications.

KEY POINTS IN THE HISTORY

- Bohn nodules and Epstein pearls are present in newborns (see Chapter 20).

- Mucoceles and ranulas arise acutely and rupture spontaneously.

- Mucoceles and ranulas are painless and asymptomatic.

- Systemic signs of infection, such as fever and throat pain, help differentiate benign swellings of the mouth from more serious infections.

- Peritonsillar abscess is generally preceded by acute tonsillopharyngitis.

- Patients with Ludwig's angina have a history of high fever and inability to handle their secretions.

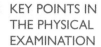

KEY POINTS IN THE PHYSICAL EXAMINATION

- Epstein pearls are smooth, translucent, pearly white, 1- to 3-mm cysts on the palate at the roof of the mouth. When such lesions occur on the gums, they are referred to as Bohn nodules.

- Mucoceles and ranulas are nontender, mobile, glistening, and have a bluish hue.

- Mucoceles are most common on the lower lip.

- Ranulas are found on the floor of the mouth.

- Trismus, or difficulty opening the mouth, is a frequent finding in patients with peritonsillar abscess and Ludwig's angina.

- Peritonsillar abscess is characterized by swelling of tissues lateral and superior to the tonsil, anterior and medial displacement of the tonsil, and displacement of the uvula toward the contralateral side.

- Patients with peritonsillar abscess have a muffled, or "hot potato," voice.

- Ludwig's angina always has bilateral involvement of the submandibular spaces.

- Ludwig's angina is characterized by tongue elevation and an inability to depress the tongue.

PHOTOGRAPHS OF SELECTED DIAGNOSES

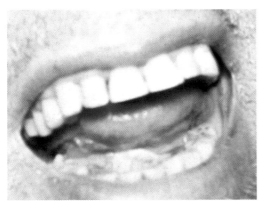

Figure 25-1 Ludwig's angina. Note elevation of tongue secondary to swelling of the floor of the mouth. (Used with permission from Greenberg MI. *Greenberg's atlas of emergency medicine.* Philadelphia: Lippincott Williams & Wilkins; 2005:7.)

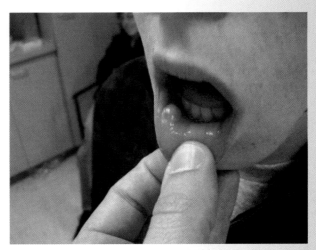

Figure 25-2 Mucocele. (Courtesy of Paul S. Matz, MD.)

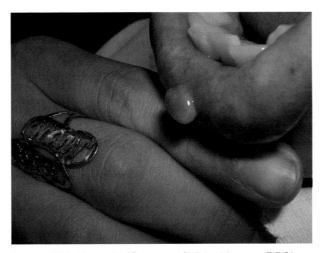

Figure 25-3 Mucocele. (Courtesy of Michael Lemper, DDS.)

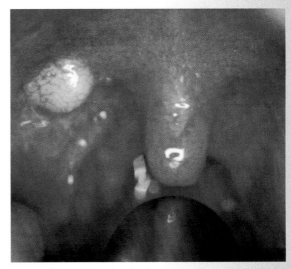

Figure 25-4 Mucocele of soft palate. (Used with permission from Handler SD, Myer CM. *Atlas of ear, nose and throat disorders in Children.* Ontario: BC Decker; 1998:85.)

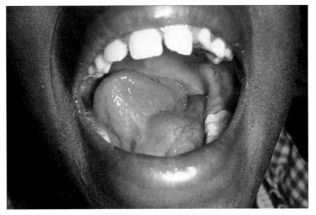

Figure 25-5 Ranula. (Courtesy of Kathleen Cronan, MD.)

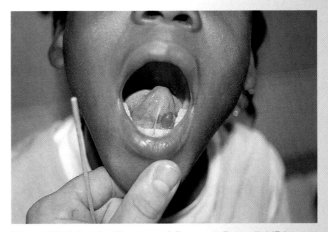

Figure 25-6 Ranula. (Courtesy of George A. Datto, III, MD.)

DIAGNOSIS	ICD-9	DISTINGUISHING CHARACTERISTICS	DISTRIBUTION
Peritonsillar Abscess with Uvular Deviation	475	Throat pain, fever, dysphagia, "hot potato voice," and drooling Occurrence of trismus in 63% of cases Tonsil—erythematous, enlarged, and covered with exudates	Swelling of the tissues lateral and superior to the tonsil with medial and anterior displacement of the tonsil
Ludwig's Angina with Tongue Elevation	528.3	Acute life-threatening cellulitis Trismus, high fever, halitosis, unable to handle secretions Feels woody on palpation Unable to depress tongue Caused by gingival bacteria (anaerobic streptococci, bacteroides species, fusobacteria, and spirochetes)	Bilateral involvement of the submandibular spaces
Mucocele	527.6	Pseudocyst resulting from mucus extravasation into the surrounding tissues Minor salivary gland in origin Acute onset of painless, asymptomatic swelling May fluctuate in size May rupture spontaneously	Most common on the lower lip Less common on the upper lip, palate, buccal mucosa, tongue, or the floor of the mouth
Ranula	527.6	Pseudocyst resulting from mucus extravasation into the surrounding tissues Most arise from sublingual gland Nontender, mobile, glistening, broad-based enlargement Bluish hue May fluctuate in size May rupture spontaneously	Floor of the mouth

DURATION/ CHRONICITY	ASSOCIATED FINDINGS	COMPLICATIONS	PREDISPOSING FACTORS
Develops over several days after acute tonsillopharyngitis Recurrence rates of 6% to 36%	Tender cervical adenopathy	Airway compromise Aspiration, if spontaneous rupture of abscess Spread of infection resulting in retropharyngeal abscess, parapharyngeal abscess, mediastinitis Septic thrombi leading to metastatic spread and resulting in osteomyelitis, meningitis, or brain abscess	Acute tonsillopharyngitis
Develops over several days	Overlying skin erythema, pitting edema, and tenderness	Spread of infection resulting in mediastinitis Laryngeal or subglottic edema Respiratory distress Difficult intubation	Poor oral hygiene Dental extractions Sialadenitis
Recurrence rate of 14% Can be present for weeks to months before rupture	None	None	Trauma to the salivary gland and excretory duct Obstruction to salivary gland duct flow Trauma to salivary glandular parenchymal cells
Recurrence rate of 14% Can be present for weeks to months before rupture	None	Large ranulas—may interfere with speech, swallowing, or respiration	Trauma to the salivary gland excretory duct Obstruction to salivary gland duct flow Trauma to salivary glandular parenchymal cells

- Hemangioma

- Lymphangioma

- Fibroma

- Parulis (gum abscess)

SUGGESTED READINGS
Bluestone CD, Casselbrant ML, Stool SE, et al, eds. *Pediatric otolaryngology.* 4th ed. Philadelphia: WB Saunders; 2003:1261,1272,1688–1699.
Delaney, J, Keels MA. Pediatric oral pathology. *Pediatr Clin North Am.* 2000;47(5):1125–1147.
Greenberg MI. *Greenberg's atlas of emergency medicine.* Philadelphia: Lippincott Williams & Wilkins; 2005:7.
Handler SD, Myer CM. *Atlas of ear, nose and throat disorders in Children.* Ontario: BC Decker; 1998:85.
Patel NJ, Sciubba J. Oral lesions in young children. *Pediatr Clin North Am.* 2003;50:469–486.
Pinkham JR, Casamassimo PS, McTigue DJ, et al, eds. *Pediatric dentistry: infancy through adolescence.* 4th ed. St. Louis: Elsevier Science; 2005:9–60.
Wetmore RF, Muntz HR, McGill TJ, eds. *Pediatric otolaryngology: principles and practice pathways.* New York: Thieme Medical Publishers; 2000:555–614.

ROBERT L. BONNER, JR.

Throat Redness

26

APPROACH TO THE PROBLEM

Erythema of the posterior oropharynx suggests an inflammatory process, most commonly caused by infection. In most cases, the inflammation may be attributed to viral pharyngitis. Bacterial pharyngitis from group A beta-hemolytic streptococcus is very common in school-aged children. These disorders may present with or without exudates. Obtaining a throat culture is important when considering the diagnosis of strep throat or scarlet fever. Noninfectious causes of pharyngeal erythema are rare, but they should be considered in patients with a prolonged course or with treatment failure.

KEY POINTS IN THE HISTORY

• Throat redness associated with upper respiratory tract symptoms such as rhinorrhea, cough, and conjunctivitis is characteristic of a viral infection and rarely represents a bacterial infection.

• Throat redness in association with conjunctivitis, otitis media, or both suggests infection with adenovirus.

• Infectious mononucleosis—Epstein-Barr virus (EBV) infection—should be considered in adolescents with fever, throat pain, swollen lymph nodes, and significant fatigue.

• Streptococcal pharyngitis, which peaks in the late winter and early spring, presents with a sudden onset of pain, fever, and redness in the throat.

• Children fewer than 3 years of age with throat redness and exudates are less likely to have a streptococcal infection.

• Throat redness with progressive unilateral throat pain and dysphagia may suggest a peritonsillar abscess.

• Children with pharyngitis may complain of neck pain and stiffness.

KEY POINTS IN THE PHYSICAL EXAMINATION

- Severe viral pharyngitis and streptococcal pharyngitis may be clinically indistinguishable, because both may present with fever, pharyngeal erythema, and cervical lymphadenopathy.

- Infectious mononucleosis may present with pharyngeal and tonsillar erythema, fever, and posterior cervical lymphadenopathy.

- Children with a peritonsillar abscess may have pharyngeal erythema accompanied by unilateral tonsillar hypertrophy, uvular deviation toward the unaffected side, fever, and trismus. In addition, they typically have a "hot potato" voice.

- Ulcerations typically are seen with viral pharyngitis and stomatitis. Ulcerations on the tonsillar pillars suggest the diagnosis of herpangina, typically caused by coxsackie virus.

- Drooling occurs from the inability to swallow one's secretions, and it typically occurs as a result of pain. Drooling may be seen with severe pharyngitis, pharyngeal ulcerations, and retropharyngeal abscess.

- Sitting in a tripod position, inspiratory stridor, difficulty breathing, and dehydration are findings that may accompany pharyngeal erythema and require prompt attention and evaluation.

- Retropharyngeal cellulitis/abscess should be considered in an ill-appearing, young child with pharyngeal erythema and drooling.

DIFFERENTIAL DIAGNOSIS

DIAGNOSIS	ICD-9	DISTINGUISHING CHARACTERISTICS	DISTRIBUTION	ASSOCIATED FINDINGS	COMPLICATIONS
Strep Pharyngitis	034.0	Posterior pharyngeal erythema Palatal petechiae Tonsillar enlargement and erythema	Posterior oropharynx	Fever Throat pain Cervical adenopathy Abdominal pain	Rheumatic fever Glomerulonephritis Cervical adenitis Peritonsillar and retropharyngeal abscesses
Viral Pharyngitis	462.0	Mild to severe pharyngeal erythema Vesicles or ulcers	Posterior oropharynx	Cough Coryza Conjunctivitis Hand and foot papulovesicles in hand-foot-and-mouth disease	None
Herpangina	074.0	Discrete erythematous ulcers Painful gray ulcers on an erythematous base	Posterior oropharynx	Fever Headache Malaise	None
Infectious Mononucleosis	075	Pharyngeal and tonsillar erythema	Posterior oropharynx	Fever Fatigue Cervical lymphadenopathy	Splenomegaly Hepatomegaly Jaundice Splenic rupture
Peritonsillar Abscess	475.0	Unilateral tonsillar enlargement Uvular deviation	Tonsils	Fever Trismus "Hot potato voice"	Cellulitis

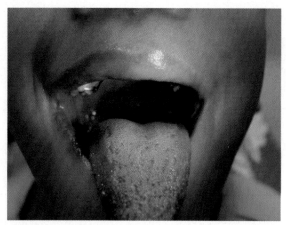

Figure 26-1 Group A strep pharyngitis. Note the marked erythema posteriorly in this patient with scarlet fever. (Courtesy of Esther K. Chung, MD.)

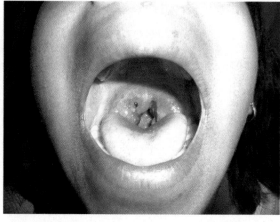

Figure 26-2 Viral pharyngitis. (Courtesy of Paul S. Matz, MD.)

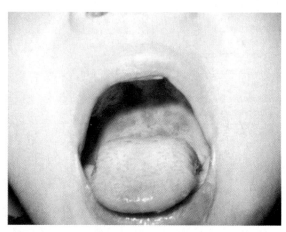

Figure 26-3 Herpangina. (Courtesy of Philip Siu, MD.)

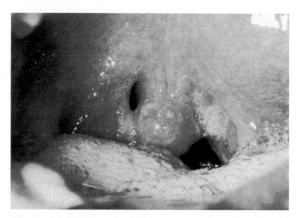

Figure 26-4 Peritonsillar abscess of the left tonsil. (Used with permission from Handler SD, Myer CM. *Atlas of ear, nose and throat disorders in children.* Ontario: BC Decker; 1998:90.)

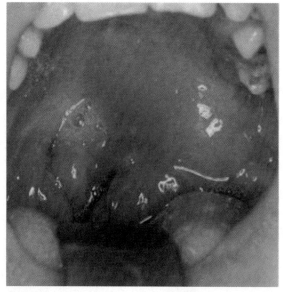

Figure 26-5 Peritonsillar abscess. Note the erythema and swelling on the left and the right deviation of the uvula. (Courtesy of Seth Zwillenberg.)

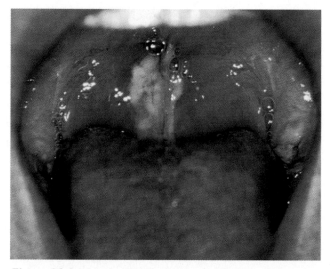

Figure 26-6 Acute tonsillitis secondary to infectious mononucleosis. Note the marked tonsillar enlargement with erythema and the large white-gray patches. (Used with permission from Handler SD, Myer CM. *Atlas of ear, nose and throat disorders in children.* Ontario: BC Decker; 1998:91.)

OTHER
DIAGNOSES TO
CONSIDER

- Pharyngitis resulting from *Neisseria gonorrheoeae*

- Diphtheria

- Pharyngitis resulting from *Mycoplasma pneumoniae*

SUGGESTED READINGS

Attia MW, Bennett JE. Pediatric pharyngitis. *Pediatr Case Rev.* 2003;3(4):203–210.

Bisno AL. Acute pharyngitis. *N Engl J Med.* 2001;344(3):205–211.

Feldman WE. Pharyngitis in children. *Postgrad Med.* 1993;93(3):141–145.

Handler SD, Myer CM. *Atlas of ear, nose and throat disorders in children.* Ontario: BC Decker; 1998:90,91.

McCracken GH. Diagnosis and management of children with streptococcal pharyngitis. *Pediatr Infect Dis J.* 1986;5(6):754–759.

Steyer TE. Peritonsillar abscess: diagnosis and treatment. *Am Fam Physician.* 2002;65(1):93–96.

Vincent MT, Celestin N, Hussain AN. Pharyngitis. *Am Fam Physician.* 2004;69(6):1465–1470.

Section

SEVEN

Neck

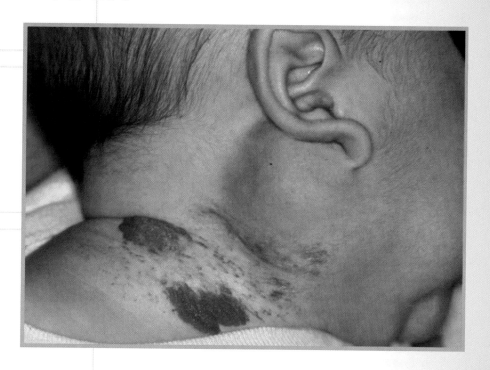

Neck Masses and Swelling

27

APPROACH TO THE PROBLEM

The major causes of childhood neck masses, the majority of which are benign, may be categorized as congenital, inflammatory, neoplastic, and trauma-related. Many neck masses represent cervical adenopathy or adenitis. To determine the etiology of a neck mass, it is helpful to determine whether the swelling is acute versus chronic, unilateral versus bilateral, or associated with focal versus generalized lymphadenopathy. Though malignancies are uncommon, one should be able to recognize the signs and symptoms of these lesions so that an early diagnosis may be made.

KEY POINTS IN THE HISTORY

• A history of a painless mass noted at birth or shortly after birth suggests a congenital etiology.

• Acute onset of erythema, tenderness, and rapid progression in size suggest an inflammatory etiology, particularly when these symptoms are in association with an upper respiratory tract infection.

• More than 90% of patients with cat scratch disease have a history of contact with a cat, and up to 75% of patients have a history of being scratched by a cat. Three to 10 days after inoculation, 60% to 93% of patients develop a vesicle or pustule at the inoculation site that may persist for days to months afterward. Cervical lymphadenopathy typically appears proximal to the inoculation site 2 to 4 weeks later.

• Malignant masses are typically firm and painless, and they may be associated with systemic symptoms such as weight loss.

• When a malignancy is suspected, the patient's age is an important factor when considering the differential diagnosis. Those younger than 6 years presenting with neck swelling are at greatest risk for neuroblastoma; those aged 7 to 12 years, for Hodgkin and non-Hodgkin lymphomas; and those who are adolescents, for Hodgkin lymphoma.

KEY POINTS IN THE PHYSICAL EXAMINATION

- The majority of branchial cleft sinuses and cysts present laterally, along the anterior border of the sternocleidomastoid muscle.

- Thyroglossal duct cysts usually are midline at or next to the hyoid bone. Rarely, they may be sublingual or suprasternal.

- Dermoid cysts, which contain sebaceous material, are also found in the midline. But compared to thyroglossal duct cysts, they are more superficial. In addition, they typically do not have connections to the hyoid bone or tongue.

- Congenital torticollis is associated with a hard fibrotic mass in the sternocleidomastoid muscle that may be detected at 2 to 8 weeks of life.

- Cystic hygromas are soft, mobile, non-tender, cystic masses usually found in the posterior triangle of the neck, and they transilluminate when a light source is applied.

- Hemangiomas are soft, mobile, painless masses that are initially bluish to fiery-red, then they turn gray during the involution phase.

- In children, palpable cervical lymph nodes less than 1 cm may be normal. In infants, palpable nodes are rare, and the possibility of an underlying disease should be considered.

- The chronic cervical lymphadenitis caused by *Mycoplasma tuberculosis* (often associated with fluctuance, a draining sinus, and/or supraclavicular adenopathy) usually represents an extension of primary pulmonary disease.

- The most common site of inoculation for cat scratch disease is the upper extremity, resulting in epitrochlear or axillary adenopathy, or both.

- Any of the following should raise suspicion for malignancy: overlying skin ulceration, supraclavicular adenopathy, and a nontender, fixed, rubbery cervical mass greater than 3 cm.

DIFFERENTIAL DIAGNOSIS

DIAGNOSIS	ICD-9	DISTINGUISHING CHARACTERISTICS	ASSOCIATED FINDINGS	COMPLICATIONS	PREDISPOSING FACTORS
Congenital					
Branchial Cleft Cyst	744.42	Most originate from second branchial cleft May be an associated fistula in the mid-to-lower anterior border of sternocleidomastoid muscle Cyst forms when a fistula becomes occluded	Recurrent cyst Infection	Recurrence rate following resection: 7%	N/A
Thyroglossal Duct Cyst	759.2	Most common congenital neck mass Commonly presents after age 2, when infected, and drains externally Located anywhere along line of descent of the thyroid (midline or next to hyoid bone)	Ectopic thyroid tissue Papillary adenocarcinoma	Recurrence rate after resection: <10% Previous infection or incomplete excision are risk factors for recurrence	N/A
Dermoid Cyst	229.9	Contains sebaceous material Soft, mobile, nontender, superficial mass Can be found midline over hyoid bone and confused with thyroglossal duct cyst	Infection Malignancy is rare	N/A	N/A
Congenital Torticollis	754.1	Noted at 2 to 8 weeks of age when head tilts toward affected side Fibrotic mass associated with shortening of sternocleidomastoid muscle May be associated with a difficult delivery	Congenital hip dislocation Tibial torsion	Facial hemihypoplasia	N/A
Cystic Hygroma	228.1	Twice the likelihood of presenting on left side of neck because the thoracic duct enters the left subclavian vein Soft, mobile, nontender, cystic mass associated with gradual or rapid enlargement and compression of surrounding structures Most commonly in posterior triangle of neck Transilluminates when light source applied Spontaneous resolution is rare	When infected, may become warm, erythematous, and tender	Airway compromise Dysphagia Failure to thrive	Rapid enlargement resulting from infection, trauma, or hemorrhage into lesion
Hemangioma	228.01	Most common head and neck lesion detected during early infancy Soft, mobile, nontender, bluish to fiery-red color turning to gray or beige during involution phase Proliferates during first year of life, then regresses over the next 3 to 4 years (80% resolve by age 5)	Hemangiomatosis Internal hemangiomas	Airway obstruction Hemorrhage Thrombocytopenia Congestive heart failure Infection Ulceration Necrosis Kasabach-Merritt syndrome (consumptive coagulopathy)	Females:males (3:1)

DIAGNOSIS	ICD-9	DISTINGUISHING CHARACTERISTICS	ASSOCIATED FINDINGS	COMPLICATIONS	PREDISPOSING FACTORS
Inflammatory					
Cervical Adenopathy	785.6	In children, palpable cervical lymph nodes less than 1 cm are typically benign In infants, palpable nodes are rare and should raise suspicion for an underlying disease	When recurrent, consider chronic granulomatous disease When associated with supraclavicular adenopathy, consider malignancy	N/A	Upper respiratory infections Epstein-Barr virus (EBV) Cytomegalovirus (CMV) Human immunodeficiency virus (HIV)
Cervical Adenitis	683	Tenderness Erythema Swelling Warmth May be associated with fever	Acute bilateral adenitis is most often because of viruses that infect the upper respiratory tract Acute unilateral adenitis is most often caused by *Staphylococcus aureus* and group A streptococcus Chronic adenitis is associated with EBV, CMV, mycobacteria, and *Bartonella henselae*	N/A	At 3 to 7 weeks of age, males are at greater risk of cervical adenitis because of late-onset group B streptococcal infection
Mycobacterial Cervical Adenitis	031.8	A chronic, suppurative adenitis that may develop a draining sinus Tuberculous mycobacteria presents in school-aged and adolescent years Person-to-person spread Nontuberculous mycobacteria presents in those aged <5y, no definitive person-to-person spread	Tuberculous mycobacteria: supraclavicular nodes, pulmonary infection Nontuberculous mycobacteria: no systemic symptoms (unless immunocompromised)	Scarring Otomastoiditis Sinusitis	Populations at risk for *Mycoplasma tuberculosis* include: • Contact with persons from endemic areas • Foreign-born from endemic areas • Contact with persons infected with tuberculosis, HIV, or a history of IV drug abuse and/or incarceration • Indigent or homeless
Cat Scratch Disease	078.3	Caused by *Bartonella henselae* Chronic, tender adenitis that forms 2 to 4 weeks after inoculation Papule often found at inoculation site	Mild constitutional symptoms Suppuration Parinaud's oculoglandular syndrome (resulting from conjunctival inoculation by rubbing eye after handling cat)	Dysphagia Encephalitis	A history of cat exposure is common but not always present
Neoplastic					
Lymphoma	202.81	Hodgkin and non-Hodgkin lymphoma are most common types of tumor found in the neck for children aged 7 to 12 years Hodgkin lymphoma is the most common tumor in the neck for adolescents Unilateral clusters of firm, fixed, rubbery, nontender masses	Non-Hodgkin: extranodal involvement (i.e., bone marrow, CNS) common Hodgkin: systemic signs and symptoms (i.e., anorexia, fever) common	Airway obstruction Superior vena cava syndrome Horner syndrome	Male:female (3:1)

PHOTOGRAPHS OF SELECTED DIAGNOSES

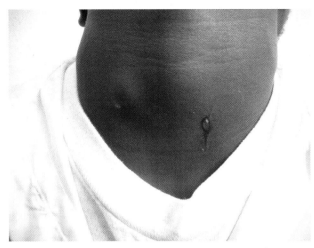

Figure 27-1 Branchial cleft cyst. Draining branchial cleft sinus. (Courtesy of Paul S. Matz, MD.)

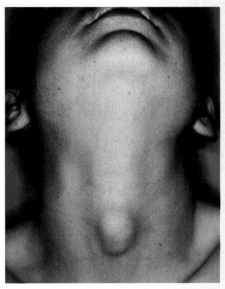

Figure 27-2 Thyroglossal duct cyst. A midline cervical mass presenting in a 6-year-old. (Used with permission from Snell RS. *Clinical anatomy*, 7th ed. Baltimore: Lippincott Williams & Wilkins; 2005:CD418.)

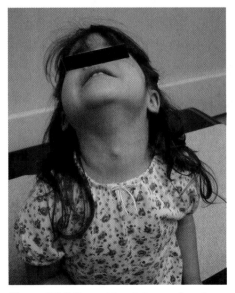

Figure 27-3 Dermoid cyst. A mass found midline overlying the hyoid bone in a 4-year-old. (Courtesy of Mary L. Brandt, MD.)

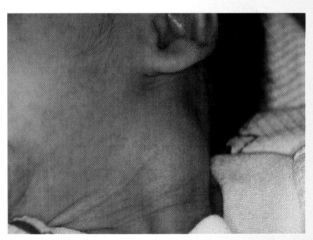

Figure 27-4 Congenital torticollis. A fibrotic mass located in the sternocleidomastoid muscle of a 1-month-old whose mother was concerned about the infant's head tilt to one side. (Courtesy of Ellen Deutsch, MD.)

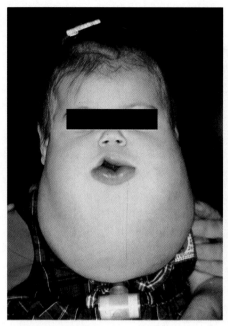

Figure 27-5 Cystic hygroma. A large, soft cervical mass in a 9-month-old. Tracheostomy was placed at birth. (Courtesy of Ellen Deutsch, MD.)

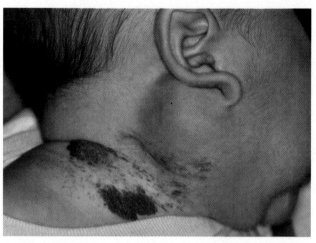

Figure 27-6 Hemangioma. A soft, nontender mass with bluish as well as bright-red aspects of color presents in this 1-month-old. (Courtesy of Ellen Deutsch, MD.)

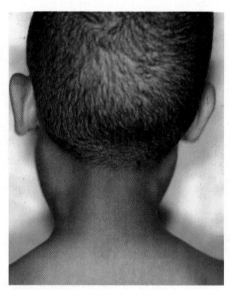

Figure 27-7 Cervical adenopathy. A posterior view of bilateral adenopathy in a 7-year-old with 1- to 2-week history of malaise, sore throat, and low-grade fevers. (Courtesy of Ellen Deutsch, MD.)

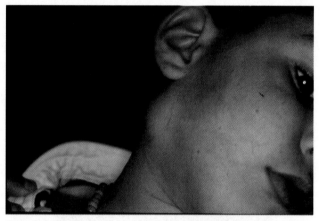

Figure 27-8 Cervical adenitis. This case of acute unilateral adenitis in a 3-year-old is most likely caused by *S. aureus* or group A streptococcus. (Courtesy of Jan E. Drutz, MD.)

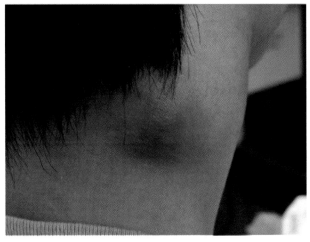

Figure 27-9 Tuberculous adenitis. Note the erythematous swelling in this 13-year-old recent immigrant from southeast Asia who presented with bilateral posterior cervical neck masses. (Courtesy of Esther K. Chung, MD.)

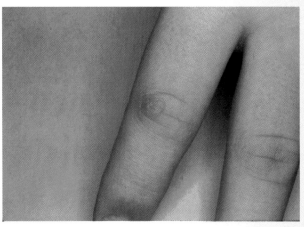

Figure 27-10 Cat scratch inoculation site on the extremity of a 9-year-old. (Courtesy of Mark A. Ward, MD.)

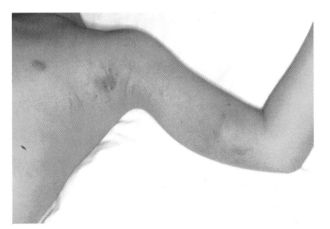

Figure 27-11 Cat scratch adenopathy. Epitrochlear and axillary adenopathy that developed proximal to the inoculation site on the finger (shown in previous photo). (Courtesy of Mark A. Ward, MD.)

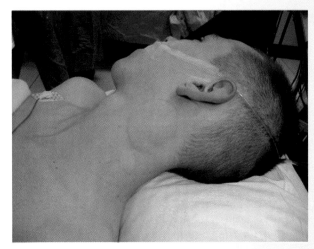

Figure 27-12 Hodgkin lymphoma. Large, fixed cervical masses in a 14-year-old with weight loss. (Courtesy of Mary L. Brandt, MD.)

OTHER
DIAGNOSES TO
CONSIDER

- Toxoplasmosis

- Kawasaki disease

- Graves disease

- Hashimoto thyroiditis

- Pyriform sinuses and cysts

- Leukemia

- Rhabdomyosarcoma

- Hematoma

SUGGESTED READINGS

Bonilla JA, Healy GB. Management of malignant head and neck tumors in children. *Pediatr Clin North Am.* 1989;36(6):1443–1450.

Brown RL, Azizkhan RG. Pediatric head and neck lesions. *Pediatr Clin North Am.* 1998;45(4):889–905.

Heroman WM, McCurley WS. Cat scratch disease. *Otolaryngol Clin North Am.* 1982;15(3):649–657.

Margileth AM. 1996. Cat scratch disease. In: Nelson WE, Behrman RE, Kliegman RM, Arvin AM, eds. *Nelson textbook of pediatrics.* 15th ed. Philadelphia: WB Saunders; 1996: 865–867.

Peters TR, Edwards KM. Cervical lymphadenopathy and adenitis. *Pediatr Rev.* 2000;21(12):399–405.

Snell RS. *Clinical anatomy.* 7th ed. Baltimore: Lippincott Williams & Wilkins; 2005:CD418.

Section

EIGHT

Chest

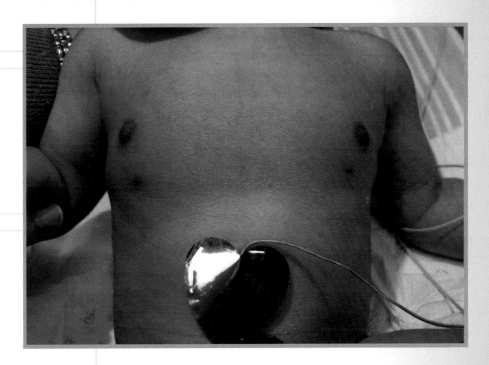

Abnormal Chest Shape

APPROACH TO THE PROBLEM

Several elements contribute to chest shape, including muscles, bones (ribs, sternum, clavicles, and spine), and underlying organs. Deficiency, hypertrophy, or malformation of any of these structures may produce abnormalities in the appearance of the chest wall. Abnormalities in lung form or function may cause changes in the chest shape; conversely, alterations in the size or shape of the thorax may significantly affect pulmonary function. Rarely, chronic cardiac enlargement may produce a prominence in the precordial chest wall. Pectus excavatum is the most common pediatric chest wall deformity; most of the others are quite rare.

KEY POINTS IN THE HISTORY

- Pectus excavatum and pectus carinatum are more common in males.

- Family history is often positive in patients with pectus excavatum.

- Asymmetry in the immediate neonatal period may be the result of intrauterine compression.

- Children who have symptoms of severe exercise intolerance with abnormal chest shape may have underlying pulmonary or cardiac disease.

KEY POINTS IN THE PHYSICAL EXAMINATION

- Tall stature, arachnodactyly, and joint laxity suggest Marfan syndrome in patients with pectus excavatum or pectus carinatum.

- Syndactyly and brachydactyly are associated with Poland syndrome.

- Short stature and webbed neck with shield chest (broad, with widely spaced nipples) may be seen in Turner or Noonan syndrome. Patients with Noonan syndrome also may have pectus excavatum or pectus carinatum.

- Narrow shoulders with various anomalies of the clavicles and upper extremities occur in Holt-Oram syndrome (which is also associated with cardiac and sternal defects), and cleidocranial dysostosis (in which delays in fontanel closure and tooth eruption also may be seen).

- A narrow or bell-shaped thorax is associated with many osteochondrodysplasias, such as achondroplasia, cleidocranial dysostosis, and Jeune thoracic dystrophy. It may also be seen in patients with neuromuscular disorders.

- Skin overlying a sternal cleft may be thin, scarlike, and hyperpigmented.

PHOTOGRAPHS OF SELECTED DIAGNOSES

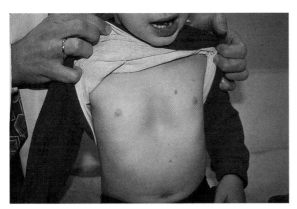

Figure 28-1 Pectus excavatum. Anterior view of child with pectus excavatum. (Courtesy of George A. Datto, III, MD.)

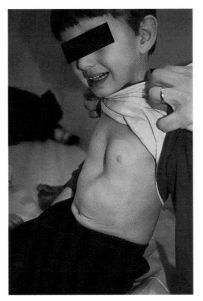

Figure 28-2 Pectus excavatum. Lateral view of child with pectus excavatum. (Courtesy of George A. Datto, III, MD.)

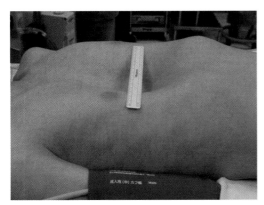

Figure 28-3 Pectus excavatum. Severe pectus in an adolescent with significant exercise intolerance. (Courtesy of Christopher Derby, MD.)

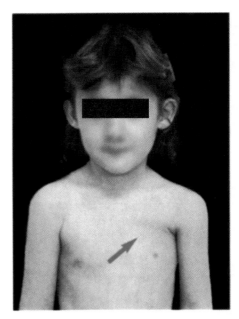

Figure 28-4 Poland sequence. Absence of pectoralis major muscle. (Used with permission from Staheli LT. *Practice of pediatric orthopedics.* Philadelphia: Lippincott Williams & Wilkins; 2001:192.)

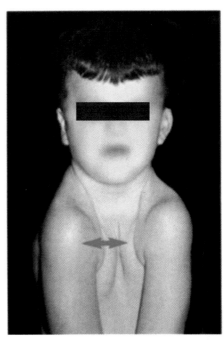

Figure 28-5 Cleidocranial dysostosis. Narrow chest with drooping shoulders. (Used with permission from Staheli LT. *Practice of pediatric orthopedics.* Philadelphia: Lippincott Williams & Wilkins; 2001:192.)

DIFFERENTIAL DIAGNOSIS

DIAGNOSIS	ICD-9	DISTINGUISHING CHARACTERISTICS	ASSOCIATED FINDINGS
Pectus Excavatum	754.81	Sternal depression Sternum may rotate to right, making right-sided structures smaller Deformity worsens during puberty	Increased incidence of scoliosis, congenital heart disease May be associated with Marfan syndrome, homocystinuria, Noonan syndrome, and other genetic disorders
Pectus Carinatum	754.82	Sternal protrusion Generally noted later in childhood than pectus excavatum	As for pectus excavatum
Barrel Chest	738.3	AP diameter of chest increased relative to transverse diameter (Normal ratio is 1:1 in infancy, with transverse diameter increasing with age)	Digital clubbing
Shield Chest	754.89	Wide chest with broadly spaced nipples	Turner syndrome Noonan syndrome
Poland Sequence	756.81	Unilateral deficiency of pectoralis muscles and breast structures Usually right-sided	May also have rib defects Ipsilateral syndactyly of hand
Sternal Cleft	756.3	Complete or partial separation of sternum May manifest as U-shaped or V-shaped depression, or with bulge from underlying structures May change with respiration Pulsations of heart may be visible. If there is overlying skin, it is often thin and hyperpigmented.	Usually an isolated anomaly Ectopia cordis Pentalogy of Cantrell Facial hemangiomas Cleft lip or palate
Cleidocranial dysostosis	755.59	Absent or hypoplastic clavicles resulting in abnormal shoulder movement Narrow thorax	Variety of other skeletal anomalies Abnormal teeth Delayed tooth eruption Deafness

COMPLICATIONS	PREDISPOSING FACTORS
Rarely interferes with cardiac or respiratory function, though some children have exercise limitations May be a significant cosmetic problem Can give false appearance of cardiomegaly on chest x-ray	Excessive growth of costal cartilage Male:female (3:1)
Rarely interferes with cardiac or respiratory function, though some children have exercise limitations May be a significant cosmetic problem	Excessive growth of costal cartilage More common in males
According to underlying cause	Severe asthma or other obstructive lung disease (e.g., Meconium aspiration syndrome) Genetic disorders such as spondyloepiphyseal dysplasia, Smith-McCort dysplasia, Costello syndrome
According to underlying cause	N/A
Respiratory problems when significant rib defects are present Breast tissue also is typically absent on affected side	Male:female (3:1) Abnormal blood flow through subclavian artery
None (unless associated defects)	None
Respiratory problems in infancy	Autosomal dominant inheritance

OTHER
DIAGNOSES TO
CONSIDER

- Vertebral deformities

- Acute or healed injuries

- Isolated rib anomalies

- Isolated clavicle anomalies

- Other genetic syndromes or congenital malformations

SUGGESTED READINGS

Grissom LE, Harcke HT. Thoracic deformities and the growing lung. *Semin Roentgenol.* 1998;33:199–208.

Jones K. *Smith's recognizable patterns of human malformation.* 5th ed. Philadelphia: WB Saunders; 1997.

Myers NA. An approach to the management of chest wall deformities. *Prog Pediatr Surg.* 1991;27:170–190.

Ravitch M. *Congenital deformities of the chest wall and their operative correction.* Philadelphia: WB Saunders; 1977.

Staheli LT. *Fundamentals of pediatric orthopedics.* 3rd ed. Philadelphia: Lippincott Williams & Wilkins; 2003:112.

Welch KJ. Chest wall deformities. In: Holder TM, Ashcraft KW, eds. *Pediatric surgery.* Philadelphia: WB Saunders; 1980:162–182.

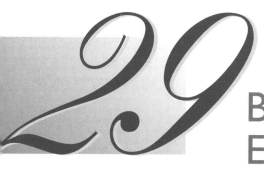

HEATHER E. NEEDHAM
AND MARIAM R. CHACKO

Breast Swelling and Enlargement

APPROACH TO THE PROBLEM

Various breast disorders may occur in children and adolescents, including breast asymmetry, gynecomastia, premature thelarche, and mastitis. It is important to consider the age of the patient at presentation when determining the cause of breast swelling or enlargement. These disorders may be classified as developmental, hormonal, or infectious.

KEY POINTS IN THE HISTORY

- Initiation of breast development is important in differentiating premature thelarche from normal pubertal development in girls. On average, normal thelarche occurs between 8 and 13 years of age.

- The onset of menses occurs approximately 2 years after breast buds appear.

- Enlarged breasts, unilaterally or bilaterally, in a young adolescent male usually suggests physiologic gynecomastia.

- Recreational or therapeutic use of certain drugs for an underlying illness may be associated with nonphysiological gynecomastia.

- Rapid growth of one breast may be associated with mammary hyperplasia or hypertrophy (or a mass).

- Chest or breast surgery, radiation to the chest, or chemotherapy before the onset of puberty may cause one breast to be smaller than the other.

- Breast asymmetry that occurs during the peripubertal period, accompanied by primary or secondary amenorrhea, may be a sign of ovarian failure.

- With asymmetric breast enlargement, pain may be reported in the larger breast whenever there is an underlying mass, cyst, or abscess.

- A history of breastfeeding may precede mastitis.

- A history of trauma to the breast or chest including nipple piercing, removal of areolar hairs, sports trauma, and abuse may precede an infectious process.

KEY POINTS IN THE PHYSICAL EXAMINATION

- In an adolescent patient with breast asymmetry, the two breasts may be at differing Tanner stages. Stretch marks and a circumferential reddish hue secondary to venous distension may be seen on the larger breast; however, a palpable mass or galactorrhea should not be present.

- With normal breast development in the female, Tanner stage I is where there is no glandular tissue and the areola conforms to the chest wall.

- Tanner stage II differs from stage I in that a breast bud is palpable, a small amount of glandular tissue exists, and the areola widens.

- In Tanner stage III, the breast tissue and areola enlarge further, and no separation is present between the contour of the breast and the areola.

- Tanner stage IV is a distinctive stage characterized by a "mound on a mound." The areola and papilla form a mound above the breast tissue.

- Tanner stage V is characterized as the adult breast. The areola is in contour with the breast, and the papilla projects above the breast.

- In a male with gynecomastia, the breast is prominent and breast tissue is palpable.

- In a male with pseudogynecomastia, no breast tissue is palpable. The prominence in the breast is soft because of obesity or is hard because of well-developed pectoralis muscles.

- Erythema, warmth, and tenderness of breast tissue are symptoms suggestive of an infectious process.

- Evidence of nipple piercing, removal, or shaving of areolar hair may be noted in patients with mastitis.

DIFFERENTIAL DIAGNOSIS

DIAGNOSIS	ICD-9	DISTINGUISHING CHARACTERISTICS	DURATION	ASSOCIATED FINDINGS	PREDISPOSING FACTORS
Breast Asymmetry	757.0	Breasts may be at the same or different Tanner staging Mass not palpable in the larger breast	Common in early and mid-puberty Usually self-limited Surgery may be necessary when there is marked asymmetry after pubertal development is completed	Common for left breast to be larger than right May be stretch marks or a circumferential reddish hue because of overlying venous distension in the larger breast	Usually unknown May have history of previous chest or breast surgery, radiation, or chemotherapy
Gynecomastia	611.1	Firm breast tissue palpated in males Three types: • Type I—one or more subareolar nodules • Type II—breast nodules beneath the areola and extending beyond the perimeter of the areola • Type III—resembles Tanner III female breast	Physiologic gynecomastia usually resolves in 12 to 24 months Nonphysiologic gynecomastia resolves after the precipitating factor is discontinued or treated	Physiologic gynecomastia commonly occurs during Tanner stage II–III in males Nonphysiologic gynecomastia may also occur in the postpubertal male Gynecomastia usually bilateral but may be unilateral Testicular mass may be palpable if a hormone-secreting tumor is present	Puberty is a precipitating factor for physiologic gynecomastia Recreational or therapeutic drug use, liver disease, and Klinefelter syndrome are precipitating factors for nonphysiologic gynecomastia
Premature Thelarche	259.1	Females Breast development under 8 years of age, specifically <6 years in non-obese black females and <7 years in non-obese white females Other signs of puberty absent No evidence of infection	Usually self-limited	Isolated breast budding—may be the first sign of true precocious puberty	Majority of cases idiopathic Use of exogenous estrogen has been reported
Mastitis	611.0	Symptoms include pain, tenderness, and induration +/- Fever Unilateral	Responds to antibiotic treatment Incision and drainage may be necessary for an abscess	Occurs in neonates (males and females) and adolescent females	In neonates, streptococcus usually causes cellulitis of the breast; cellulitis with an abscess is usually caused by staphylococcus In adolescent females, mastitis is associated with breastfeeding, nipple piercing, and removal or shaving of areolar hair

PHOTOGRAPHS OF SELECTED DIAGNOSES

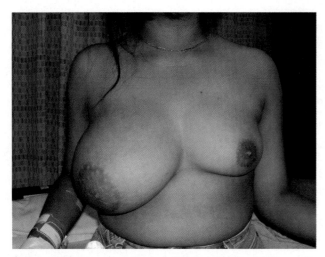

Figure 29-1 Breast asymmetry. Adolescent female with Tanner III breast development and significantly asymmetric breasts. (Courtesy of Mary L. Brandt, MD.)

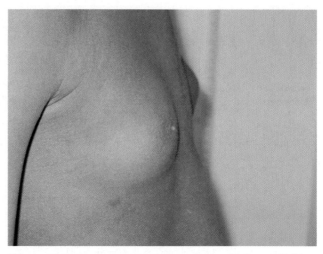

Figure 29-2 Gynecomastia. Adolescent male with Tanner III–IV genital staging and bilateral breast development with palpable breast buds, side view. (Courtesy of Christine Finck, MD.)

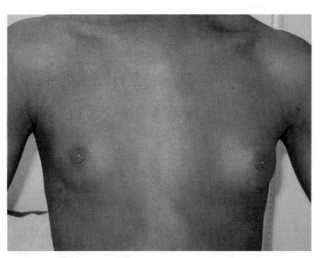

Figure 29-3 Gynecomastia. Adolescent male with Tanner III–IV genital staging and bilateral breast development with palpable breast buds, front view. (Courtesy of Christine Finck, MD.)

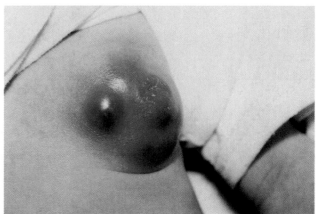

Figure 29-4 Mastitis. Ten-day-old female with swelling and erythema of the left breast. (Used with permission from Fleisher GR, Ludwig S, Baskin MN, et al. *Pictorial review of pediatrics.* Baltimore: Lippincott Williams & Wilkins; 1998:185.)

OTHER
DIAGNOSES TO
CONSIDER

- Fibroadenoma

- Breast cyst

- Breast abscess

SUGGESTED READINGS

Boepple PA. Overview of precocious puberty. In: *UpToDate* ONLINE 12.3;2005. http://www.uptodate.com.

Fleisher GR, Ludwig S, Baskin MN, et al. *Pictorial review of pediatrics.* Baltimore: Lippincott Williams & Wilkins; 1998:185.

Goldstein DP, Emans SJ, Laufer MR. The breast: examination and lesions. In: Emans SJ, Laufer MR, Goldstein DP, eds. *Pediatric and adolescent gynecology.* 4th ed. Philadelphia: Lippincott Williams & Wilkins; 1998:587–610.

Kaplowitz PB, Slora EJ, Wasserman RC, et al. Earlier onset of puberty in girls: relation to increased body mass index and race. *Pediatrics.* 2001;108:347–353.

Neinstein LS. Breast disease in adolescents and young women. *Pediatr Clin North Am.* 1999;46:607–629.

Neinstein LS. Breast disorders. In: Neinstein LS, ed. *Adolescent health care: a practical guide.* 4th ed. Philadelphia: Lippincott Williams & Wilkins; 2002:1063–1082.

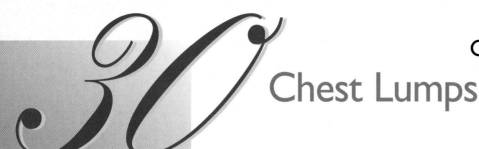

GEORGE A. DATTO, III

Chest Lumps

APPROACH TO THE PROBLEM

Lumps on the chest wall usually originate from bony structures of the chest cavity. With the exception of a prominent xyphoid process, which is often noticed in the neonatal period, all chest lumps should have a thorough evaluation to determine their etiology. The most common cause of an acquired chest lump is traumatic injury to the ribs or the clavicle from either accidental injury or child abuse. Less common causes include congenital rib anomalies, metabolic bone disease, infection, and malignancy. A chest radiograph is often helpful in determining the etiology of the chest lump.

KEY POINTS IN THE HISTORY

- Any acquired chest wall lump that is painful or is associated with other systemic complaints needs a careful investigation; congenital asymptomatic lumps are more likely to be benign developmental variations.

- A chest wall lump that increases in size over time raises concern for malignant, infectious, or traumatic etiologies.

- A child who is physically abused presents with a rib fracture between 5% and 25% of the time. Any rib fracture in a child should raise the suspicion of child abuse or an underlying metabolic bone disease such as rickets or osteogenesis imperfecta.

- Clavicular fractures are seen in newborns from birth trauma and in older children who fall onto an outstretched arm from accidental trauma.

- A child with a midclavicular mass in the absence of a history of trauma may represent a callus from a missed clavicular fracture or pseudoarthrosis of the clavicle.

- Dark skinned and premature infants who are breastfed are at risk for rickets when they are not supplemented with vitamin D.

- Adolescent males may complain of a chest lump that may simply represent physiologic male gynecomastia.

KEY POINTS IN THE PHYSICAL EXAMINATION

- When evaluating an infant with an acquired chest wall lump, other signs of child abuse such as scalp edema, bruises, and retinal hemorrhages should be sought and considered.

- Rib fractures of child abuse are usually bilateral and tend to involve the posterior ribs.

- Enlargement of the costochondral junction, "the rachitic rosary," craniotabes, and widening of the wrists and ankles are the osseous manifestations of rickets.

- Supernumerary nipples are always present in the nipple (or mammary or milk) line and are usually at least 50% smaller than the normal nipple and areola tissue.

- Erythema, soft tissue swelling, and pain on palpation are concerning signs for traumatic, infectious, or malignant causes of a child's chest wall lump.

- An asymmetric nontender prominence along the chest wall may be noted in a child with a bifid rib anomaly.

DIFFERENTIAL DIAGNOSIS

DIAGNOSIS	ICD-9	DISTINGUISHING CHARACTERISTICS	DISTRIBUTION
Supernumerary Nipple	757.6	Small, pigmented, umbilicated spot	Embyronic milk line
Clavicular Fracture with Callus	810.0	Hard callus at site of fracture	Clavicle
Pseudoarthrosis of Clavicle	733.82	Painless mass over clavicle	Clavicle
Prominent Xyphoid Process	756.3	Lump at inferior margin of the sternum	Midline Inferior sternum
Bifid Rib	756.3	Nontender prominence of anterior chest wall	Third, fourth, or fifth rib anteriorly
Rib Fracture	807.0	Painful chest swelling at site of trauma	Posterior ribs
Rickets	268.0	Small lumps at costochondral junction, "rachitic rosary"	Costochondral junction

ASSOCIATED FINDINGS	COMPLICATIONS	PREDISPOSING FACTORS
None	Cosmetic concerns	None
Neonates—asymmetric Moro reflex, clavicular crepitus, pain to palpation Child—pain with arm movement	Pneumothorax Brachial plexus injury Vascular injury	Neonates—large baby Child—fall onto outstretched arm
None	None	Congenital failure of ossification of the central portion of clavicle
None	None	None
Gorlin syndrome	None	None
Other signs of child abuse: other fractures, scalp edema, bruises, retinal hemorrhages Ineffective respirations	Respiratory compromise Pneumothorax	Child abuse Blunt trauma Penetrating injury
Craniotabes Widened wrists and ankles Bowed tibia	Respiratory infections Pulmonary atelectasis	Infants who are primarily breastfed with dark skin and/or minimal sun exposure

PHOTOGRAPHS OF SELECTED DIAGNOSES

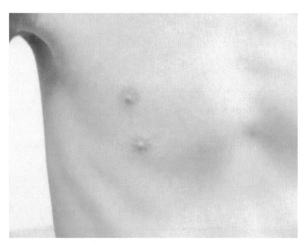

Figure 30-1 Supernumerary nipple. Fully developed nipple in embryonic milk line. (Courtesy of Philip Siu, MD.)

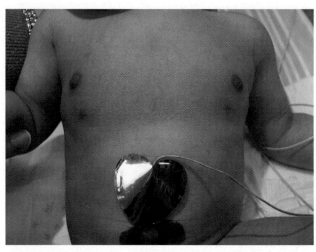

Figure 30-2 Supernumerary nipples. Bilateral supernumerary nipples in a newborn. (Courtesy of Esther K. Chung, MD.)

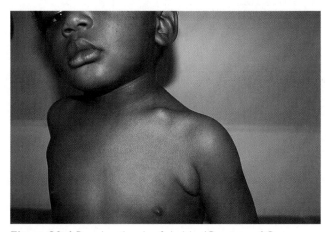

Figure 30-3 Clavicular fracture. Distal clavicular fracture with swelling over child's acromioclavicular joint. (Used with permission from Fleisher GR, Ludwig S, Baskin MN, eds. *Atlas of pediatric emergency medicine.* Philadelphia: Lippincott Williams & Wilkins; 2004:362.)

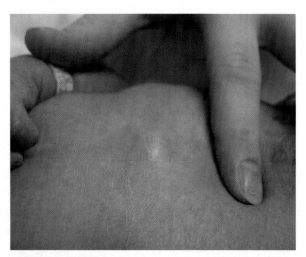

Figure 30-4 Pseudoarthrosis of clavicle. (Courtesy of George A. Datto, III, MD.)

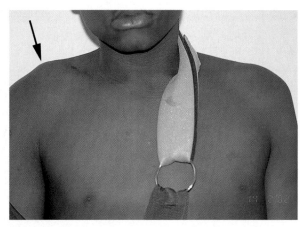

Figure 30-5 Prominent xyphoid process. (Courtesy of Esther K. Chung, MD.)

- Ewing sarcoma

- Rhabdomyosarcoma

- Neuroblastoma

- Osteochondroma

- Osteomyelitis

SUGGESTED READINGS

Balint JP. Physical findings in nutritional deficiencies. *Pediatr Clin North Am*. 1998;45:245–260.
Epps HR. Orthopedic conditions of the cervical spine and shoulder. *Pediatr Clin North Am*. 1996;43:919–931.
Fefferman NR, Pinkney LP. Imaging evaluation of chest wall disorders in children. *Radiol Clin North Am*. 2005;43:355–370.
Fleisher GR, Ludwig S, Baskin MN, eds. *Atlas of pediatric emergency medicine*. Philadelphia: Lippincott Williams & Wilkins; 2004:362.
Nimkin K, Kleinman PK. Imaging of child abuse. *Pediatr Clin North Am*. 1997;44:615–635.

NINE

Abdomen

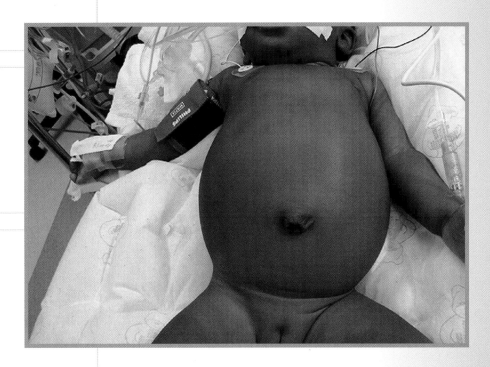

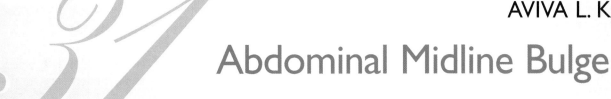

AVIVA L. KATZ

Abdominal Midline Bulge

APPROACH TO THE PROBLEM

There exists a variety of midline bulges that can be seen in the newborn. These bulges generally represent either abnormal or incomplete fetal development or complications involving a fetal remnant. These disorders of the umbilical region generally represent persistence of structures, which usually obliterate before birth, or failure of closure of the umbilical ring. Bulges range from entirely benign lesions, such as diastasis recti, to an acutely life-threatening anomaly, such as gastroschisis.

KEY POINTS IN THE HISTORY

- Umbilical hernias are more common in African American children and are usually present shortly after cord separation.

- The presence of a persistent draining umbilical cord should raise the suspicion of a patent urachus.

- Urachal cysts and sinuses may present at any age, generally secondary to infection including abscess formation.

- Visible anomalies related to vitelline/omphalomesenteric duct remnants include umbilical fistula, umbilical polyp, and sinus enteric cyst. An umbilical fistula, and frequently an umbilical polyp, will be apparent in the newborn period, while a sinus enteric cyst may not be apparent until it is secondarily infected later in childhood.

- Omphalocele and gastroschisis frequently present antenatally because of the broad use of maternal quadruple screens and Level II ultrasounds. Omphalocele and gastroschisis are apparent at birth.

KEY POINTS IN THE PHYSICAL EXAMINATION

- Diastasis recti, separation of the rectus abdominis muscles that manifests as a midline bulge from the xiphoid process to the umbilicus, is a common finding in newborns.

- In contrast to inguinal hernia, it is extremely rare to have an incarcerated umbilical hernia. A tender erythematous, irreducible umbilical hernia is a surgical emergency.

- A patent urachus will present with urine visibly draining from the umbilical cord. A patent vitillene/omphalomesenteric fistula will present with meconium and stool drainage at the umbilicus.

- Urachal cysts and enteric sinus cysts usually present after they have become secondarily infected, appearing as a tender, erythematous, infraumbilical midline mass.

- Gastroschisis and omphalocele are generally easily distinguishable antenatally and at birth. A sac is always present in omphalocele, though it may be somewhat disrupted because of the birth process; however, no sac is present in gastroschisis, which consists of extruded bowel loops with some element of fibrous peel.

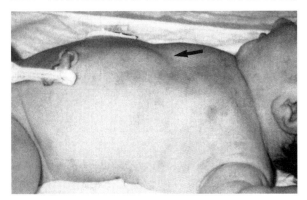

Figure 31-1 Diastasis recti. (Used with permission from Fletcher MA. *Physical diagnosis in neonatology.* Philadelphia: Lippincott–Raven Publishers; 1998:357.)

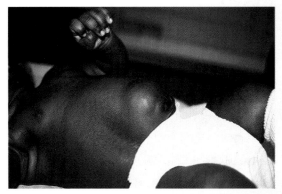

Figure 31-2 Umbilical hernia and diastasis recti. (Courtesy of George A. Datto, III, MD.)

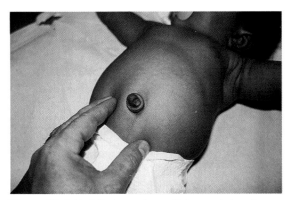

Figure 31-3 Umbilical granuloma. Pink granulation tissue at the base of the umbilicus. (Courtesy of George A. Datto, III, MD.)

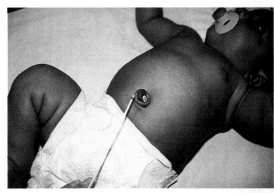

Figure 31-4 Umbilical granuloma. Umbilical granuloma after treatment with silver nitrate. (Courtesy of George A. Datto, III, MD.)

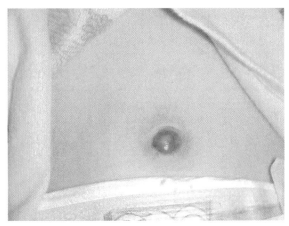

Figure 31-5 Urachal cyst. Infected urachal cyst in a 3-month-old infant. (Courtesy of Ben Alouf, MD.)

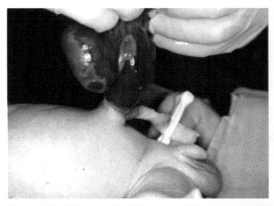

Figure 31-6 Gastroschisis. (Courtesy of Douglas Katz, MD.)

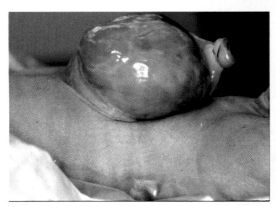

Figure 31-7 Omphalocele. (Courtesy of Douglas Katz, MD.)

DIAGNOSIS	ICD-9	DISTINGUISHING CHARACTERISTICS	DISTRIBUTION	ASSOCIATED FINDINGS
Diastasis Recti	728.84	Valsalva maneuvers and flexion of the abdominal muscles reveal this midline bulge Common in newborns May be seen in women during or following pregnancy	From xiphoid process to umbilicus	None
Umbilical Hernia	553.1	Skin-covered protrusion at umbilicus Fascial edge felt circumferentially	Replaces normal umbilicus	Diastasis recti
Umbilical Granuloma	771.4	Mass of pink granulation tissue at the base of the umbilicus Seropurulent secretions	Umbilicus	None
Urachal Cyst	753.7	Most asymptomatic unless infected Red, tender infraumbilical mass If there is a patent sinus, there may be drainage at the umbilicus	As with the patent urachus, presents deep in the anterior abdominal wall, in the midline, in the infraumbilical area, above the dome of the bladder	Fever, tenderness, and purulent drainage when infected
Gastroschisis	756.79	Evisceration of gastrointestinal tract through relatively small abdominal wall defect to the right of the umbilical cord No covering sac; cord intact otherwise	Stomach through to and including sigmoid colon may be found in continuity	Testes, ovaries, and fallopian tubes may be found eviscerated alongside the intestine Generally no other solid organs are involved Intestinal atresia: 10%
Omphalocele	756.79	Sac-covered bulge, with cord extending from near its center, replacing the normal umbilicus Sac composed of amnion and peritoneum	Fascial defect may range in diameter from 4 to 14 cm Intestinal loops and liver may be herniated into the sac	Trisomy 13, 14, 15, 18, and 21. Beckwith-Wiedemann syndrome Associated cardiac, renal, and limb anomalies

COMPLICATIONS	PREDISPOSING FACTORS
None	None
Incarceration rare, but should be suspected if not easily reducible	Low birth weight Female/gender/ African American race/ethnicity
May epithelialize, but not completely resolve, after treatment with silver nitrate, leading to excision	Unknown
Rare reported cases of urachal carcinoma from urachal remnants	Persistence of allantoic duct
Risk of third trimester in utero fetal death (IUFD) Most series report a 10% to 15% mortality rate, mostly related to short bowel syndrome and its associated complications of sepsis and liver failure	Vascular accident or atrophy involving the right umbilical vein
May be technical difficulties in achieving abdominal wall closure in the larger omphalocele In large or giant omphalocele, may be pulmonary hypoplasia with associated respiratory distress because of the associated narrow thoracic cavity	Defective development in the formation of the umbilical ring

<table>
<tr><td>

OTHER
DIAGNOSES TO
CONSIDER

</td><td>

- Abdominal wall hernia

- Omphalomesenteric cyst

- Patent vitelline/omphalomesenteric fistula

- Patent urachus

</td></tr>
</table>

SUGGESTED READINGS

Fletcher MA. *Physical diagnosis in neonatology.* Philadelphia: Lippincott–Raven Publishers; 1998:357.

Katz DA. Evaluation and management of inguinal and umbilical hernias. *Pediatr Ann.* 2001;30:729–735.

Weber TR, Au-Fliegner M, Downard CD, et al. Abdominal wall defects. *Curr Opin Pediatr.* 2002;14:491–497.

Wilson RD, Johnson MP. Congenital abdominal wall defects: an update. *Fetal Diagn Ther.* 2004;19:385–398.

VANI GOPALAREDDY AND
DEVENDRA I. MEHTA

Enlarged/Distended Abdomen

APPROACH TO THE PROBLEM

Distension of the abdomen can occur because of feces, flatus, fluid, fat, full urinary bladder, tumors, cysts, organomegaly, and pregnancy. Ileus from many causes or reduced intestinal motility from drugs or metabolic derangements may also lead to acute abdominal distension. Intestinal obstruction of any etiology can lead ultimately to diffuse distension. Lumbar lordosis, whether physiologic in a prepubescent child or pathologic in neuromuscular disorders, will cause the child to have the appearance of abdominal distension. Rapid recognition of abdominal distension in an ill-appearing child is essential to reduce morbidity and mortality. Imaging studies have their role in determining the etiology of a child's enlarged abdomen.

KEY POINTS IN THE HISTORY

- Failure to thrive or acute weight loss may be a marker for significant pathology causing the enlarged abdomen.

- A child usually will complain of minimal pain with an ileus but will complain of significant pain with an intestinal obstruction.

- Severe infections (including gastrointestinal infections, pneumonia, and peritonitis) and abdominal surgeries may be associated with paralytic ileus and abdominal distension.

- Prior abdominal surgery puts a child at risk for adhesions and small-bowel obstruction.

- Bilious vomiting should be presumed to be secondary to intestinal obstruction until proven otherwise.

- A thorough history assessing for frequency, consistency, and difficulty with stool passage is important for diagnosing constipation.

- Often, bezoars are found in neurologically or psychologically impaired children with pica.

- Children with diseases associated with hemolysis are at risk for splenomegaly.

- Hematemesis, melena, and jaundice can be seen with portal hypertension.

- Parents often note abdominal tumors when their child is in the bathtub.

- Increased flatus suggests that the abdominal distension may be from increased intestinal air.

- Pregnancy should be considered and ruled out in a postpubertal female with secondary amenorrhea and lower abdominal distension.

KEY POINTS IN THE PHYSICAL EXAMINATION

- The overall health and habitus of a child will suggest whether the condition is acute or chronic.

- To detect abdominal organomegaly on palpation, it is important to examine the lower abdomen close to the groin then proceed upward toward the chest.

- Pallor and nail clubbing are physical findings that suggest chronic malabsorption.

- Ascites, flatus, and ileus present with symmetrical abdominal distension.

- Malignancy, constipation, pregnancy, and organomegaly may present with localized abdominal distension.

- Skin findings of chronic liver disease include spider nevi, palmar erythema, and jaundice.

- Visible peristaltic waves may be seen with intestinal obstruction.

- Bowel sounds are often absent in ileus, but they are hyperactive in intestinal obstruction.

- A child with peritonitis often resists any movement and has involuntary guarding on abdominal examination.

- A large fecal mass palpable in the left lower quadrant with hard stool on rectal exam is suggestive of functional constipation, while constipation with an empty rectal vault is suggestive of Hirschsprung disease.

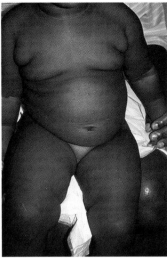

Figure 32-1 Obesity. Enlarged abdomen from increased adiposity. (Courtesy of George A. Datto, III, MD.)

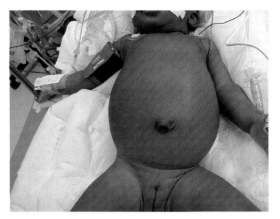

Figure 32-2 Ascites. (Courtesy of Vani Gopalareddy, MD.)

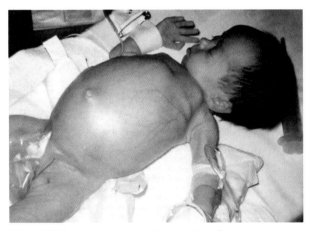

Figure 32-3 Abdominal distention resulting from hepatomegaly in a child with untreated galactosemia. Note the distention is more prominent in the upper abdomen. (Used with permission from Fletcher MA. *Physical diagnosis in neonatology.* Philadelphia: Lippincott–Raven Publishers; 1998:353.)

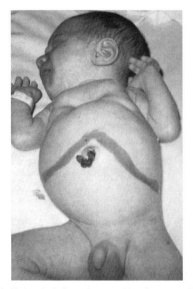

Figure 32-4 Abdominal distention resulting from massive hepatosplenomegaly in an infant with congenital cytomegalovirus infection. Note the distention is more prominent in the upper abdomen. (Used with permission from Fletcher MA. *Physical diagnosis in neonatology.* Philadelphia: Lippincott–Raven Publishers; 1998:354.)

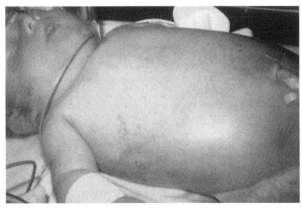

Figure 32-5 Abdominal distention in an infant with anasarca. Note that the distention is more prominent in the flanks. (Used with permission from Fletcher MA. *Physical diagnosis in neonatology.* Philadelphia: Lippincott–Raven Publishers; 1998:355.)

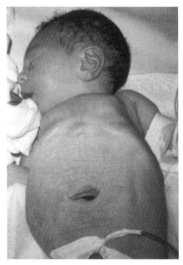

Figure 32-6 Abdominal distention at the flanks in an infant with Prune Belly syndrome. (Used with permission from Fletcher MA. *Physical diagnosis in neonatology.* Philadelphia: Lippincott–Raven Publishers; 1998:355.)

DIFFERENTIAL DIAGNOSIS

DIAGNOSIS	ICD-9	DISTINGUISHING CHARACTERISTICS	DISTRIBUTION
Obesity	278.0	Increased subcutaneous fat	Generalized
Constipation	564.0	Indentable abdominal mass Hard stool in rectum	Left lower quadrant and suprapubic pain and enlargement May be generalized if more severe
Flatus	787.3	Resonant percussion note	Generalized
Ascites	789.5	Dull percussion note Fluid wave Fullness of flanks	Generalized
Hepatomegaly	789.1	Enlarged liver span determined by palpation or percussion	Right upper quadrant, but if severe may appear to be generalized enlargement of the abdomen
Splenomegaly	789.2	Palpable edge in left upper quadrant	Left upper quadrant
Intestinal Obstruction	560.9	Acute abdominal distension	Generalized
Wilms Tumor	189.0	Asymptomatic flank mass Median age of presentation: 3y	Flank
Neuroblastoma	194.0	Large abdominal mass Lymphadenopathy Median age: 2y	Flank or abdominal
Prune Belly Syndrome	756.71	Wrinkled abdominal wall skin with abdominal distension	Generalized

DURATION/ CHRONICITY	ASSOCIATED FINDINGS	COMPLICATIONS	PREDISPOSING FACTORS
Chronic	Acanthosis nigricans Polycystic ovarian syndrome	Hypertension Diabetes Obstructive sleep apnea	Excessive caloric intake Inactivity
Chronic—often begins in toddler age	External or internal hemorrhoid Anal fissures	Encopresis Psychologic distress	Diet low in fiber Psychologic factors
Chronic	Periumbilical pain	Psychologic distress	Consumption of lactose in lactose intolerant patient Certain foods
Acute or nonacute	Ankle swelling	Patient at risk for developing spontaneous bacterial peritonitis	Liver disease Cardiac disease Infections Lymphoma Ovarian pathology
Acute or nonacute	Jaundice Pruritus Skin findings Ascites	Portal hypertension Liver failure Encephalopathy Renal failure	Infection Storage disease Malignancy Autoimmune Vascular disease
Acute or nonacute	Superficial abdominal venous distension when associated with portal hypertension Pallor	Cytopenias Splenic rupture	Infection Hematological Neoplasm Storage diseases Congestion Autoimmune
Acute	Bilious vomiting Obstipation	Peritonitis	Prior abdominal surgery
Acute	Hypertension Hematuria Abdominal pain Vomiting	Dependent on stage of tumor	Beckwith-Wiedemann syndrome WAGR syndrome
Acute	Bone pain Proptosis and ecchymosis Opsoclonus myoclonus Horner syndrome	Dependent on stage of tumor	N/A
Chronic	Urethral obstruction Pulmonary hypoplasia Undescended testes Renal dysplasia Congenital cardiac disease	One third of children are stillborn or die in the first 3 months of life Renal failure	Male

OTHER
DIAGNOSES TO
CONSIDER

- Intussusception

- Volvulus

- Pancreatic pseudocyst

- Mesenteric cysts

- Necrotizing enterocolitis

SUGGESTED READINGS

Fletcher MA. *Physical diagnosis in neonatology.* Philadelphia: Lippincott–Raven Publishers; 1998:353–355.

Squires RH Jr. Abdominal masses. In: Walker WA, Durie PR, Hamilton JR, et al., eds. *Pediatric gastrointestinal disease.* 3rd ed. Ontario: B.C. Decker; 2000:150–163.

Youssef NN, Di Lorenzo C. Childhood constipation: evaluation and treatment. *J Clin Gastroenterol.* 2001;33:199–205.

Back

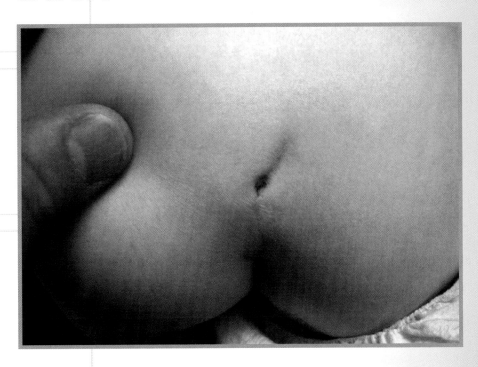

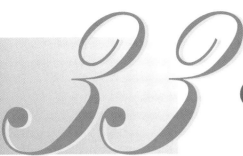

SHAREEN F. KELLY

Curvature of the Back

APPROACH TO THE PROBLEM

Curvature of the spine is described by the plane of curvature and the position of the curve relative to the spine. Kyphosis is an exaggerated curve of the thoracic spine in the sagittal plane with the apex of the curve directed posteriorly. Lordosis refers to a marked curvature that occurs in the sagittal plane of the lumbar spine, the apex of which is directed anteriorly. The term *scoliosis* describes lateral spinal curvature in the coronal plane and necessarily involves a rotational component as well. The rotational component is visualized most often as a rib hump viewed posteriorly. Curvature of the spine can present with varying severity and may progress with age and time. Beyond skeletal maturity, scoliosis generally does not progress; however, kyphosis and lordosis may progress into older adulthood.

KEY POINTS IN THE HISTORY

- Family history of scoliosis is present in approximately 30% of new cases of scoliosis.

- Complaints of back pain are not characteristic of idiopathic scoliosis and should prompt the physician to rule out other treatable diseases.

- Sports participation and day-to-day functioning usually are not affected by the curvature of scoliosis unless it is very severe.

- Nonambulatory patients are more likely to have progressive scoliosis than ambulatory patients.

- Fixed kyphosis may cause pain with neck motion.

- Radicular pain, changes in bowel or bladder function, sensory abnormalities, and problems with balance and/or coordination all point to an underlying neurologic problem.

- Constitutional symptoms—including prolonged fever, weight loss, night sweats, and malaise—may provide clues regarding malignancies or inflammatory diseases.

- Rapidly progressing curves are more likely to require treatment.

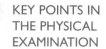

KEY POINTS IN THE PHYSICAL EXAMINATION

- Bony deformities detected upon palpation along the spine suggest vertebral anomalies or spinal dysraphism.

- Skin overlying the lumbar spine marked with hemangiomas, hair tufts, clefts, and/or other macular discolorations may be the only clinical clue to occult spinal dysraphism.

- The most common presentation of idiopathic scoliosis is that of a thoracic curve with a right thoracic rib hump when viewed from behind.

- Lower extremity muscular weakness, tightness of hamstrings, and decreased deep tendon reflexes are indicative of a neurologic abnormality.

- Patients with more advanced sexual maturity ratings are less likely to have progression of their spinal curvature.

- Range of motion assessment is critical in children with kyphosis or lordosis.

PHOTOGRAPHS OF SELECTED DIAGNOSES

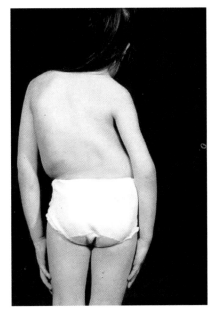

Figure 33-1 Scoliosis. (Used with permission from SIU/Biomedical Communications/Custom Medical Stock Photography.)

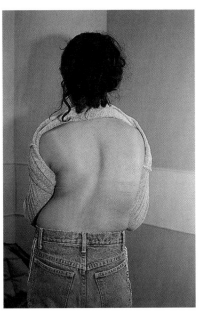

Figure 33-2 Scoliosis, standing. (Courtesy of George A. Datto, III, MD.)

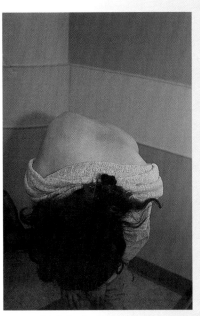

Figure 33-3 Scoliosis, bending forward. Note the marked asymmetry of the back. (Courtesy of George A. Datto, III, MD.)

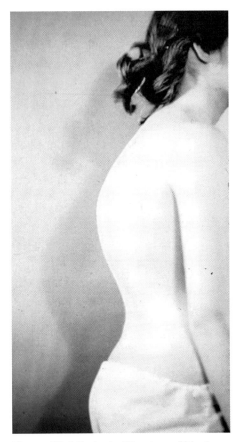

Figure 33-4 Kyphosis. (Courtesy of Martin Herman, MD.)

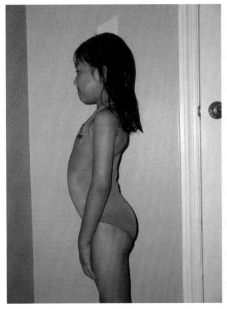

Figure 33-5 Lordosis. Note the thoracolumbar curvature on side view of this child in her normal stance. (Courtesy of Esther K. Chung, MD.)

DIFFERENTIAL DIAGNOSIS

DIAGNOSIS	ICD-9	DISTINGUISHING CHARACTERISTICS	DISTRIBUTION
Scoliosis	737.30	Lateral curvature of the spine Right (most often) thoracic rib hump on Adams forward bend test	Females:males (4:1) Idiopathic presents most often in adolescence
Kyphosis	737.10	Convex curvature of the upper thoracic spine Best viewed from the side with the child standing	Postural more common in prepubertal children Structural may affect any age
Lordosis	737.20	Concave curve of the lumbar spine Best viewed from the side while child is standing or when child is lying supine on a firm, flat surface	All age groups

DURATION/ CHRONICITY	ASSOCIATED FINDINGS	COMPLICATIONS	PREDISPOSING FACTORS
Curve progresses through puberty Usually no decrease in function	Asymmetry of clavicles and/or scapulae Asymmetry of back skin folds Leg length discrepancy Asymmetric iliac crests	Severe cases (mostly nonambulatory) may result in restrictive lung disease and/or cor pulmonale	Most often idiopathic Congenital scoliosis may result from vertebral anomalies
Postural corrects with physical therapy Structural may progress into old age	Postural often seen with compensatory lordosis Fixed kyphosis is often painful	When associated with osteoporosis, painful and may cause symptoms of compression	Postural: poor posture Scheurman's disease, has no known etiology
Physical therapy may be all that is needed to correct flexible lordosis	Buttocks appear more prominent Curve may correct with forward bending	Pain Decreased flexibility and movement	Poor posture, obesity Congenital: vertebral or neuromuscular problems Acquired: diskitis or spondylolisthesis

OTHER
DIAGNOSES TO
CONSIDER

- Marfan syndrome

- Ehlers Danlos syndrome

- Bone dysplasias

- Metabolic diseases, including rickets, osteoporosis, homocystinuria, osteogenesis imperfecta, may be associated with scoliosis

- Spinal tumors

- Neuromuscular disorders

- Spondylolisthesis

SUGGESTED READINGS

Chen AL. Lordosis. *Medline Plus. A Service of the U.S. National Library of Medicine and the National Institutes of Health.* Available at: http://www.nlm.nih.gov/médlineplus/ency/article/003278.htm. Accessed October 6, 2005.

Chin KR, Price JS, Zimbler S. A guide to early detection of scoliosis. *Contemp Pediatr.* 2001;18:77–103.

Killian JT, Mayberry S, Wilkinson L. Current concepts in adolescent idiopathic scoliosis. *Pediatr Ann.* 1999;28:755–761.

Marsh JS. Screening for scoliosis. *Pediatr Rev.* 1993;14:297–298.

Ward T, Davis HW, Hanley EN. Orthopedics. In: *Atlas of pediatric physical diagnosis.* 2nd ed. New York: Gower Medical Publishing; 1992:21.25–27.30.

PAUL S. MATZ

34 Midline Back Pits, Skin Tags, Hair Tufts, and Other Lesions

APPROACH TO THE PROBLEM

Up to 5% of children have congenital back dimples, pits, skin tags, or hair tufts. Additionally, lipomas and hemangiomas may occur along the midline area of the back. The history and physical examination should focus on the location of the lesion and associated neurologic symptoms and signs. A small percentage of these lesions are associated with underlying spinal pathology, which includes spinal dysraphism, or failure of the neural folds to fuse in utero (such as myelomeningocoele or spina bifida), or other abnormalities, such as tethered spinal cord or spinal lipomas. A tethered cord occurs when the spinal cord is abnormally fixed to a mass, the meninges, a vertebra, or the skin. As a child with tethered cord grows, excess tension is placed on the spinal cord and its blood vessels, leading to damage to the nerve fibers. It is important to remember that delayed diagnosis can lead to permanent neurologic damage in these conditions. Early diagnosis and treatment is associated with a better prognosis. In the absence of underlying spinal pathology, superficial back lesions other than infected pilonidal cysts rarely require treatment.

Spina bifida and sacrococcygeal teratoma are distinct from the other midline lesions. They usually present as sacral masses prenatally or at birth and require immediate intervention.

KEY POINTS IN THE HISTORY

- Nearly all midline back skin tags, pits, and tufts are congenital.

- Presence of neurologic symptoms, such as bowel or bladder incontinence in older children or lower extremity weakness, toe walking, pain, or paresthesias strongly suggests a spinal dysraphism or other spinal pathology.

- Long-standing tethered cord may result in asymmetric lower extremity growth.

- A family history of neural tube defects may increase the likelihood that a midline defect will be associated with occult spinal dysraphism.

- Symptoms of localized inflammation, such as pain and redness, in an older child could signify an infected pilonidal cyst.

- Spina bifida and sacrococcygeal teratoma are congenital lesions that are apparent prenatally or in the delivery room.

- A large sacrococcygeal teratoma may be associated with a history of hydrops fetalis during pregnancy.

- Folic acid supplementation in pregnant women greatly reduces the incidence of spinal cord defects.

KEY POINTS IN THE PHYSICAL EXAMINATION

- High thoracolumbar lesions are more likely than low lumbosacral lesions to be associated with underlying spinal cord lesions.

- Pilonidal sinuses or cysts are located below the superior margin of the gluteal cleft and are rarely associated with spinal cord defects.

- Sacral dimples are located above the superior margin of the gluteal cleft and can be associated with spinal cord defects.

- Midline lesions have an increased risk of spinal cord involvement; nonmidline lesions, such as skin tags, may also be associated with underlying spinal cord lesions.

- It is important to distinguish shallow dimples, which require no further workup, from deep ("bottomless") pits. The latter require further evaluation to rule out occult spinal pathology.

- The presence of any neurologic abnormality, such as weakness of the lower extremities, abnormal reflexes, or abnormal gait, suggests spinal cord involvement.

- While an abnormal neurologic exam strongly suggests a spinal cord abnormality, a normal exam cannot rule it out.

- Defects may sometimes be palpated along the spine when there is spinal dysraphism.

- Deviation of the gluteal cleft suggests an underlying mass, such as a lipoma or myelomeningocoele.

- Spina bifida and sacrococcygeal teratoma are sacral masses that may be covered by skin or have exposed membranes and spinal cord.

- Deep pilonidal sinuses may become blocked with hair, skin, or other debris and may become cystic and infected.

- Signs of acute inflammation, including redness, warmth, and tenderness, suggest an infected pilonidal cyst.

- Many newborns are born with hair on their backs. Further evaluation is warranted only for distinct hair tufts or patches.

DIFFERENTIAL DIAGNOSIS

DIAGNOSIS	ICD-9	DISTINGUISHING CHARACTERISTICS	LOCATION	ASSOCIATED FINDINGS	PREDISPOSING FACTORS
Sacral Dimple or Pit	685	Small indentation of the skin, often circular; may be shallow or deep ("bottomless"); located above the superior margin of the gluteal cleft	Mid or lower back, midline or lateral	Potential for occult spinal pathology with deep, midline dimples	Unknown
Skin Tag	757.39	Small outgrowth of skin	Mid or lower back	Potential for occult spinal pathology	Unknown
Hair Tufts/Patches	757.4	Cluster of hair, often dark	Mid or lower back	Potential for occult spinal pathology	Unknown
Pilonidal Sinus/Cyst	685	Small indentation or sinus tract in the skin containing hair; located below the superior margin of the gluteal cleft May appear inflamed if infected	Intergluteal, usually lateral	Rare occult spinal pathology with deep, midline tracts Infection	Sex hormones, obesity, local trauma, and poor hygiene increase the risk of obstruction, which may lead to cyst formation and infection
Hemangioma	228.0	Benign neoplasms of proliferating vascular endothelium Rapid growth in infancy followed by involution	May occur anywhere on the back and on other parts of the body	May be associated with spina bifida, meningomyelocele, tethered cord	Unknown
Spina Bifida	741	Sacral mass that may have exposed mucous membranes or spinal cord or may be covered by skin	Midline, lower back	Weakness or paralysis of legs May be associated with hydrocephalus or Arnold-Chiari malformation	Inadequate folic acid supplementation during pregnancy
Sacrococcygeal Teratoma	215.6	Large sacral mass that may have exposed membranes or be covered by skin	Overlying the sacrum and coccyx	High output heart failure and hydrops fetalis	Unknown

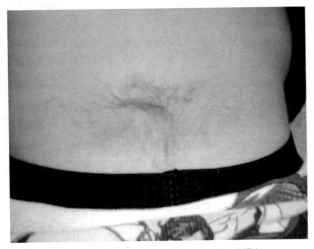

Figure 34-1 Sacral dimple. (Courtesy of Paul S. Matz, MD.)

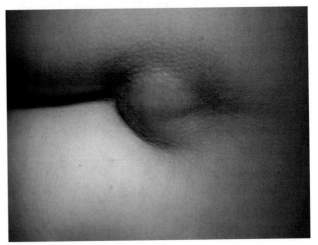

Figure 34-2 Sacral skin tag with no underlying spinal pathology. (Courtesy of Esther K. Chung, MD.)

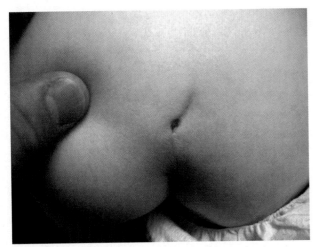

Figure 34-3 Hair tuft. (Courtesy of Joseph Piatt, MD.)

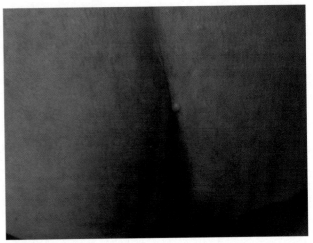

Figure 34-4 Infected pilonidal cyst. (Courtesy of Scott VanDuzer, MD.)

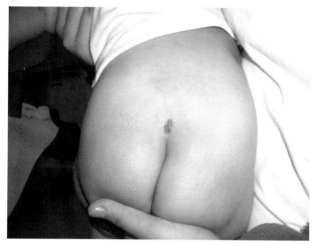

Figure 34-5 Sacral hemangioma. (Courtesy of Paul S. Matz, MD.)

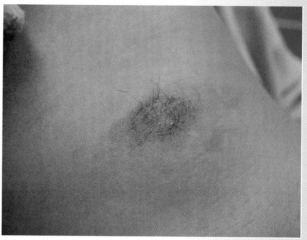

Figure 34-6 Lumbar hemangioma. This midline lesion was associated with a dermal sinus and an underlying tethered cord. (Courtesy of Esther K. Chung, MD.)

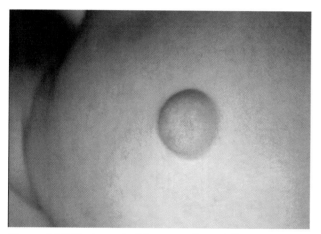

Figure 34-7 Meningocele. (Courtesy of Joseph Piatt, MD.)

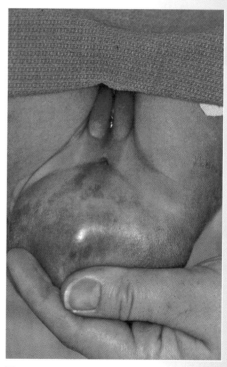

Figure 34-8 Sacrococcygeal teratoma. (Courtesy of Joseph Piatt, MD.)

SUGGESTED READINGS

Ackerman LL, Menezes AH. Spinal congenital dermal sinuses: a 30-year experience. *Pediatrics.* 2003;112:641–647.

Drolet, BA. Cutaneous signs of neural tube dysraphism. *Pediatr Clin North Am.* 2000;47(4):813–823.

Gibson PJ, Britton J, Hall DMB, et al. Lumbosacral skin markers and identification of occult spinal dysraphism in neonates. *Acta Pediatr.* 1995;84:208–209.

Howard R. Congenital midline lesions: pits and protuberances. *Pediatr Ann.* 1998;27(3):150–159.

Section
ELEVEN

Extremities

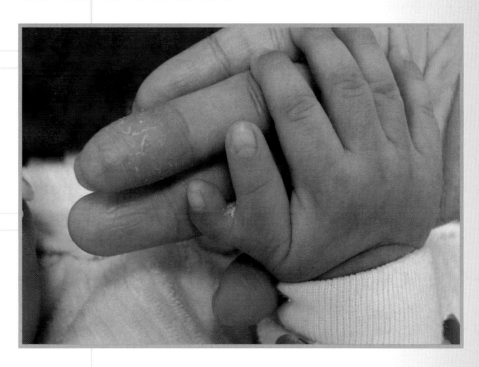

DENISE W. METRY
AND BRANDI M. KENNER

Nail Abnormalities

APPROACH TO THE PROBLEM

Abnormalities of the nail may represent a problem within the nail apparatus itself, an extension of a primary dermatologic disorder, or a systemic disease. The nail grows continuously throughout life and is extremely sensitive to changes in the body and the environment. Anything that disrupts the normal growth and development of the nail or damages its structural components will cause changes in the appearance and function of the nail. Nail abnormalities are sometimes a clue to more serious systemic illness, which may not otherwise be apparent. Most nail abnormalities, however, are benign and primarily of cosmetic concern. It is thus important for the evaluating physician to properly diagnose nail disorders, reassure anxious patients and parents when appropriate, and offer treatment suggestions when available.

KEY POINTS IN THE HISTORY

- Trauma (including nail biting, excessive manicuring, or picking) is a common contributor to abnormal nails.

- Acrocyanosis involves a persistent discoloration, distinguishing it from Raynaud's phenomenon or other transient conditions.

- Drug exposure, especially to chemotherapy, tetracycline, chloroquine, or antiretrovirals, is a frequent cause of nail discoloration.

- Longitudinal melanonychia is a common, normal finding among dark-skinned individuals.

- Malignant melanoma should be considered whenever a new, solitary nail hyperpigmentation develops in a light-skinned person or when growing or changing hyperpigmentation occurs in a person of any skin type.

KEY POINTS IN THE PHYSICAL EXAMINATION

- Leukonychia striata is characterized by white spots on the nails that are the result of trauma to the nail (such as from grooming techniques).

- Systemic diseases usually produce uniform changes that affect all nails simultaneously.

- Primary dermatologic disorders and fungal infections may affect one or more nails but rarely affect all nails at any given time.

- Schamroth's sign, seen with nail clubbing, refers to the obliteration of the normal, diamond-shaped window formed between the dorsal surfaces of opposed left and right nail bases.

- Hutchinson's sign refers to the periungal extension of longitudinal melanonychia, a potential indicator of malignant melanoma.

- Nail findings of psoriasis, such as pitting and trachyonychia, are rare in the absence of cutaneous findings.

- Nail changes associated with alopecia areata, such as pitting and trachyonychia, may appear months to years before the onset of hair loss.

DIAGNOSIS	ICD-9	DISTINGUISHING CHARACTERISTICS	DISTRIBUTION	ASSOCIATED FINDINGS	PREDISPOSING FACTORS
Onychomycosis	110.1	Most common type is distal, lateral subungal: yellow-white discoloration at distal edge near lateral nail fold, extending proximally Thickening of nail plate, may develop dark discoloration with time Less common before puberty	Toenails most frequently affected, usually affects great toenail first Fingernail infection usually associated with toenail infection	Distal subungal hyper-keratosis and onycholysis (separation of the nail plate from the nail bed) Tinea pedis and tinea cruris	Warm, moist conditions Commercial manicures and pedicures Prolonged wearing of occlusive footwear
Acrocyanosis	443.89	Cool, sometimes sweaty, dusky red or violaceous hands and/or feet No progressive color changes as with Raynaud's phenomenon Common in neonates/infants and adolescent girls	Symmetric, hands and feet May also involve nose, ears, lips, nipples	Rare edema	Unknown, although may be related to cold sensitivity in some
Nail Pitting	703.8	Punctate depressions, usually ≤1 mm	Varies from isolated pit involving one nail to uniform pitting of all nails	Randomly distributed, shallow pits are common features of psoriasis and eczema Transverse rows of regularly spaced pits are typically associated with alopecia areata	May also result from trauma
Longitudinal Melanonychia/ Pigmented Bands	709.09	Brown to black, longitudinal pigmentation	May be solitary or multiple (most commonly a result of normal ethnic pigmentation in darker-skinned persons)	Malignant melanoma (very rare) should be suspected whenever solitary streak suddenly becomes darker and/or wider, edges become blurred, and/or a family history of melanoma exists	May be caused by infection (fungal or bacterial) or melanin (nevi, normal ethnic pigmentation) Multiple pigmented bands may also be a feature of Addison disease or Cushing disease, Peutz-Jeghers syndrome, or pernicious anemia
Koilonychia/Nail Spooning	703.8	Flattened, concave nail shape Normal finding in neonates/infants, especially of the great toenails	Usually all 20 nails	Nails thin, soft	Feature of iron deficiency with/without anemia, hemochromatosis, hypothyroidism, lichen planus Can also be familial
Trachyonychia/ Nail Dystrophy	681.02 fingers 681.11 toes	Rough nails with sandpapered, opaque appearance, longitudinal ridging with adherent small scales, thinning, fragility, and distal notching Multiple small pits can make nails appear shiny Peak incidence in ages 3 to 12 years, M>F	May affect 1 to 20 nails	N/A	May be clinical manifestation of: • Alopecia areata (most commonly) • Eczema • Lichen planus • Psoriasis
Clubbing	781.5	Sponginess of proximal nail plate with thickening/swelling of distal digit; onset usually slow and painless Schamroth's sign—obliteration of diamond-shaped space between dorsal sides of opposed, corresponding R and L distal phalanges	Usually all 20 digits, but may be more obvious on thumbs, index finger, and middle fingers	Possible acral cyanosis, hypoxia, murmur	Sign of many systemic disorders In children, most commonly recognized in association with cyanotic congenital heart disease, cystic fibrosis, or inflammatory bowel disease

PHOTOGRAPHS OF SELECTED DIAGNOSES

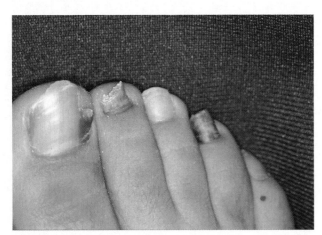

Figure 35-1 Onychomycosis. Note the yellow discoloration and thickening of the nail bed. (Courtesy of Denise W. Metry, MD.)

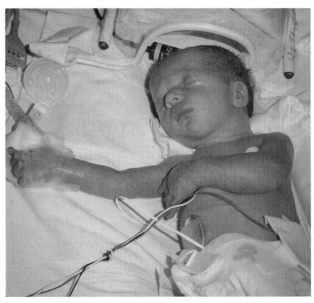

Figure 35-2 Acrocyanosis. A newborn with acrocyanosis of the forearms and hands. (Courtesy of Gerardo Cabrera-Meza, MD.)

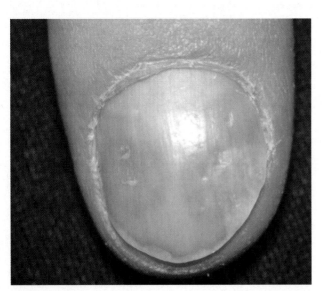

Figure 35-3 Longitudinal melanonychia. Note the longitudinal band of hyperpigmentation with no extension onto surrounding skin. (Courtesy of Moise L. Levy, MD.)

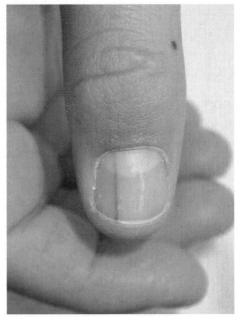

Figure 35-4 Psoriatic nail pitting. The punctate lesions arise from the nail matrix and appear as the nail plate grows. (Used with permission from Goodheart HP. *Goodheart's photoguide to common skin disorders.* 2nd ed. Philadelphia: Lippincott Williams & Wilkins; 2003:101.)

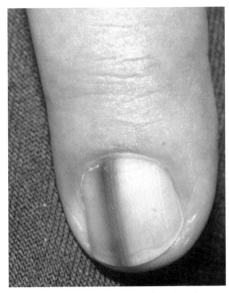

Figure 35-5 Junctional nevus. (Used with permission from Goodheart HP. *Goodheart's photoguide to common skin disorders.* 2nd ed. Philadelphia: Lippincott Williams & Wilkins; 2003:356.)

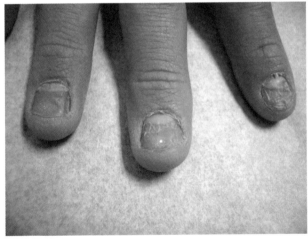

Figure 35-7 Nail dystrophy. A teenager with scaling of the nail suggestive of nail dystrophy. (Courtesy of Paul S. Matz, MD.)

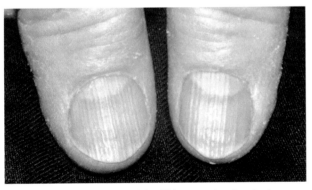

Figure 35-9 Longitudinal ridging. This normal variant is characterized by ridging in all of the nails. (Used with permission from Goodheart HP. *Goodheart's photoguide to common skin disorders.* 2nd ed. Philadelphia: Lippincott Williams & Wilkins; 2003:233.)

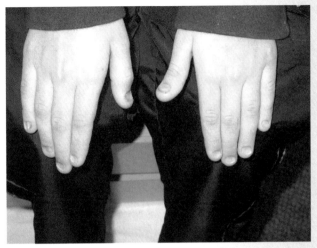

Figure 35-6 Koilonychia/nail spooning. Note the concave shape of the nail bed. (Courtesy of Moise L. Levy, MD.)

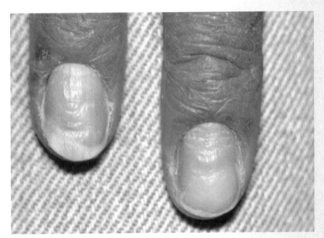

Figure 35-8 Nail dystrophy seen with atopic dermatitis. The eczema of the proximal skin affects the matrix resulting in nail dystrophy. (Used with permission from Goodheart HP. *Goodheart's photoguide to common skin disorders.* 2nd ed. Philadelphia: Lippincott Williams & Wilkins; 2003:237.)

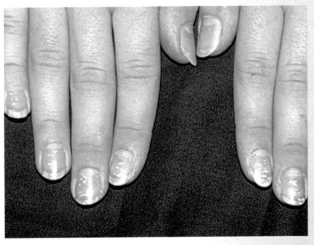

Figure 35-10 Leukonychia striata. (Used with permission from Goodheart HP. *Goodheart's photoguide to common skin disorders.* 2nd ed. Philadelphia: Lippincott Williams & Wilkins; 2003:240.)

- Lichen planus

- Yellow-nail syndrome

- Beau's lines

- Mees' lines

- Muehrcke's lines

- Habit tick deformity

SUGGESTED READINGS

Buka R, Friedman KA, Phelps RG, et al. Childhood longitudinal melanonychia: case reports and review of the literature. *Mt Sinai J Med.* 2001;68(4–5):331–335.

Fawcett RS, Linford S, Stulberg DL. Nail abnormalities: clues to systemic disease. *Am Fam Physician.* 2004;69(6):1417–1424.

Goodheart HP. *Goodheart's photoguide to common skin disorders.* 2nd ed. Philadelphia: Lippincott Williams & Wilkins; 2003:101, 233, 237, 240, 356.

Noronha PA. Nails and nail disorders in children and adults. *Am Fam Physician.* 1997;55(6):2129–2140.

Nousari HC, Kimyai-Asadi A, Anhalt GJ. Chronic idiopathic acrocyanosis. *J Am Acad Dermatol.* 2001;45(6 Suppl):S207–S208.

Scheinfeld NS. Trachyonychia: a case report and review of manifestations, associations, and treatments. *Cutis.* 2003;71(4):299–302.

Arm Displacement

APPROACH TO THE PROBLEM

Arm dislocations in children most commonly occur from trauma, but they also may be associated with an underlying abnormality. Congenital musculoskeletal abnormalities that cause joint laxity or conditions that affect nervous system development may be associated with dislocations of the upper extremity. The mechanism of injury must be kept in mind when dealing with traumatic dislocations.

KEY POINTS IN THE HISTORY

- A prior history of dislocation is important to consider because congenital and chronic dislocations are treated differently from acute dislocations.

- Congenital dislocations frequently are seen without a history of trauma and may be associated with an underlying connective tissue disorder.

- Traction injuries of the upper extremity frequently lead to acute radial head subluxation, also known as *nursemaid's elbow*.

- Traumatic shoulder dislocations, most of which are due to sports injuries, are typically the result of twisting forces of the arm that are transmitted to the shoulder. Shoulder dislocations are uncommon in young children, who will present more commonly with a proximal humeral fracture.

- Elbow dislocations occur most commonly in adolescent boys (75%) and in the left elbow (60%).

- Radial head subluxation, commonly occurring in children under 5 years of age, is seen more in girls (65%) and in the left arm (70%).

- Radial head dislocations are seen in children of all ages. These usually are caused by trauma and are often associated with fractures.

- Wrist dislocations are uncommon because of the protective cushioning effect of immature bone and usually are associated with carpal or distal radius fractures.

- Habitual dislocations occur in children who have ligamentous laxity and can voluntarily dislocate their joints (typically the shoulder).

- Brachial plexus injuries may lead to shoulder dislocations as early as 3 months of age.

- Sprengel deformity is a congenital elevation of the scapula, may have multidirectional joint instability, and frequently is associated with other abnormalities of the vertebrae and ribs.

KEY POINTS IN THE PHYSICAL EXAMINATION

- With an anterior dislocation of the shoulder, patients hold their arm abducted and externally rotated.

- With a posterior dislocation of the shoulder, the arm is held adducted and internally rotated.

- Assessment of distal nerve function and vascular supply need to be determined early in the physical examination.

- The axillary nerve can be affected in shoulder dislocations, while the ulnar nerve most commonly is involved with elbow injuries.

- Lateral proximal radial tenderness with swelling and severe limitation to range of motion of the elbow suggest a fracture.

- Radial head subluxation will typically present with an immobile arm held with slight elbow flexion. There is no point tenderness to palpation, and there is more pain on supination than pronation.

- Elbow dislocations occur when the radius and the ulna dislocate together as a unit.

- Anterior dislocations of the elbow and shoulder are seen more commonly in traumatic dislocations; whereas, posterior dislocations of the elbow and shoulder are seen more commonly in children with a history of congenital dislocations.

- Sprengel deformity may lead to loss of abduction of the shoulder.

DIFFERENTIAL DIAGNOSIS

DIAGNOSIS	ICD-9	DISTINGUISHING CHARACTERISTICS	DEMOGRAPHICS	PREDISPOSING FACTORS	SPECIAL CONSIDERATIONS
Radial Head Subluxation (also Nursemaid's Elbow)	832.00	Elbow held slightly flexed	Up to 5 years of age	Traction of extended arm	Rapid return of function when reduced by flexion and supination
Brachial Plexus Injury	953.4 (newborn) 767.6	Painless Displaced humeral head may be palpated posteriorly	Shoulder dislocation can occur by 3 months of age	Birth injury leads to imbalance of musculature, pulling the shoulder posteriorly	Diagnosis may require MRI as the humeral head may not be ossified
Shoulder Dislocation	(anterior) 831.0 (posterior) 831.02	Anterior dislocation—arm held abducted and externally rotated. Posterior dislocation—arm adducted and internally rotated	Rare in young children	Twisting of arm or direct trauma to humerus and shoulder Dislocations from neurologic disorders (such as brachial plexus injury) tend to be posterior	May be associated with axillary nerve injury
Elbow Dislocation	832.00	Both ulna and radius dislocate as a unit	Usually adolescent boys	Hyperextension of elbow	Ulnar nerve may be affected
Radial Head Dislocation	831.01	Pain (typically proximal ulna) Swelling Severe limitation of range of motion	N/A	Hyperextension of elbow, fall on outstretched arm, direct trauma to posterior forearm	Typically associated with ulnar fracture or ulnar nerve injury
Wrist Dislocation	833.00	None	Rare	Severe trauma to distal radius or carpals	Suspect ligamentous injury when pain persists
Sprengel Deformity	755.52	Elevation of scapula	N/A	None	Rib or vertebral anomalies

PHOTOGRAPHS OF SELECTED DIAGNOSES

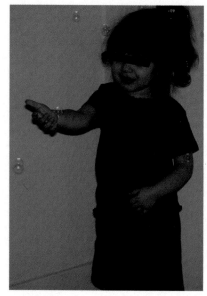

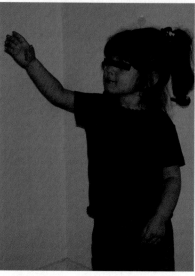

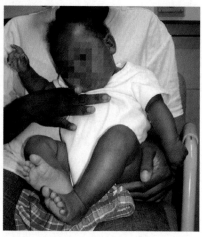

Figure 36-1 Nursemaid's elbow. Child holding left arm slightly flexed and pronated toward body. Note child reaching for bubbles freely with right arm, but not with affected arm. (Courtesy of Jeoffrey K. Wolens, MD.)

Figure 36-2 Nursemaid's elbow. Child holding left arm slightly flexed and pronated at side. Note child reaching for bubbles freely with right arm over head, but not with affected arm. (Courtesy of Jeoffrey K. Wolens, MD.)

Figure 36-3 Brachial plexus injury. An infant with left arm held in adduction with internal rotation of the arm and pronation of the forearm. (Courtesy of Joseph Piatt, MD.)

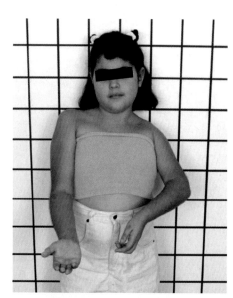

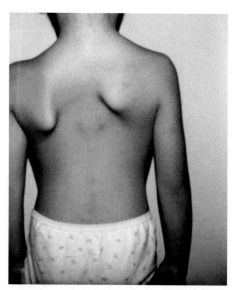

Figure 36-4 Brachial plexus injury. Patient attempting to extend and supinate arms. Compare to normal movement of right arm. (Courtesy of Shriners Hospitals for Children, Houston, Texas.)

Figure 36-5 Sprengel deformity. Note right-sided deformity with elevation of scapula and asymmetry of shoulders and neck when compared to normal left side. (Courtesy of Shriners Hospitals for Children, Houston, Texas.)

<table>
<tr><td>

OTHER
DIAGNOSES TO
CONSIDER

</td><td>

- Cerebral palsy

- Ehlers-Danlos syndrome

- Larsen syndrome

- Familial joint instability syndrome

- Marfan syndrome

- Radioulnar synostosis

</td></tr>
</table>

SUGGESTED READINGS

Cramer CE, Scherl SA, eds. *Pediatrics: orthopedic surgery essentials.* Philadelphia: Lippincott Williams & Wilkins; 2004:104–135.

Moukoko D, Ezaki M, Wilkes D, et al. Posterior shoulder dislocations in infants with neonatal brachial plexus palsy. *J Bone Joint Surg Am.* 2004;86-A(4):787–793.

Pizzutillo PD, ed. *Pediatric orthopedics in primary practice.* New York: McGraw-Hill; 1997:9–12, 29–32, 37–44, 51–54, 61–64, 325–328.

Schuck JE. Radial head subluxation: epidemiology and treatment of 87 episodes. *Ann Emerg Med.* 1990;19(9):1019–1023.

Staheli L. *Practice of pediatric orthopedics.* Philadelphia: Lippincott Williams & Wilkins; 2001:183–201, 216–219, 244–262.

Young K, Sarwark JF. Proximal humerus, scapula, and clavicle. In: Beaty JH, Kassar JR, eds. *Rockwood and Wilkins fractures in children.* 5th ed. Philadelphia: Lippincott Williams & Wilkins; 2001:741–806.

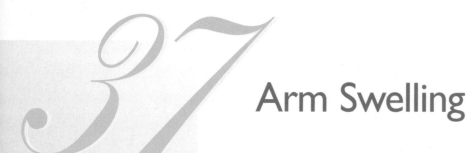

TERESIA O'CONNOR

Arm Swelling

APPROACH TO THE PROBLEM	Swelling of a child's arm may be an alarming situation for parents. Arm swelling is often the result of an injury to the arm and may represent a fracture, sprain, or hematoma. The most common fractures of childhood occur in the forearm, with those in the distal radius and ulna accounting for 55% of all pediatric fractures. Other causes of arm swelling include tumors and cysts, which can cause discrete masses in the forearm or wrist. Systemic illnesses, such as juvenile rheumatoid arthritis, may also cause joint swelling. Complications of injuries such as compartment syndrome, deep vein thrombosis, or vascular aneurysm may also result in arm swelling. To correctly identify the etiology of arm swelling, obtain a history of associated systemic symptoms, elicit a plausible mechanism for recent trauma, and have an accurate description of the location and appearance of the arm swelling.
KEY POINTS IN THE HISTORY	• Falling on an outstretched hand is the most common cause of a distal radial (Colles) fracture.
	• A fall with forward momentum, such as from a bicycle, is more likely to result in a displaced fracture of the distal radius.
	• A nonpainful mass that gradually appears at the wrist may represent a ganglion cyst, which usually resolves on its own within a year of onset, but may recur.
	• If the arm swelling is explained by a vague or inconsistent history, the practitioner should consider the possibility of physical abuse.
	• Pain out of proportion to the type of injury may indicate the presence of a compartment syndrome, a rare complication of a fracture.
	• Involvement of multiple joints, with or without systemic symptoms, such as fever and malaise, may indicate the onset of juvenile rheumatoid arthritis or systemic lupus erythematosus (SLE).
	• Deficiency of vitamin D or C should be suspected in a child with wrist swelling and a history of a poor or unbalanced diet.

KEY POINTS IN THE PHYSICAL EXAMINATION

- The most sensitive predictors of an upper extremity fracture in children are gross deformity and point tenderness.

- In the absence of a clear and consistent history for localized trauma to the arm, a thorough physical examination should be performed to rule out other areas of trauma that may be the result of accidental or nonaccidental trauma.

- A ganglion cyst is a discrete, fluid-filled, nonmobile, firm mass at the volar or dorsal area of the wrist, arising from synovial fluid of the wrist joint.

- A wrist mass that does not transilluminate or is solid should be further investigated and is unlikely to be a ganglion cyst.

- A bony mass may indicate a bone tumor.

- Muscle tenderness or pain on passive stretching of forearm muscles raises the suspicion for a compartment syndrome.

- A pulsating mass of the wrist may represent an aneurysm or other arteriovenous malformation.

DIFFERENTIAL DIAGNOSIS

DIAGNOSIS	ICD-9	DISTINGUISHING CHARACTERISTICS	DISTRIBUTION
Wrist Sprain	842.00	Generalized swelling, pain, and nonspecific tenderness Injury resulting from overstretching of a ligament	Region of wrist over the affected ligament
Colles Fracture	813.41 (closed) 813.51 (open)	Distal fracture of the radius confirmed by radiographs	Forearm
Ganglion Cyst	727.43	Firm, single or multiloculated mass of the wrist that is fixed Transilluminates	Volar wrist Dorsal wrist Retinacular area of wrist (arises from the flexor tendon sheath)
Hemangioma	228.00	Soft, boggy Bright red, papular (superficial); or blue, nodular (deep); or combination (mixed) Size varies	Varies Intradermal: superficial, mixed, or deep
Benign Bone Tumors (Osteo-chondroma, Enchondroma)	213.4 (upper extremity long bone) 213.5 (upper extremity short bone)	Hard mass, often painless and nontender Does not transilluminate Can be deforming (eg ulnar deviation with distal ulnar osteochondromas)	Varies—ulna, radius, metacarpals, digits

DURATION	COMPLICATIONS	ASSOCIATED FINDINGS
Acute event Heals with rest, ice, compression, and elevation (RICE) within 3 weeks	N/A	Ecchymosis
Acute event	Compartment syndrome Nerve damage Vascular damage	Distal ulnar fracture Injury to radial-ulnar joint Injury to annular ligament
Often regresses or ruptures by 12 months (if it has not spontaneously resolved, may consider surgical drainage or excision)	N/A	N/A
Appears with rapid growth at 2 to 4 weeks of age Usually slowly involutes starting at 2 years of age, but within first decade	Bleeding Ulceration and infection	N/A
Needs excision and curettage for removal	Malignant degeneration (rare) Pathologic fracture	Pathologic fracture Multiple enchondromas, also known as *Ollier disease*

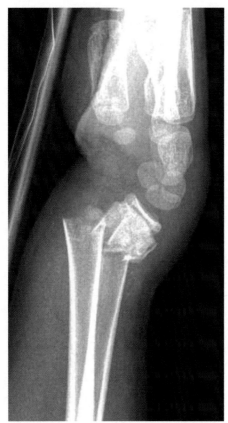

Figure 37-1 Distal radial fracture. Fracture of the left distal radius with obvious visual deformity and swelling. (Courtesy of William Phillips, MD.)

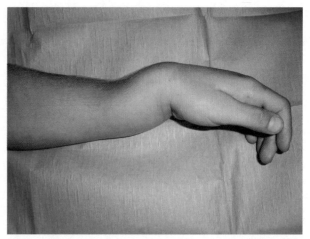

Figure 37-2 Colles fracture. (Courtesy of William Phillips, MD.)

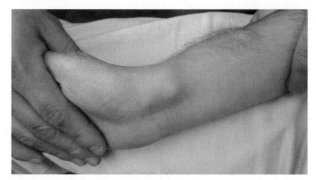

Figure 37-3 Ganglion cyst. Swelling over the volar surface of the right wrist in a school-aged child. (Courtesy of Mary L. Brandt, MD.)

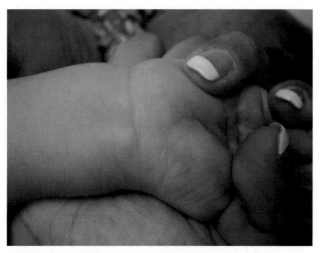

Figure 37-4 Ganglion cyst in infant. Swelling over the volar surface of the right lateral wrist in an infant. (Courtesy of Mary L. Brandt, MD.)

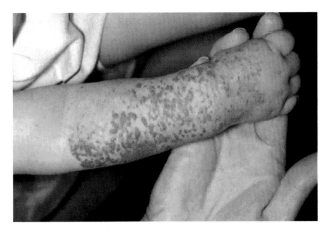

Figure 37-5 Large hemangioma of right forearm of an infant. Swelling with raised areas of vascular prominence are present. (Courtesy of Moise L. Levy, MD.)

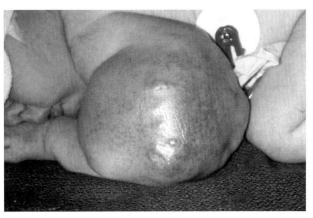

Figure 37-6 Cavernous hemangioma of the arm. (Courtesy of Jan E. Drutz, MD.)

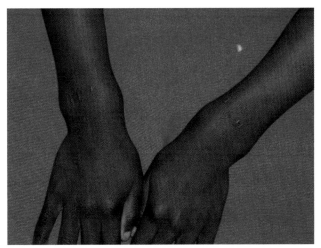

Figure 37-7 Rickets. This 4-year-old presents with wrist enlargement because of vitamin D deficiency rickets. (Courtesy of Tom Thacher, MD.)

OTHER
DIAGNOSES TO
CONSIDER

- Juvenile rheumatoid arthritis

- Septic arthritis

- Deep vein thrombosis

- Osteosarcoma

- Compartment syndrome

- Rickets

SUGGESTED READINGS
Eiff M, Hatch R. Boning up on common pediatric fractures. *Contemp Pediatr.* 2003;20:30–59.
Huurman W, Ginsburg G. Musculoskeletal injury in children. *Pediatr Rev.* 1997;18(12):429–440.
Rivera F, Parish RA, Mueller B. Extremity injuries in children: predictive value of clinical findings. *Pediatrics.* 1986;78(5):803–807.
Tumors of the upper limb. In: Herring J, ed. *Tachdjian's pediatric orthopaedics.* 3rd ed, vol. 1. Philadelphia: WB Saunders; 2002:487–503.
Wang A, Hutchinson D. Longitudinal observation of pediatric hand and wrist ganglia. *J Hand Surg.* 2001;26A(4):599–602.
Weston W, Lane A, Morelli J. Vascular lesions. In: *Color textbook of pediatric dermatology.* 3rd ed. St. Louis:Mosby; 2002:187–201.

38 Hand Swelling

SERENA YANG

APPROACH TO THE PROBLEM

The differential diagnoses of hand swelling may be divided into infectious and noninfectious etiologies. Infections from various organisms may manifest as arthritis, synovitis, osteomyelitis, and cellulitis. Hand swelling may result from viral, bacterial, or fungal infections. Noninfectious causes of hand swelling include reactive arthritis, arthritis as part of a systemic vasculitis, metabolic joint disease, sickle-cell disease, trauma, and malignancy.

KEY POINTS IN THE HISTORY

- Viral arthritis commonly presents in a polyarticular fashion, while bacterial arthritis frequently is monoarticular.

- When septic (or pyogenic) arthritis is suspected, the bacteria responsible for the infection vary by age of the child. *Staphylococcus aureus* is the most common causative agent in children younger than 2 months and older than 5 years. Disseminated gonococcal infection and subsequent arthritis may occur in newborns and adolescent females (particularly during menstruation or pregnancy); more rarely in males.

- Osteomyelitis is most often caused by hematogenous spread. Nonhematogenous osteomyelitis occurs through direct inoculation, such as from a puncture wound, or from a contiguous focus of infection.

- A history of chronic arthritis is seen with infection resulting from mycobacteria or fungi.

- A history of migratory or recurrent arthritis is seen in juvenile rheumatoid arthritis (JRA).

- A Boxer's fracture, or a fracture at the neck of the fifth metacarpal, is usually the result of a closed fist striking against a hard, immobile object.

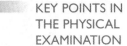

KEY POINTS IN THE PHYSICAL EXAMINATION

- Septic arthritis in older children is often monoarticular, but in infancy, it commonly presents in multiple joints.

- Viral arthritis often involves the interphalangeal-metacarpal joints with other commonly affected joints being the knee, wrist, ankle, and elbow.

- Blistering distal dactylitis characteristically appears on the distal volar fat pad of a finger as a medium-to-large, tender blister with an erythematous base.

- Dactylitis, a sausage-shaped swelling of the fingers resulting from synovitis of inter-phalangeal joints and tenosynovium, may be the presenting sign of sickle-cell disease. Dactylitis may also be seen with juvenile rheumatoid arthritis (JRA) or certain infections.

- Among the three types of JRA, systemic-onset and polyarticular are more likely to have wrist and hand joint involvement than pauciarticular JRA.

- Induration of the hands, accompanied by palmar erythema, is one of the six principal diagnostic criteria for Kawasaki syndrome.

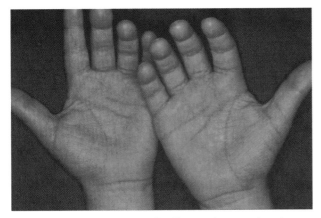

Figure 38-1 Kawasaki disease. Swelling, erythema, and tenderness develop in the hands of this 4-year-old a few days after onset of high fever. (Courtesy of Mark A. Ward, MD.)

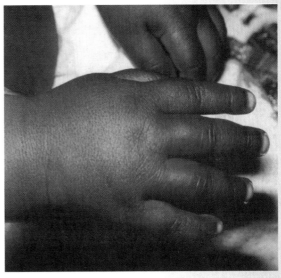

Figure 38-2 Dactylitis. This infant with sickle-cell disease presents with painful, nonerythematous, nonpitting, symmetric swelling of his hands. (Courtesy of Tom Thacher, MD.)

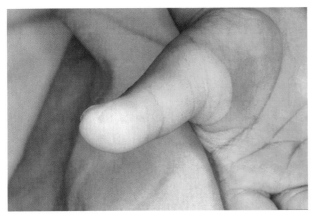

Figure 38-3 Blistering distal dactylitis. A 5-year-old presents with a superficial, tender blister on an erythematous base overlying the distal volar fat pad of his right thumb. (Courtesy of Mark A. Ward, MD.)

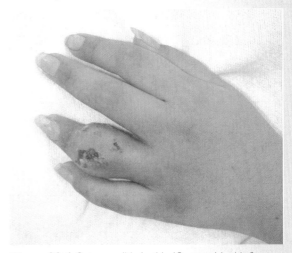

Figure 38-4 Osteomyelitis. In this 12-year-old with finger osteomyelitis, the infection has also affected the soft tissue surrounding the joint. (Courtesy of Mary L. Brandt, MD.)

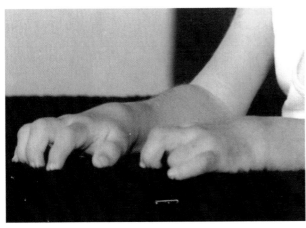

Figure 38-5 Juvenile rheumatoid arthritis. This 5-year-old with polyarticular JRA has swelling in his wrists and fingers bilaterally. Also, note the flexion contractures at his proximal and distal interphalangeal joints. (Courtesy of Shriners Hospitals for Children, Houston, Texas.)

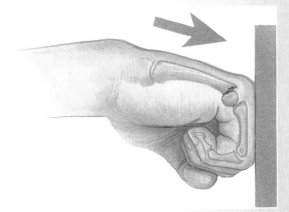

Figure 38-6 Boxer's fracture. A teenager presents with depression of his right fourth and fifth knuckles and proximal edema and discoloration after striking a hard immobile object with a closed fist. (Used with permission from the Anatomical Chart Company. ACC Systems and Structures Chart Images, p. 2.)

DIFFERENTIAL DIAGNOSIS

DIAGNOSIS	ICD-9	DISTINGUISHING CHARACTERISTICS
Kawasaki Disease	446.1	Diagnostic criteria: • Extremity swelling and tenderness • Fever for at least 5 days • Conjunctival injection • Changes in oropharyngeal mucosae • Rash • Cervical lymphadenopathy
Dactylitis (Hand-Foot Syndrome)	282.61	The first manifestation of sickle-cell disease that occurs during infancy Painful, warm, nonerythematous, nonpitting, symmetric swelling
Blistering Distal Dactylitis	681.00	Superficial tender blisters on an erythematous base Usually caused by beta-hemolytic streptococci or S. *aureus*
Septic Arthritis	711.00	***Staphylococcus aureus***—most common cause of septic arthritis in children aged less than 2 months and greater than 5 years Fever and pain with movement ***Neisseria gonorrhoeae***—disseminated gonococcal infection (DGI) occurs in 1% to 3% of all gonococcal infections and most commonly presents as acute polyarthralgias with fever, not genitourinary symptoms DGI presents as: tenosynovitis-dermatitis syndrome or suppurative arthritis syndrome
Viral Arthritis	711.54	**Rubella**—retroauricular, posterior cervical and occipital adenopathy **Hepatitis B**—joint involvement can precede jaundice by days to weeks
Osteomyelitis	730.24	Mainly caused by S. *aureus* and *Streptococcus* via hematogenous route In young infants, infection spreads rapidly through cortex and periosteum, into adjacent joint cavity and muscle, resulting in edematous fingers In older children, the infection is very focal, rarely affecting surrounding soft tissue because of the thick bony cortex
Juvenile Rheumatoid Arthritis	714.30	Transient arthritis that lasts for 3 months or more Associated with stiffness and flexion contractures Disuse of hand from arthritis leads to forearm muscle wasting
Boxer's Fracture	815.04	Fracture of neck of the fifth or fourth metacarpal associated with striking hard immobile object with closed fist Depression of knuckle(s) with proximal edema and discoloration

DISTRIBUTION	ASSOCIATED FINDINGS	PREDISPOSING FACTORS
Initially in hands and feet, but transient symmetric arthritis can occur in large and small joints	Acute phase (day 1–11): carditis, meningitis, sterile pyuria Subacute phase (day 11–21): coronary artery aneurysm, gall bladder hydrops, desquamation	All racial groups may be affected, but patients of Japanese descent appear to be particularly at risk
Metacarpals, metatarsals, and proximal phalanges of hands and/or feet	Splenic infarcts leading to "autosplenectomy" and increased susceptibility to pneumococci, *H. influenzae*, and Salmonella infections Acute splenic sequestration Acute chest syndrome	African Americans (incidence 1:600)
Usually affects the distal volar fat pad of a finger	Not associated with poststreptococcal glomerulonephritis	N/A
Usually lower extremities, rarely wrist and small joints	N/A	Bacterial upper respiratory infection Trauma or puncture wound
Tenosynovitis-dermatitis syndrome: polyarthralgias (wrists, hands, and fingers) Suppurative arthritis syndrome: monoarticular (knee, shoulder, wrist, ankle)	Dermatitis Acute endocarditis Meningitis Osteomyelitis	Neonates Adolescent females (particularly during menstruation or the second to third trimester of pregnancy)
Interphalangeal-metacarpal joints	Low-grade fevers, rash, conjunctival injection	Postpubertal females with inadequate rubella vaccination history
Interphalangeal-metacarpal joints	Urticaria Angioedema	Perinatal exposure Contaminated IV drugs or blood products Sexual contact
Most commonly found in tubular bones (femur, tibia, humerus, phalanges)	Deep venous thrombophlebitis Periosteal abscess Inadequate treatment of acute osteomyelitis can result in chronic osteomyelitis and draining sinuses	Sickle-cell disease Immunocompromised patients Puncture wounds Trauma Surgery
Pauciarticular JRA: knee, ankle, elbow, wrist Polyarticular and systemic-onset JRA: wrist, fingers	Pauciarticular JRA: iridocyclitis Polyarticular JRA: pericarditis, iridocyclitis Systemic-onset JRA: fevers, rash, hepatosplenomegaly, uveitis, pericarditis	Pauciarticular and polyarticular JRA occur more commonly in girls than boys
Lateral aspect of hand	Other injuries	Aggressive behavior

OTHER DIAGNOSES TO CONSIDER

- Systemic lupus erythematosus (SLE)

- Serum sickness

- Henoch-Schönlein purpura

- Farber disease (lysosomal storage of ceramide)

- Soft-tissue tumors

- Leukemia

SUGGESTED READINGS

Abramson H, Bertles JF, Wethers DL, eds. *Sickle-cell disease diagnosis, management, education, and research.* St. Louis: Mosby; 1973:245.

Feigin RD, Cherry JD, eds. *Textbook of pediatric infectious disease.* 4th ed. Philadelphia: WB Saunders; 1998:321.

Laxer RM, Clarke HM. Rheumatic disorders of the hand and wrist in childhood and adolescence. *Hand Clin.* 2000;16(4):659–671.

Nelson WE, Behrman RE, Kliegman RM, Arvin AM, eds. *Nelson textbook of pediatrics.* 15th ed. Philadelphia: WB Saunders; 1996:728–731.

Simmons BP, Nutting JT, Bernstein RA. Juvenile rheumatoid arthritis. *Hand Clin.* 1996;12(3):573–589.

39

Finger Abnormalities

ROBERT L. ZARR

APPROACH TO THE PROBLEM

Congenital finger abnormalities may present as failure of formation (brachydactyly), failure of differentiation (syndactyly), duplication (polydactyly), overgrowth (macrodactyly), or undergrowth (hypoplasia). Syndactyly and polydactyly are the most common hand deformities seen in children. It is important to distinguish between isolated abnormalities and those that occur as part of a syndrome. Deficiencies that may occur include: radial (thumb), ulnar (fifth finger), central (second, third, and fourth fingers), and transverse deficiencies. Ulnar deficiencies generally are not associated with syndromes or associations; however, radial deficiencies warrant further evaluation. Central deficiencies can be typical (bilateral, familial inheritance) or atypical (unilateral, spontaneous). Transverse deficiencies are usually unilateral, spontaneous, and rarely occur with other abnormalities.

KEY POINTS IN THE HISTORY

- Familial syndactyly can be transmitted through autosomal dominant inheritance.

- Syndactyly occurs commonly in Poland syndrome (synbrachydactyly) and Apert syndrome (acrocephalosyndactyly).

- Preaxial (radial) polydactyly, more commonly seen in Caucasians, is often unilateral, sporadic, and isolated.

- Postaxial (ulnar) polydactyly as an isolated finding is seen more commonly in African Americans. When seen in Caucasians, postaxial polydactyly often occurs as part of a syndrome as with Ellis-van Creveld syndrome.

- Central polydactyly (second, third, and fourth digits) is often bilateral and inherited by autosomal dominant transmission.

- Camptodactyly, a painless flexion contracture, may present during infancy as an isolated finding limited to the small finger; during preadolescence as an isolated finding that may progress to a severe flexion deformity of the proximal interphalangeal joint; or as part of a syndrome.

- Maternal ingestion of thalidomide is associated with brachydactyly.

- Maternal use of certain vasoactive substances, such as cocaine, is associated with isolated limb abnormalities.

- The family history can be useful in identifying autosomal dominant inheritance.

KEY POINTS IN THE PHYSICAL EXAMINATION

- Syndactyly is characterized by webbing between the fingers, most commonly the third and fourth fingers.

- Syndactyly may be complete (entire length of adjacent fingers), incomplete (syndactyly ends proximal to the fingertip), simple (only skin and fibrous tissue involvement), or complex (includes bone).

- Camptodactyly most often occurs in the proximal interphalangeal joint of the fifth finger.

- Brachydactyly is absent or short digits.

- Clinodactyly is characterized by a deviation of a finger toward the radial or ulnar bones (a deviation of fewer than 10 degrees may be considered normal).

DIFFERENTIAL DIAGNOSIS

DIAGNOSIS	ICD-9	DISTINGUISHING CHARACTERISTICS	DISTRIBUTION	ASSOCIATED FINDINGS	COMPLICATIONS
Polydactyly/ Supernumerary Digit	755.1	Duplication of fingers	Preaxial-radial side (thumb); Central—second, third, fourth digits; Postaxial—ulnar side (fifth digit)	Familial polydactyly (inherited trait) Ellis-van Creveld syndrome (chondroectodermal dysplasia) Carpenter syndrome Trisomy 13 Rubinstein Taybi syndrome Smith-Lemli-Opitz syndrome Laurence-Moon-Biedl syndrome Greig Cephalopolysyndactyly Syndrome	None
Brachydactyly	755.5	Shortened or absent digit	May affect any digit	Turner syndrome Pseudohypoparathyroidism Thrombocytopenia absent radius syndrome (TAR) VATER syndrome Poland syndrome	Decreased functionality
Syndactyly	755.2	Webbing between the fingers	Most commonly occurs between the third and fourth fingers	Apert syndrome Carpenter syndrome Poland syndrome	Decreased function Inability to fully extend fingers
Clinodactyly	755.59	Deviation of finger	Usually involves fifth digit	Trisomy 28, 21 Brachydactyly Klinefelter syndrome Holt-Oram syndrome Turner syndrome Cornelia de Lange syndrome	None
Macrodactyly	755.65	Overgrowth of all structures of the finger	May affect one or more fingers but more commonly radial fingers	Neurofibromatosis Klippel-Trenaunay-Weber syndrome	Decreased function secondary to progressive stiffness

PHOTOGRAPHS OF SELECTED DIAGNOSES

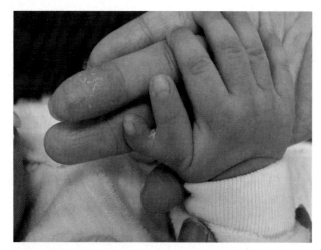

Figure 39-1 Polydactyly. An infant with a preaxial thumb duplication. (Courtesy of Esther K. Chung, MD.)

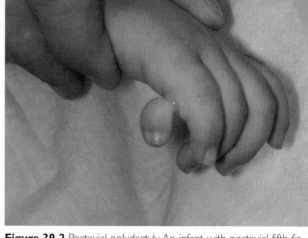

Figure 39-2 Postaxial polydactyly. An infant with postaxial fifth finger duplication on the right hand. (Courtesy of Paul S. Matz, MD.)

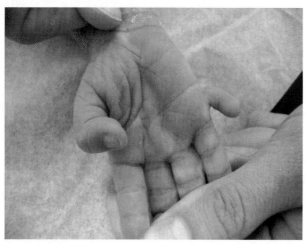

Figure 39-3 Postaxial polydactyly. A newborn with postaxial fifth finger duplication of the right hand. (Courtesy of Paul S. Matz, MD.)

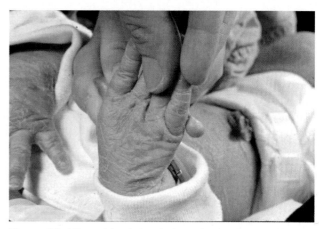

Figure 39-4 Postaxial polydactyly. A newborn with right fifth finger duplication. Note the partially formed digit is conceded by a thin band of tissue. (Courtesy of Kenneth Rosenbaum, MD.)

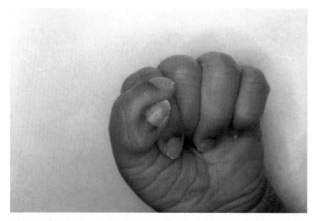

Figure 39-5 Preaxial polydactyly. A newborn with left preaxial duplication of the thumb. (Courtesy of Gerardo Cabrera-Meza, MD.)

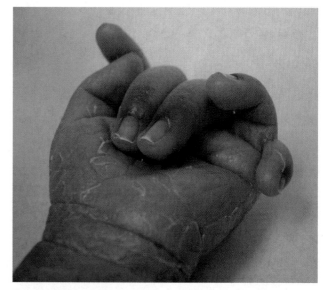

Figure 39-6 Polydactyly. A postaxial duplication of the left fifth finger in an African American infant. (Courtesy of Mary L. Brandt, MD.)

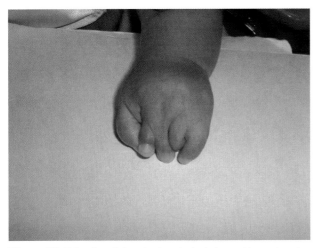

Figure 39-7 Syndactyly/brachydactyly. An infant with syndactyly and brachydactyly of the second, third, fourth and fifth left fingers in a child with Poland syndrome. (Courtesy of Robert L. Zarr, MD.)

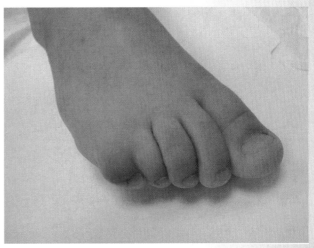

Figure 39-8 Syndactyly. A child with syndactyly of the right fourth and fifth toe. (Courtesy of Robert L. Zarr, MD.)

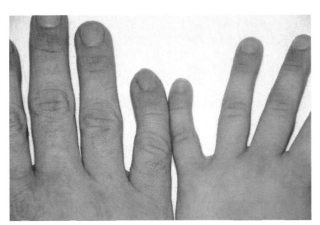

Figure 39-9 Clinodactyly. Inherited clinodactyly in a father (left) and son (right). (Courtesy of Julie A. Boom, MD.)

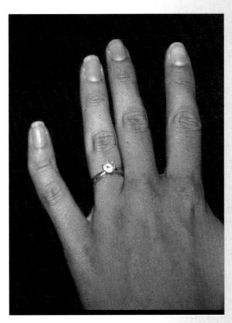

Figure 39-10 Clinodactyly. (Courtesy of George A. Datto, III, MD.)

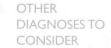   OTHER   • Constriction band syndrome
         DIAGNOSES TO
         CONSIDER   • Congenital trigger thumb

SUGGESTED READINGS

Canale ST, ed. *Campbell's operative orthopaedics.* 10th ed. St. Louis: Mosby; 2003:3860–3861.

Graham TJ, Ress AM. Finger polydactyly. *Hand Clin.* 1998;14(1):49–63.

Kozin SH. Upper-extremity congenital anomalies. *J Bone Joint Surg Am.* 2003;85-A(8):1564–1576.

Townsend CM, ed. *Sabiston textbook of surgery.* 16th ed. Philadelphia: WB Saunders; 2001:2224–2225.

Van Heest AE. Congenital disorders of the hand and upper extremity. *Pediatr Clin North Am.* 1996;43(5):1113–1129.

Wolpert L. Vertebrate limb development and malformations. *Pediatr Res.* 1999;46(3):247–253.

40 Fingertip Swelling

APPROACH TO THE PROBLEM

Most cases of fingertip swelling in young patients result from trauma or infection. Trauma to the hand, specifically the fingertip, is the most frequent injury among children under 5 years of age. These injuries may cause damage to the soft tissue, nail bed, and distal phalanx. Trauma to the fingertip provides a portal of entry for pathogens, which may result in infection of any component of the nail complex or distal pulp of the fingertip.

KEY POINTS IN THE HISTORY

- Crush injuries (from a door slamming, for example) are the most common cause of fingertip trauma.

- Common penetrating injuries that may lead to an abscess of the distal finger pulp, a felon, include splinters, shards of glass, abrasions, and minor puncture wounds.

- Children at high risk for fingertip swelling from an infectious etiology tend to bite their nails or suck their thumbs.

- The herpetic whitlow occurs as a complication of primary oral or genital herpes lesions.

KEY POINTS IN
THE PHYSICAL
EXAMINATION

- Angulation of the fingertip can be detected by comparing the planes of the fingernails of both hands with the fingers flexed.

- The swelling associated with a felon will not extend proximal to the distal interphalangeal joint.

- Fluctuance and pain are rare in cases of chronic paronychia but are common in acute paronychia.

- With herpetic whitlow, the pain may be out of proportion to the physical exam findings.

DIFFERENTIAL DIAGNOSIS

DIAGNOSIS	ICD-9	DISTINGUISHING CHARACTERISTICS	DURATION	ASSOCIATED FINDINGS	PREDISPOSING FACTORS
Acute Paronychia	681.02	Swelling, erythema, and pain along nail fold	Onset within 2 to 5 days after cuticle trauma; resolution often requires antibiotics	Abscess along nail fold	Bacterial invasion from trauma to the cuticle
Chronic Paronychia	112.3	Swelling and boggy-appearing along nail fold; tenderness is mild or absent	Longer than 6 weeks duration; resolution often requiring antifungal agent	Fingernail dystrophy	Chronic dermatitis or frequent exposure to water leading to candidal infection
Felon	681.01	Throbbing pain with redness and swelling of the distal pulp of the finger	Onset within 2 to 5 days after trauma; resolution requires antibiotics and/or incision and drainage	May be associated with osteomyelitis or a foreign body	Bacterial invasion from penetrating trauma to fingertip
Herpetic Whitlow	054.6	Grouped, painful vesicles on an erythematous base	Abrupt onset with resolution in 2 to 3 weeks without medications	Fever, malaise, and regional lymphadenopathy. Herpetic lip or mouth lesions	Primary infection with herpes simplex virus type 1
Fracture	816.0	Swelling, tenderness, and often angulation	Abrupt onset	May be associated with nail avulsion or nail bed laceration	Acute trauma to the fingertip, usually from a crush injury
Subungal Hematoma	923.3	Brown, black, or purplish discoloration under the nail bed	Abrupt onset Resolution often requires evacuation of blood collection	May be associated with a fracture of the distal phalanx	Acute trauma to nail bed, usually from a crush injury

PHOTOGRAPHS OF SELECTED DIAGNOSES

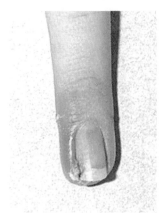

Figure 40-1 Acute paronychia. Visible swelling, erythema, and discharge along the nail fold, yet the nail itself is intact. (Courtesy of Mary L. Brandt, MD.)

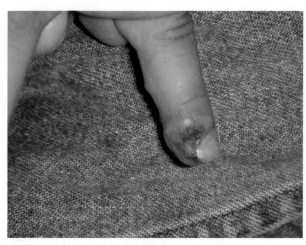

Figure 40-2 Acute paronychia. Swelling, erythema, and discharge along the lateral nail edge. (Courtesy of Larry H. Hollier Jr, MD.)

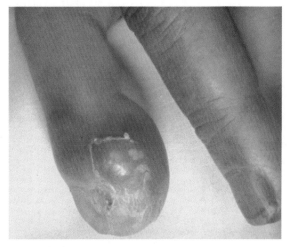

Figure 40-3 Felon. (Used with permission from Greenberg MI. *Greenberg's atlas of emergency medicine.* Philadelphia: Lippincott Williams & Wilkins; 2005:458.)

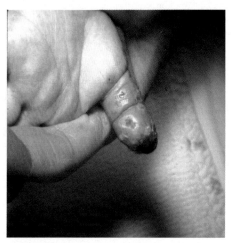

Figure 40-4 Herpetic whitlow. Ulcers where previously there were vesicles along the ventral thumb. (Courtesy of Mark A. Ward, MD.)

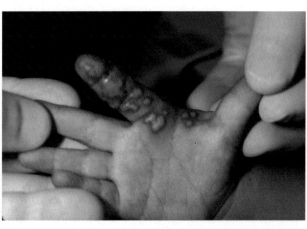

Figure 40-5 Herpetic whitlow. Grouped vesicles on an erythematous base along the ventral surface of the finger. (Courtesy of Mark A. Ward, MD.)

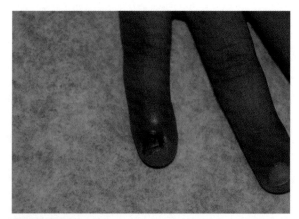

Figure 40-6 Subungual hematoma. A 2-year-old with a subungual hematoma that resulted from a fall with a plate in his hand. (Courtesy of Julie A. Boom, MD.)

- Sprain of the distal interphalangeal joint

- Osler nodes (embolic infectious lesions in the finger pulp)

- Subungual melanoma

SUGGESTED READINGS

Clark DC. Common acute hand infections. *Am Fam Physician.* 2003;68:2167–2176.

Doraiswamy, NV, Baig H. Isolated finger injuries in children—incidence and etiology. *Injury.* 2000;31:571–573.

Greenberg MI. *Greenberg's atlas of emergency medicine.* Philadelphia: Lippincott Williams & Wilkins; 2005:458.

Hart RG, Kleinert HE. Fingertip and nail bed injuries. *Emerg Med Clin North Am.* 1993;11:755–765.

Ljungberg E, Rosberg HE, Dahlin LB. Hand injuries in young children. *J Hand Surg.* 2003;28B:376–380.

Rockwell PG. Acute and chronic paronychia. *Am Fam Physician.* 2001;63:1113–1116.

Shmerling RH. Finger pain. *Prim Care.* 1988;15:751–766.

Zitelli BJ, Davis HW. *Atlas of pediatric physical diagnosis.* 4th ed. Philadelphia: Mosby; 2002:312–313, 405.

SERENA YANG

Newborn Physical Findings: Lower Extremity Abnormalities

APPROACH TO THE PROBLEM

To understand torsional and angular deformities of the newborn lower extremity, one must first recognize the typical positioning of the lower extremities in utero, where the feet are in contact with the posterolateral portion of the contralateral thigh. In addition, the feet are in slight equinus and are supinated; the knees are flexed with the lower legs internally rotated; and the hips are flexed, abducted, and externally rotated.

Abnormal positional deformities result when the fetus is unable to kick, which is crucial to the normal development of the lower extremities. Deformities may result from intrinsic factors such as central nervous system defects and muscle degeneration or extrinsic factors related to fetal crowding that occurs with breech presentation or oligohydramnios.

KEY POINTS IN THE HISTORY

- Infants who were breech in utero are at increased risk of hip dislocation and valgus abnormalities of the foot.

- The frequency of caudal regression (which includes sacral agenesis) in infants of mothers with insulin-dependent diabetes mellitus has been estimated to be 200 times that of infants in the general population.

- When a skeletal dysplasia is suspected in a newborn, it is essential to obtain a family history that assesses for skeletal dysplasias, consanguinity, and short stature.

- Heterozygous achondroplasia is the most common form of chondrodysplasia and follows an autosomal dominant inheritance pattern.

KEY POINTS IN THE PHYSICAL EXAMINATION

- The newborn lower extremity may appear bowed because of the combination of an externally rotated hip and an internally rotated tibia.

- The calcaneovalgus deformity, typically self-correcting in the first 2 to 3 months of life, is characterized by hyperdorsiflexion, hindfoot valgus, and forefoot abduction.

- Congenital vertical talus (also known as "rockerbottom foot" or congenital convex pes valgus) presents with a convex plantar surface, forefoot abduction, and dorsiflexion. Most of these infants may have additional findings, such as multiple joint contractures consistent with arthrogryposis multiplex or an underlying neurologic disorder such as a meningomyelocele.

- The examination findings of sacral agenesis vary depending on the severity of the agenesis (unilateral versus bilateral, partial versus complete, extent of spinal cord involvement). The most severely affected infants may have lack of growth in the caudal region, hip flexion and abduction, and popliteal webs because of lack of movement.

DIFFERENTIAL DIAGNOSIS

DIAGNOSIS	ICD-9	DISTINGUISHING CHARACTERISTICS	DURATION/ CHRONICITY	ASSOCIATED FINDINGS	PREDISPOSING FACTORS
Physiologic Bowing of Legs	754.43	Legs appear bowed because of a combination of externally rotated hips and internally rotated tibia	Resolves after 6 to 12 months of independent walking	N/A	Secondary to in utero positioning
Pes Calcaneovalgus	754.69	Hyperdorsiflexion, forefoot abduction, and hindfoot valgus	Resolves during first 6 months of life	External tibial torsion	Secondary to in utero positioning
Congenital Vertical Talus (Rockerbottom Foot)	754.79	Convex plantar surface, forefoot abduction, and dorsiflexion	Most require surgical correction	Arthrogryposis multiplex Meningomyelocele Trisomy 18	N/A
Lower Limb Abnormalities Associated with Breech Presentation	763.0	Developmental dysplasia of the hip Valgus foot deformities	Varies with diagnosis	Breech deformation sequence also includes torticollis, facial asymmetry, and bathrocephaly (a step-like posterior projection of the skull)	N/A
Sacral Agenesis	756.13	Partial, symmetric sacral agenesis (the most common type of agenesis); bilateral hip subluxation and foot deformities because of loss of lower sacral innervation Complete sacral agenesis (absent sacrum); flattened buttocks, shortened gluteal cleft, narrowed pelvis	N/A	Bowel and/or urinary incontinence and lower extremity neurologic deficits Renal anomalies Imperforate anus Cleft lip and palate Microcephaly Meningomyelocele	Infants of mothers with insulin-dependent diabetes mellitus
Achondroplasia (Heterozygous)	756.4	Tibial bowing Rhizomelia (the proximal limb segment is shorter than the distal segment) Brachydactyly (short fingers)	Increased mortality in first 5 years of life (particularly in first year) because of sudden death from cervicomedullary compression	Frontal bossing and head circumference greater than 97th percentile Hypotonia Normal intelligence	Autosomal dominant inheritance 80% of cases arise de novo, likely to be exclusively inherited from the father and associated with advanced paternal age

PHOTOGRAPHS OF SELECTED DIAGNOSES

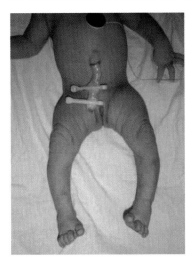

Figure 41-1 Physiologic bowing of legs. Legs of a newborn appear bowed because of externally rotated hips and internally rotated tibia. (Courtesy of Gerardo Cabrera-Meza, MD.)

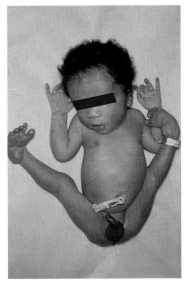

Figure 41-4 Hip flexion contracture. A newborn presents with bilateral hip flexion contracture after breech presentation. (Courtesy of Gerardo Cabrera-Meza, MD.)

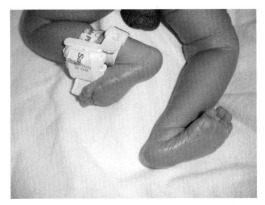

Figure 41-2 Calcaneovalgus foot. Right foot is in hyperdorsiflexion, with the forefoot abducted. (Courtesy of Gerardo Cabrera-Meza, MD.)

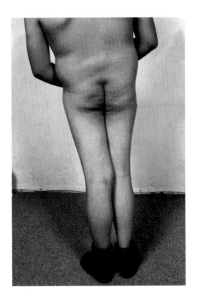

Figure 41-5 Sacral agenesis. This 8 year old with complete sacral agenesis (absent sacrum) has flattened buttocks, a shortened gluteal cleft, and a narrowed pelvis. (Courtesy of Shriners Hospitals for Children, Houston, Texas.)

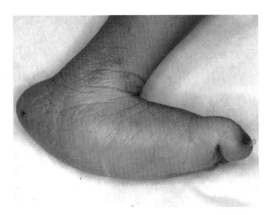

Figure 41-3 Congenital vertical talus (rockerbottom foot). Forefoot is abducted and dorsiflexed and has a convex plantar surface. (Courtesy of Gerardo Cabrera-Meza, MD.)

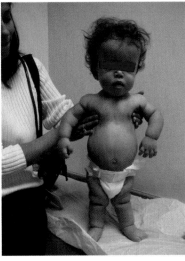

Figure 41-6 Achondroplasia. This infant with achondroplasia has tibial bowing, frontal bossing, rhizomelia (the proximal limb segment is shorter than the distal segment), and brachydactyly (short fingers). (Courtesy of Paul S. Matz, MD.)

OTHER
DIAGNOSES TO
CONSIDER

- Steinert myotonic dystrophy

- Werdnig-Hoffman disease

- Congenital posteromedial tibial angulation

- Congenital anterolateral tibial angulation

SUGGESTED READINGS

Jones KL. *Smith's recognizable patterns of human malformation.* 5th ed. Philadelphia: WB Saunders; 1997:635.

Dugoff L, Thieme G, Hobbins JC. Skeletal anomalies. *Clin Perinatol.* 2000;27(4):979–1005.

Hunter AG, Bankier A, Rogers JG, et al. Medical complications of achondroplasia: a multicentre patient review. *J Med Genet.* 1998;35(9):705–712.

Raffel LJ, Scheuner MT, Rimoin DL, et al. Diabetes mellitus. In: Rimon DL, Connor JM, Pyeritz RE, eds. *Emery and Rimoin's principles and practice of medical genetics.* 3rd ed. New York: Churchill Livingstone; 1996:1401–1440.

Sharrard WJW. *Pediatric orthopaedics and fractures.* 3rd ed. Cambridge, MA: Blackwell Science; 1993:556–718.

Thompson GH, Scoles PV. Torsional and angular deformities. In: Nelson WE, Behrman RE, Kliegman RM, Arvin AM, eds. *Nelson textbook of pediatrics.* 15th ed. Philadelphia: WB Saunders; 1996:1925–1933.

Leg Asymmetry

JEOFFREY K. WOLENS

APPROACH TO THE PROBLEM	Asymmetry between the lower extremities has a wide range of etiologies. Discrepancies in length can be caused by structural bone abnormalities or by alterations in rates of bone growth. Variations in the overall size of the lower extremities can be caused by neurologic disorders, vascular or lymphatic abnormalities, or processes that restrict growth. Understanding the etiology of the discrepancy is important because some conditions need to be followed closely for associated conditions.
KEY POINTS IN THE HISTORY	• A birth history of oligohydramnios, constriction bands, or peripheral localized perinatal infections suggests an isolated problem, while prematurity, birth trauma, or a central perinatal infection may be associated with a neurologic etiology.
	• Congenital leg length discrepancy can be the result of aplasia, hypoplasia, or hyperplasia or conditions that change normal anatomic relationships, such as clubfoot or hip dysplasia.
	• Physeal injury can lead to shortening of a limb, while fractures in other locations can cause overgrowth of the bone.
	• Neurologic causes of leg length discrepancy tend to cause an overall small-sized limb because of disuse and joint contractures.
	• Vascular ischemia can lead to shortening of a limb, while arteriovenous fistulas may lead to overgrowth.
	• Infections and tumors may lead to either shortening or overgrowth of bones.
	• Family history is important to consider for hemihypertrophy, development dysplasia of the hip (DDH), clubfoot, and bone dysplasias.

KEY POINTS IN THE PHYSICAL EXAMINATION

- Leg length discrepancies are considered significant when the difference is more than 1 cm.

- A positive Galeazzi sign indicates developmental dysplasia of the hip.

- Children compensate for leg length differences by flexing the hip and knee on the long side or walking on the toes of the short side.

- Hemihypertrophy associated with café-au-lait (CAL) spots suggests neurofibromatosis type I, while hemihypertrophy associated with macroglossia and an omphalocele is seen in Beckwith-Wiedemann syndrome.

- Hemihypertrophy with large cutaneous hemangiomas suggests Klippel-Trenaunay-Weber syndrome, while Proteus syndrome is associated with deeper cutaneous growths (lipomatosis).

- When examining a patient with lower leg asymmetry, inspection of the back is essential to rule out a midline back lesion, such as a skin tag or a mass that may be associated with spinal dysraphism and a tethered cord.

- The presence of an abdominal mass in a patient with hemihypertrophy should raise suspicion for a tumor, especially a Wilms or hepatic tumor.

- Localized edema, caused by surgery, burns, infection, allergic reactions, trauma, or lymphatic obstruction can cause asymmetry between the legs.

- Restriction of growth can be caused by burns or scarring of the dermis.

DIFFERENTIAL DIAGNOSIS

DIAGNOSIS	ICD-9	DISTINGUISHING CHARACTERISTICS	ASSOCIATED FINDINGS	COMPLICATIONS	PREDISPOSING FACTORS
Developmental Dysplasia of the Hip (DDH)	754.30	Leg(s) adducted and externally rotated Limited abduction of the hip, if the hip dislocated Involved side appears shorter	Positive Galeazzi sign Asymmetric thigh and buttocks folds when unilateral	Recurrent dislocation Avascular necrosis of femoral head Early degenerative joint disease with pain and stiffness in hip Shortening of affected limb	Positive family history History of breech birth Newborns with restriction of motion in the hips and legs as can be seen with oligohydramnios More common in girls than boys
Hemihypertrophy	759.89	Rarely apparent at birth	Skin and hair are thicker on the affected side Ipsilateral organs may also be affected Contralateral macroglossia common Wilms tumor, hepatoblastoma, adrenal carcinoma	Compensatory scoliosis may develop	May be isolated or part of a syndrome (see Other Diagnoses to Consider)
Lymphedema of Lower Extremity	457.1 acquired 757.0 congenital	Edema may be pitting or nonpitting	May be associated with vascular abnormalities	Verrucous hypertrophy of skin Recurrent infections	Unilateral causes of lymphedema typically acquired by congenital abnormalities, surgery, trauma or postinflammatory scarring (burns, infections, radiation)
Hemiatrophy of Leg	728.2	Neurologic exam may show flaccid paralysis Scarring of the skin may be present	Hip and back pain	Hip and back pain	Polio was a common etiology in the prevaccine era Tethered cord
Leg Length Discrepancy	736.81 acquired 755.30 congenital	Asymmetry of posterior superior iliac crest Difference ≥1 cm between legs as measured from iliac crest to lateral malleolus Lift placed under shorter leg alleviates discrepancies	Previous physeal injury Flexion contractures of the long side Toe walking on short side	Limp with or without pain	Previous physeal injury
Legg-Calves-Perthes Disease	732.1	Avascular necrosis caused by impairment of blood supply to the femoral head Antalgic limp with mild to no pain initially Examination finds pain on internal rotation and abduction of the hip Typical age 4 to 11y Unable to maintain pelvis level when standing on involved side	May have flexion contracture of affected hip and limb May be associated with hypercoagulable states	Hip dislocation Early degenerative joint disease	More common in boys
Slipped Capital Femoral Epiphysis	732.2	Painful limp after jumping No history of significant trauma Limb held externally rotated	May have flexion contracture of affected hip and limb may appear shorter than other side Endocrinopathies may be found in patients with bilateral involvement	Avascular necrosis of femoral head Early degenerative joint disease	Occurs around puberty typically in obese males

PHOTOGRAPHS OF SELECTED DIAGNOSES

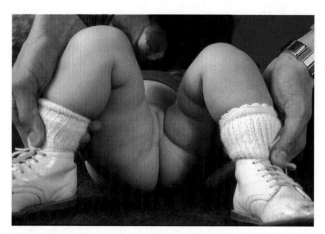

Figure 42-1 Positive Galaezzi sign. Note asymmetry in femoral heights. (Courtesy of Douglas A. Barnes, MD.)

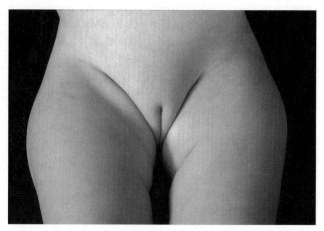

Figure 42-2 Asymmetric thigh folds in young infant. Note asymmetry between overall configuration in number and location of thigh folds. (Courtesy of Douglas A. Barnes, MD.)

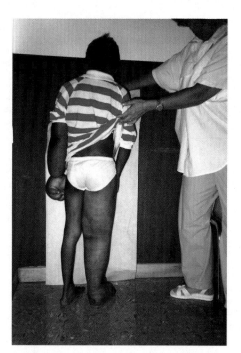

Figure 42-3 Hemihypertrophy of right lower extremity in a child with Proteus syndrome. Also note contralateral hemihypertrophy of left upper extremity. (Courtesy of Shriners Hospitals for Children, Houston, Texas.)

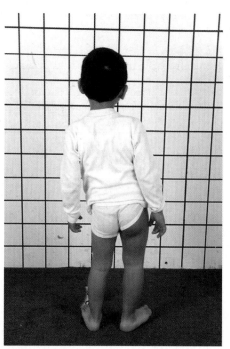

Figure 42-4 Isolated hemihyertrophy of the right lower extremity. (Courtesy of Shriners Hospitals for Children, Houston, Texas.)

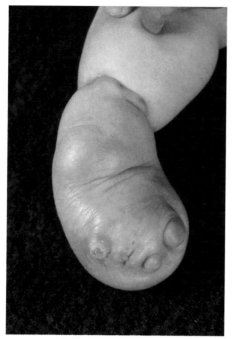

Figure 42-5 Lymphedema of foot caused by constriction band syndrome. (Courtesy of Douglas A. Barnes, MD.)

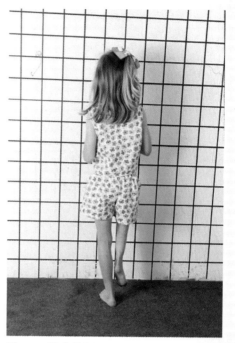

Figure 42-6 Child with hemiatrophy of the right leg. Note the overall decrease in length and bulk of leg compared to normal side. (Courtesy of Shriners Hospitals for Children, Houston, Texas.)

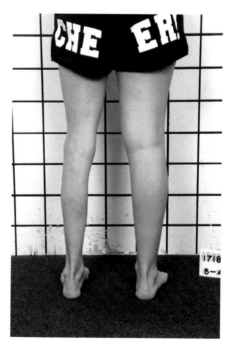

Figure 42-7 Hemiatrophy of left leg because of linear scleroderma. Note normal appearing size, muscle mass, and overall bulk of normal right leg. (Courtesy of Shriners Hospitals for Children, Houston, Texas.)

OTHER DIAGNOSES TO CONSIDER

- Congenital absence or shortening of the tibia, fibula, or femur

- Burns or dermal scarring

- Local swelling because of envenomation or allergic reaction

- Bone tumors and cysts

- Silver Russel syndrome

- Klippel-Trenaunay-Weber syndrome

- Ollier disease

- Radiation therapy

SUGGESTED READINGS

Ballock RT, Weisner GL, Myers MT, Thompson GH: Hemihypertrophy—concepts and controversies. *J Bone Joint Surg Am.* 1997;79(11):1731–1738.

Finch GD, Dawe CJ. Hemiatrophy. *J Pediatr Orthop.* 2003;23:99–101.

Guidera K. Leg length inequality. In: Cramer CE, Scherl SA, eds. *Pediatrics: orthopedic surgery essentials.* Philadelphia: Lippincott Williams & Wilkins; 2004:74–80.

Percy AK. Static encephalopathy. In: McMillan JA, DeAngelis CD, Feigin RD, Warshaw JB, eds. *Oski's pediatrics principles and practice.* 3rd ed. Philadelphia: Lippincott Williams & Wilkins; 1999:1923–1925.

Shapiro BK, Capute AJ. Cerebral palsy. In: McMillan JA, DeAngelis CD, Feigin RD, Warshaw JB, eds. *Oski's pediatrics principles and practice.* 3rd ed. Philadelphia: Lippincott Williams & Wilkins; 1999:1910–1917.

Staheli L. *Practice of pediatric orthopedics.* Philadelphia: Lippincott Williams & Wilkins; 2001:24,68,76–79,146–151,297.

43

SUJATA R. TIPNIS

Leg Bowing and Knock Knees

APPROACH TO THE PROBLEM

Leg bowing (genu varum) and knock knees (genu valgum) are angular deformities. Typically, a physiologic progression from genu varum to valgum occurs between infancy and early childhood. It is important to distinguish physiologic from pathologic deformities. Features that may suggest pathology include pain, asymmetry, progressive deformity, signs of nutritional deficiencies, or constitutional symptoms such as fever, weight loss, or rash. When evaluating a child with an angular deformity, it is important to obtain a thorough history and a careful physical exam. This will assist the practitioner in deciding whether the child has a physiologic deformity for which reassurance may be provided or whether further evaluation for pathologic conditions is necessary.

KEY POINTS IN THE HISTORY

- The incidence of genu varum peaks between ages 2 and 3 and gradually decreases.

- Genu valgum appears by age 3 and resolves by age 7.

- Children who have Blount disease are often early walkers.

- Children who have rickets, renal disease, or dysplasias such as achondroplasia and enchondromatosis, are often late walkers.

- Infantile physiologic bowing is present at birth, but it may not be brought to medical attention until later.

- Blount disease and untreated vitamin D deficiency are angular deformities that do not improve with age.

- Poor diet may suggest vitamin D deficiency as a cause of angular deformities.

- Children living in climates in which there is a paucity of sun exposure are at risk for developing vitamin D deficiency.

- Asymmetric angular deformities and pain are suggestive of pathologic causes of angulation that include infection, malignancy, and trauma.

- Blount disease is more likely to present with pain than asymmetry.

- Blount disease is often associated with obesity, black race, and male gender.

- Children with metabolic disorders (such as vitamin D deficiency, vitamin D resistance, hypophosphatemia, and renal osteodystrophy), as well as genetic disorders associated with angular deformities (such as achondroplasia, enchondromatosis, and cerebral palsy) tend to be small for their age.

- Children with Blount disease are often large for their age.

KEY POINTS IN THE PHYSICAL EXAMINATION

- An asymmetric and/or painful deformity may indicate pathology such as infection, malignancy, or trauma.

- Genu varum can be followed by measuring the distance between the knees with the ankles held together.

- Genu valgum can be followed by measuring the distance between the ankles with the knees held together.

- Minimal internal tibial torsion, mild medial collateral ligament laxity, and mild lower extremity length discrepancy can be seen in Blount disease.

- Genu varum associated with signs of malnutrition may indicate nutritional rickets.

- Craniotabes resulting from thinning of the outer skull and detected by a "ping pong ball sensation" elicited by pressing over the occiput or parietal bone, outside the newborn period, is a sign of rickets.

- Boney prominences felt by palpation of the costochondral junctions (rachitic rosary) and wrist and ankle widening suggest rickets.

- Associated findings of trauma, such as abrasions or ecchymoses, may suggest unintentional or intentional trauma as the cause of genu varum.

PHOTOGRAPHS OF SELECTED DIAGNOSES

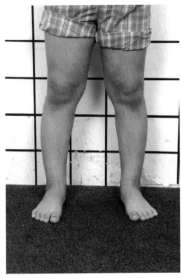

Figure 43-1 Genu varum. Outward angulation of the knees in a child. (Courtesy of Shriners Hospitals for Children, Houston, Texas.)

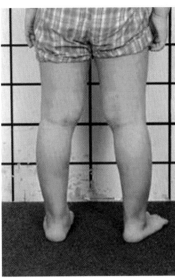

Figure 43-2 Genu varum. Posterior view of a child with genu varum. (Courtesy of Shriners Hospitals for Children, Houston, Texas.)

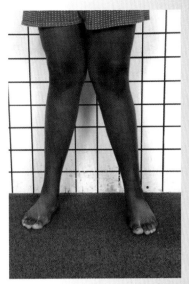

Figure 43-3 Genu valgum. Inward angulation of the knees seen in this child. (Courtesy of Shriners Hospitals for Children, Houston, Texas.)

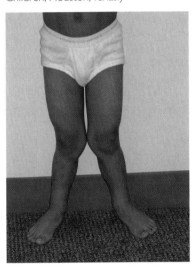

Figure 43-4 Genu valgum. A toddler with notable inward angulation of the knees. (Courtesy of Bettina Gyr, MD.)

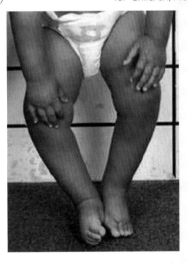

Figure 43-5 Infantile tibial bowing. Outward angulation of the tibia bilaterally in an infant. (Courtesy of Shriners Hospitals for Children, Houston, Texas.)

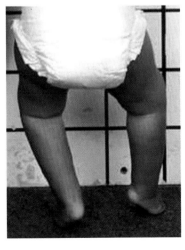

Figure 43-6 Infantile tibial bowing. Outward angulation of the tibia is also notable in the posterior view of the infant with tibial bowing. (Courtesy of Shriners Hospitals for Children, Houston, Texas.)

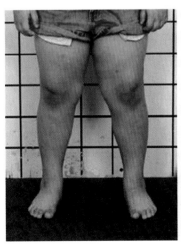

Figure 43-7 Blount disease. Genu varum deformity is seen in this obese male with Blount disease. (Courtesy of Shriners Hospitals for Children, Houston, Texas.)

DIFFERENTIAL DIAGNOSIS

DIAGNOSIS	ICD-9	DISTINGUISHING CHARACTERISTICS	DURATION/ CHRONICITY	ASSOCIATED FINDINGS
Genu Varus	755.64	Bow legs Medial malleoli touch leaving separation at knees	Peaks at 2 to 3 years, then decreases	N/A
Genu Valgus	755.64	Knock knees Knees touch leaving separation at ankles	Develops by 3 years, resolves by 7 years	N/A
Blount Disease (Tibia Vara)	732.4	Pain prior to onset of visual deformity Minimal internal tibial torsion Mild medial collateral ligament laxity Mild lower extremity length discrepancy	Infantile and adolescent forms Present until surgical correction by osteotomy to realign the tibia	Early walker Obesity
Infantile Physiologic Tibial Bowing	732.4	Usually bilateral Metaphyseal break Internal tibial torsion Leg length discrepancy	Infancy to age 2 or 3	N/A
Vitamin D Deficiency (Rickets)	268	Genu varus or genu valgus	Symptomatic until treated	Enlarged epiphyses (especially wrists and ankles) Craniotabes Enlargement of costochondral junctions (rachitic rosary)

COMPLICATIONS	PREDISPOSING FACTORS
If persistent, can cause cosmetic concerns and pain or damage to medial part of knee joint	Secondary to normal in utero positioning
Cosmetic concerns, if persists	N/A
Can lead to persistent pain, limp, and/or degenerative arthritis	N/A
Blount disease	Positional deformity
Short stature Failure to thrive Pathologic fractures Developmental delay	Vitamin D deficiency

OTHER DIAGNOSES TO CONSIDER

- Asymmetric growth related to fracture, osteosarcoma, or osteomyelitis

- Congenital patellar dislocation

- Achondroplasia or other chondrodysplasias

- Renal osteodystrophy

- Cerebal palsy

SUGGESTED READINGS

Dietz FR. Intoeing—fact, fiction, and opinion. *Am Fam Physician.* 1994;50:1249–1259.

McCrea JD. *Pediatric orthopedics of the lower extremity: an instructional handbook.* Mount Kisco, NY: Futura Publishing; 1985:345–348.

Nelson WE, ed. *Nelson textbook of pediatrics.* Philadelphia: WB Saunders; 1996:1929–1933.

Sass P, Hassan G. Lower extremity abnormalities in children. *Am Fam Physician.* 2003;68:461–468.

Scherl SA. Common lower extremity problems in children. *Pediatr Rev.* 2004;5:52–61.

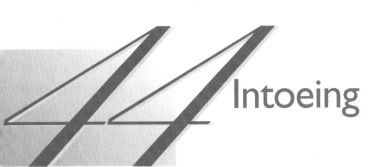

Intoeing

SUJATA R. TIPNIS

APPROACH TO THE PROBLEM

Intoeing is a common lower extremity complaint seen in pediatrics. The causes of intoeing vary by age and can be distinguished by careful examination of the feet, lower extremities, and gait. The three main areas from which intoeing originates are the foot, the area between the ankle and knee, and the area between the knee and hip. Most causes of intoeing are believed to be "packaging defects," related to the infant's intrauterine position. Most intoeing corrects spontaneously and does not require surgical intervention.

KEY POINTS IN THE HISTORY

- Tibial torsion and femoral torsion are usually first noticed when the child begins ambulating.

- Metatarsus adductus, tibial torsion, and femoral torsion—entities that typically improve with time as the child begins to ambulate—are not associated with developmental delay.

- Metatarsus adductus and clubfoot (metatarsus adductus, equinus, hindfoot varus) are present at birth.

- Clubfoot may be associated with neuromuscular diseases, such as cerebral palsy and spina bifida.

KEY POINTS IN THE PHYSICAL EXAMINATION

- A heel bisector that touches or is lateral to the third toe suggests metatarsus adductus.

- A gait in which the patellae point forward while the feet point inward suggests tibial torsion.

- A negative foot progression angle is seen in metatarsus adductus, tibial torsion, and femoral torsion.

- A negative thigh-foot angle indicates tibial torsion.

- A gait in which the patellae and feet point inward suggests femoral torsion.

- Children with femoral torsion comfortably sit in the "W" position.

- Increased internal hip rotation and decreased external hip rotation suggest femoral torsion.

- Hypertonia or hypotonia may suggest a neuromuscular cause of the intoeing.

- Metatarsus adductus corrects when the infant's foot is tickled; clubfoot does not.

PHOTOGRAPHS OF SELECTED DIAGNOSES

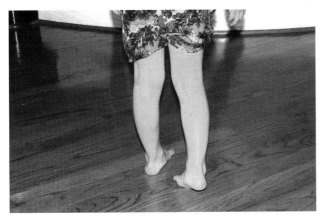

Figure 44-1 Foot progression angle. A 4-year-old with a negative foot progression angle. (Courtesy of Julie A. Boom, MD.)

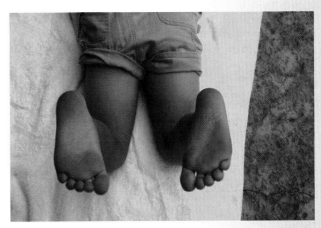

Figure 44-2 Tibial torsion. A 4-year-old with a negative thigh foot angle. (Courtesy of Julie A. Boom, MD.)

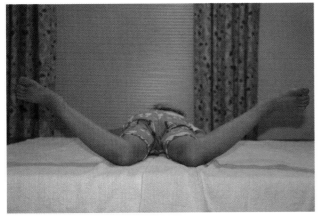

Figure 44-3 Femoral torsion. A 5-year-old girl with increased medial rotation of the hips because of femoral torsion. (Courtesy of Julie A. Boom, MD.)

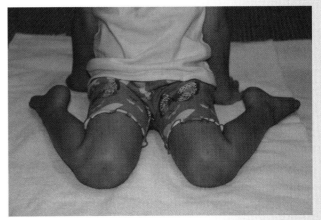

Figure 44-4 Femoral torsion. A 5-year-old girl comfortably "W" sitting. (Courtesy of Julie A. Boom, MD.)

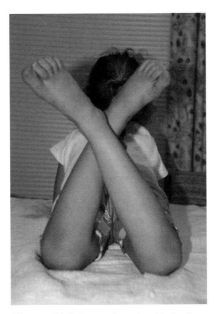

Figure 44-5 Femoral torsion. Limited lateral hip rotation in a 5-year-old girl with femoral torsion. (Courtesy of Julie A. Boom, MD.)

DIFFERENTIAL DIAGNOSIS

DIAGNOSIS	ICD-9	DISTINGUISHING CHARACTERISTICS	DURATION/ CHRONICITY	ASSOCIATED FINDINGS
Tibial Torsion	736.89	Foot-progression angle less than 10 degrees Thigh-foot angle greater than 20 to 30 degrees	Present at birth Usually resolves by 3 years of age	None
Femoral Torsion	755.63	Decreased hip abduction to approximately 15 degrees Increased hip adduction of approximately 80 degrees "W" position sitting	Resolves by age 8 to 10	None
Metatarsus Adductus	754.53	Medial border of the foot is concave ("C" shape) Transverse crease between midfoot and forefoot Heel bisector touching or lateral to third toe	Usually resolves by age 1	Approximately 10% of children have associated developmental dysplasia of the hip
Clubfoot	754.7	Metatarsus adductus with plantar flexion and foot inversion	Requires bracing, casting or surgical correction	Spina bifida Sacral agenesis Spinal muscular atrophy Arthrogryposis

COMPLICATIONS	PREDISPOSING FACTORS
None	Related to positioning in utero Part of normal physiologic development
Cosmetic deformity or gait abnormality when unresolved by age 10	Controversial as to congenital or acquired secondary to sitting habits
Very little functional limitation If persists, may have cosmetic concerns or difficulty fitting shoes	Related to positioning in utero
Cosmetic deformity or gait abnormality if left untreated	Multifactorial inheritance with major influence from a single autosomal dominant gene Inherited 20% to 30% for offspring of affected parents Inherited 3% for subsequent siblings

<table>
<tr><td>OTHER
DIAGNOSES TO
CONSIDER</td><td>• Pronation of feet

• Cerebral palsy or any neuromuscular disorder leading to spasticity

• Genu valgum (knock knees)</td></tr>
</table>

SUGGESTED READINGS

Benjamin DR, Hyman J, Royce DP. Congenital idiopathic talipes equinovarus. *Pediatr Rev.* 2004;25:124–129.

Dietz FR. Intoeing—fact, fiction, and opinion. *Am Fam Physician.* 1994;50:1249–1259.

McCrea, JD. *Pediatric orthopedics of the lower extremity: an instructional handbook.* Mount Kisco, NY: Futura Publishing; 1985:345–348.

Nelson WE, ed. *Nelson textbook of pediatrics.* Philadelphia: WB Saunders; 1996:1925–1929.

Sass P, Hassan G. Lower extremity abnormalities in children. *Am Fam Physician.* 2003;68:461–468.

Scherl SA. Common lower extremity problems in children. *Pediatr Rev.* 2004;5:52–61.

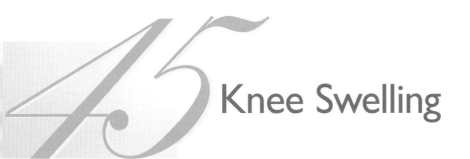

JULIE A. BOOM

Knee Swelling

APPROACH TO THE PROBLEM

Knee swelling in the pediatric patient suggests a broad differential diagnosis including musculoskeletal, rheumatic, and infectious processes. Knees are large joints commonly involved in juvenile rheumatoid arthritis. Because there are many soft tissue structures within it, the knee may be injured in almost every type of sport. The knee is involved in approximately 90% of cases of joint swelling associated with Lyme disease.

KEY POINTS IN THE HISTORY

- An acute onset of knee swelling suggests trauma, septic arthritis, rheumatic fever, or Lyme disease. Chronic knee swelling suggests juvenile rheumatoid arthritis (JRA) or malignancy.

- The mechanism of trauma may provide clues to the most likely structures injured; for example, a history of knee hyperextension may suggest an anterior cruciate ligament (ACL) injury.

- An audible pop may be concerning for a serious ligamentous injury or fracture.

- Knee instability or "giving way" may indicate a ruptured anterior cruciate ligament or patellar instability.

- Knee locking with limited extension may indicate a torn meniscus, avulsed cruciate ligament, or bony fragment.

- Extremely painful migratory polyarthritis involving the knees, elbows, wrists, and ankles and prior strep infection warrant consideration of rheumatic fever.

- Pain in septic arthritis is constant, and it generally worsens over time.

- Fever may be suggestive of an infectious or rheumatologic process; high intermittent fevers (≥39.5°C) that occur once or twice daily may indicate systemic-onset JRA.

- An evanescent rash (small, pale red macules with central clearing) that occurs during periods of temperature elevation is suggestive of systemic-onset JRA.

- Consider Lyme disease when knee arthritis with an erythema migrans rash follows a tick bite or exposure to a Lyme-endemic area.

KEY POINTS IN THE PHYSICAL EXAMINATION

- Site of bruising may provide a clue to the direction of force that may have caused the swelling.

- An effusion, indicated by asymmetry of the suprapatellar pouches, may indicate synovitis—the hallmark of late Lyme disease.

- Effusion immediately following trauma may suggest acute bleeding into the knee.

- Fluid palpated over the center of the patella suggests a prepatellar bursitis.

- Pain with palpation over the tibial tuberosities suggests Osgood-Schlatter disease.

- A mass palpated in the popliteal area suggests the presence of a popliteal cyst.

- Discovery of a new heart murmur, especially one consistent with mitral or aortic insufficiency, may suggest acute rheumatic fever.

- Excruciating knee pain with bright erythema or dramatic warmth is characteristic of acute rheumatic fever or septic arthritis.

- Knee swelling accompanied by urticarial wheals, erythematous maculopapules, or purpura involving primarily the lower extremities with gastrointestinal symptoms suggests Henoch-Schönlein purpura.

- The presence of a mass with severe pain, refusal to use limb, or abnormal hematologic findings may suggest malignancy.

PHOTOGRAPHS OF SELECTED DIAGNOSES

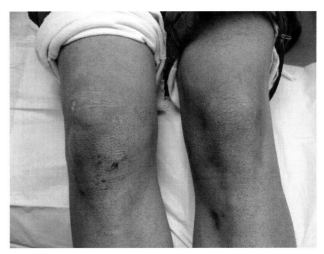

Figure 45-1 Knee effusion. Clinically obvious effusion of the right knees. (Used with permission from Fuchs MA. Hemarthrosis. In: Greenberg MI, ed. *Greenberg's atlas of emergency medicine.* Philadelphia: Lippincott Williams & Wilkins; 2005:525.)

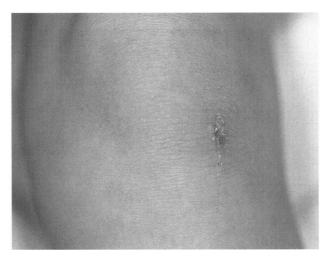

Figure 45-2 Knee cellulitis. Localized erythema suggestive of cellulitis overlying the knee. (Used with permission from Fleisher GR, Ludwig S, Baskin MN, eds. *Atlas of pediatric emergency medicine.* Philadelphia: Lippincott Williams & Wilkins; 2004:202.)

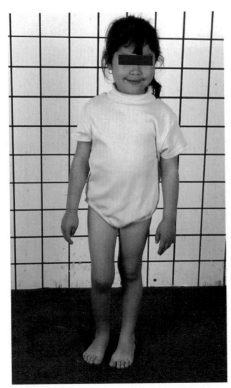

Figure 45-3 Juvenile rheumatoid arthritis. Unilateral swelling of the right knee in a young girl with juvenile rheumatoid arthritis. (Courtesy of Shriners Hospitals for Children, Houston, Texas.)

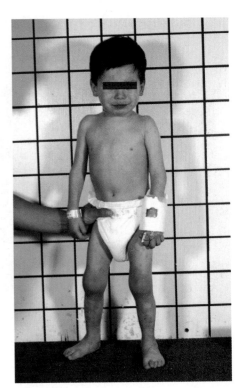

Figure 45-4 Juvenile rheumatoid arthritis. A toddler with bilateral knee swelling because of juvenile rheumatoid arthritis. (Courtesy of Shriners Hospitals for Children, Houston, Texas.)

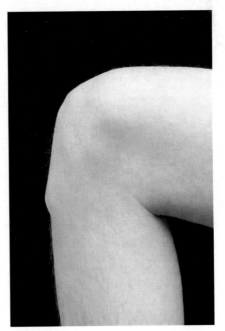

Figure 45-5 Osgood-Schlatter disease. Lateral view demonstrating prominence of the tibial tuberosity. (Courtesy of Julie A. Boom, MD.)

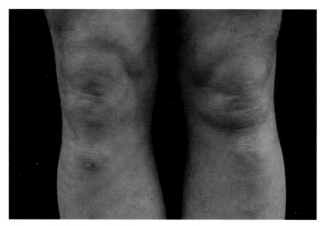

Figure 45-6 Osgood-Schlatter disease. Pain with palpation over the tibial tuberosity is suggestive of Osgood-Schlatter disease. (Courtesy of Julie A. Boom, MD.)

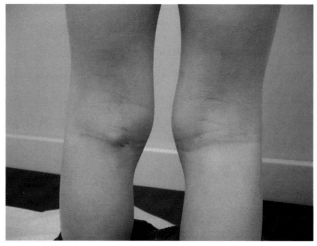

Figure 45-7 Baker's cyst. Discrete swelling in the left popliteal fossa without overlying erythema. (Courtesy of Mary L. Brandt, MD.)

DIFFERENTIAL DIAGNOSIS

DIAGNOSIS	ICD-9	DISTINGUISHING CHARACTERISTICS	DISTRIBUTION	ASSOCIATED FINDINGS
Trauma	959.7	Asymmetry with bruising and point tenderness Decreased ROM depending on location of trauma	Unilateral	Usually none
Septic Arthritis	711.06	Warmth, swelling, tenderness, or an effusion with decreased ROM in all directions Swelling after several days of decreased movement Limp or refusal to walk in a previously ambulatory child	Usually monoarticular	Irritability Poor oral intake Fever in children >12 to 18 months Crying with passive movement Voluntary splinting to prevent movement
Rheumatic Fever	390	Painful polyarthritis Arthritis presents early and lasts <4 weeks	Polyarticular (elbows, wrists, and ankles)	Carditis Erythema marginatum Subcutaneous nodules Sydenham chorea
Juvenile Rheumatoid Arthritis (JRA)	714.30	Joint swelling lasting ≥6 weeks May limp or may refuse to walk	Ankle, wrist and elbow swelling Polyarticular ≥5 joints Pauciarticular ≤4 joints	Fatigue High regularly spiking fevers Pleuritis Pericarditis Anemia Leukocytosis Rash Lymphadenopathy Uveitis
Lyme Disease	088.81	Migratory, painful arthritis of sudden onset	Monoarticular or oligoarticular Usually large joints, but all can be affected	Most commonly, expanding skin rash, erythema migrans Malaise Fatigue Neck stiffness Arthralgia Low grade fevers

COMPLICATIONS	PREDISPOSING FACTORS
Intra-articular fractures, injury to more than one ligament, or neurovascular compromise require(s) immediate orthopedic or vascular surgical consultation	Fall or blow to the knee Hyperextension or twisting injury
Permanent decreased range of motion because of tissue destruction, scarring or necrosis Impaired growth if epiphysis involved	Penetrating trauma causing direct inoculation Hematogenous spread from another location
Carditis Valvulitis (especially mitral) leading to vascular insufficiency Reoccurrence can occur unless secondary prophylaxis is instituted	History of recent streptococcal infection
Joint degeneration Contractures Leg length discrepancies Loss of vision because of chronic uveitis	HLA-B27 positivity ANA positivity
Cardiovascular abnormalities including AV block, pericarditis, cardiomegaly and left ventricular dysfunction Neurologic abnormalities including meningitis, cranial neuropathy and peripheral radiculopathy	Tick bite of the Ixodes genus, the deer tick that is infected with the spirochete Borrelia burgdorferi Lyme endemic areas in the United States include: the Northeast, Mid-Atlantic region, upper North-Central region, and northwestern California 92% of cases occur in the following states: CT, RI, NJ, NY, PA, DE, MD, MA, and WI

OTHER
DIAGNOSES TO
CONSIDER

- Osgood-Schlatter disease

- Osteochondritis dissecans

- Serum sickness

- Systemic lupus erythematosus (SLE)

- Osteomyelitis

- Viral arthritis because of parvovirus, rubella, mumps, varicella, adenovirus, hepatitis B

- Malignancy including leukemia, neuroblastoma, lymphoma, Hodgkin's disease, malignant histiocytosis, rhabdomyosarcoma, osteogenic sarcoma, and Ewing sarcoma

SUGGESTED READINGS

Barron SA. Index of suspicion. *Pediatr Rev.* 2000;21:67–71.

Baskin MN. Injury—knee. In Fleisher GR, Ludwig, S. eds. Textbook of pediatric emergency medicine. 3rd ed. Baltimore: Williams & Wilkins; 1993:276–285.

Fleisher GR, Ludwig S, Baskin MN, eds. *Atlas of pediatric emergency medicine.* Philadelphia: Lippincott Williams & Wilkins; 2004:202.

Greenberg MI, ed. *Greenberg's atlas of emergency medicine.* Philadelphia: Lippincott Williams & Wilkins; 2005:525.

Koutures CG, Landry GL. The acutely injured knee. *Pediatr Ann.* 1997;26:50–55.

Mirkinson L. The diagnosis of rheumatic fever. *Pediatr Rev.* 1998;19:310–311.

Schaller JG. Juvenile rheumatoid arthritis. *Pediatr Rev.* 1997;18:337–349.

Schwartz MW, Bell, LM, Bingham, P, et al, eds. The 5-minute pediatric consult. 3rd ed. Philadelphia: Lippincott Williams & Wilkins; 2003:134–135,716–717,748–479.

Shapiro ED. Lyme disease. *Pediatr Rev.* 1998;19:147–154.

Foot Deformities

SUJATA R. TIPNIS

APPROACH TO THE PROBLEM

Foot deformities are common concerns brought to the attention of health professionals caring for children. One of the first things to consider when obtaining a history is the child's age at presentation. Metatarsus adductus and clubfoot are deformities typically noticed at birth. While metatarsus adductus is a positional deformity that often resolves spontaneously, clubfoot is a fixed, inherited deformity that requires bracing, surgical treatment, or both. Pes planus (flatfeet) typically is noticed when a child begins walking. Initially, parents may describe the child as walking with his or her "ankles caving in." Children can have flexible or rigid flatfeet. Flexible flatfeet usually do not require treatment. Rigid flatfeet, however, may require immobilization or surgery whenever a tarsal coalition is present. Some foot deformities may occur in isolation, but others may occur as part of the constellation of findings in certain syndromes, such as Patau syndrome and Edward syndrome.

KEY POINTS IN THE HISTORY

- Foot deformities that present at birth include metatarsus adductus and clubfoot.

- Metatarsus adductus typically improves over time.

- Rigid pes planus may be associated with pain.

- Metatarsus adductus, clubfoot, and flexible pes planus usually are not associated with pain.

- Pes planus are occasionally inherited deformities.

- Clubfoot, metatarsus adductus, and pes planus are not associated with constitutional symptoms, such as fever and weight loss.

- Constitutional symptoms may be associated with other etiologies of foot deformities, such as osteomyelitis, malignancies, and joint infections.

- Metatarsus adductus and pes planus do not delay ambulation in children.

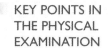

KEY POINTS IN THE PHYSICAL EXAMINATION

- A crease over the medial midfoot suggests metatarsus adductus.

- The forefoot easily corrects to midline with gentle pressure in metatarsus adductus.

- Movement of the subtalar joint is normal in metatarsus adductus.

- The combination of metatarsus adductus, equinus positioning (plantar flexion), and hindfoot varus (inversion) suggests clubfoot.

- A smaller calf may be associated with clubfoot on the affected side.

- Callus and hyperpigmentation may be present on the dorsolateral clubfoot.

- Flatfeet that develop an arch when the child stands on his or her toes are consistent with flexible pes planus; however, if there is no arch when the child stands on his or her toes, rigid pes planus should be considered.

- Flexible flatfeet will have an arch in the non–weight-bearing position that disappears with standing.

- A tight heel cord may lead to compensatory flatfoot.

- Stiffness during inversion and eversion of the subtalar joint suggests tarsal coalition.

PHOTOGRAPHS OF SELECTED DIAGNOSES

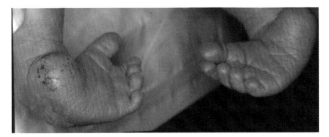

Figure 46-1 Clubfeet. Bilateral clubfeet in an infant with notable metatarsus adductus. (Courtesy of Gerardo Cabrera-Meza, MD.)

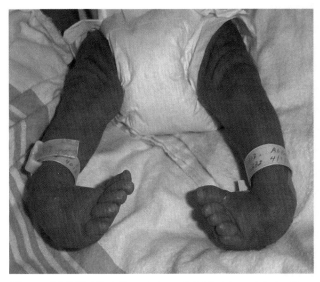

Figure 46-2 Clubfeet. Dorsal view of clubfeet in an infant with plantar flexion and foot inversion. (Courtesy of Gerardo Cabrera-Meza, MD.)

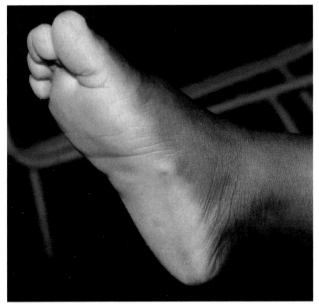

Figure 46-3 Pes planus. Arch absent in non–weight-bearing position in this child with rigid pes planus. (Courtesy of Tom Thacher, MD.)

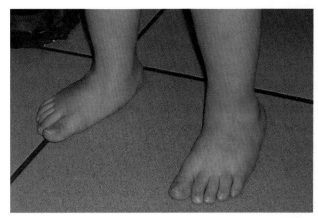

Figure 46-4 Pes planus. Mild pronation noted in this child with pes planus. (Courtesy of Sujata R. Tipnis, MD.)

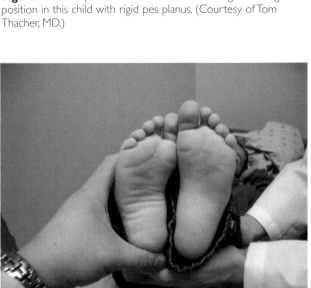

Figure 46-5 Metatarsus adductus. The convex ("C") shape of the child's right foot suggests metatarsus adductus. (Courtesy of Paul S. Matz, MD.)

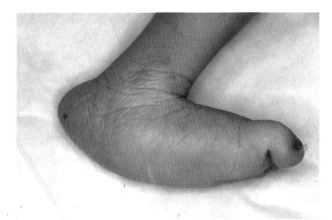

Figure 46-6 Rockerbottom feet. Gentle curvature to the bottom of this infant's feet is typical of rockerbottom feet and may be associated with Patau syndrome or Edward syndrome. (Courtesy of Gerardo Cabrera-Meza, MD.)

DIFFERENTIAL DIAGNOSIS

DIAGNOSIS	ICD-9	DISTINGUISHING CHARACTERISTICS	DURATION/ CHRONICITY	ASSOCIATED FINDINGS
Clubfoot	754.7	Metatarsus adductus with plantar flexion and foot inversion	Requires bracing, casting, or surgical correction	Spina bifida Sacral agenesis Spinal muscular atrophy Arthrogryposis
Flexible Pes Planus	734	Arch present in non–weight-bearing position Pronated foot Slightly increased subtalar motion	Usually resolves spontaneously by 6 years of age	None
Rigid Pes Planus	734	Arch absent in all positions Rigid subtalar joint	Becomes symptomatic in early adolescence	None
Metatarsus Adductus	754.53	Medial border of foot is concave Transverse crease between midfoot and forefoot	Usually resolves by 1 year of age	In 10% of cases associated with developmental dysplasia of the hip

COMPLICATIONS	PREDISPOSING FACTORS
Cosmetic deformity or gait abnormality if left untreated	Multifactorial inheritance with major influence from a single autosomal dominant gene Inherited 20% to 30% for offspring of affected parents Inherited 3% for subsequent siblings
None	Inherited, autosomal dominant Ligamentous laxity
Pain Gait dysfunction	Tarsal coalition
Very little functional limitation If persists can have cosmetic concerns Difficulty fitting shoes	Related to positioning in utero

OTHER
DIAGNOSES TO
CONSIDER

- Foot sprain following trauma

- Occult foot fracture

- Osteomyelitis

- Cellulitis

- Foreign body

- Osteosarcoma

- Cavus foot (high-arched foot)

- Rockerbottom foot

SUGGESTED READINGS

Benjamin DR, Hyman J, Royce DP. Congenital idiopathic talipes equinovarus. *Pediatr Rev.* 2004;25:124–129.

Dietz FR. Intoeing—fact, fiction, and opinion. *Am Fam Physician.* 1994;50:1249–1259.

McCrea JD. *Pediatric orthopedics of the lower extremity: an instructional handbook.* Mount Kisco, NY: Futura Publishing; 1985:171–188,228–248.

Nelson WE, ed. Nelson textbook of pediatrics. Philadelphia: WB Saunders; 1996:1918–1925.

Sass P, Hassan G. Lower extremity abnormalities in children. *Am Fam Physician.* 2003;68:461–468.

Scherl SA. Common lower extremity problems in children. *Pediatr Rev.* 2004;5:52–61.

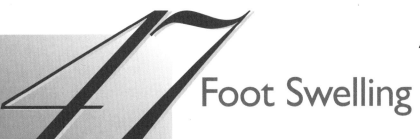

Foot Swelling

APPROACH TO THE PROBLEM

Swelling, or edema, occurs when fluid from within the blood vessels moves into the surrounding soft tissues. The presence or absence of pain will help to determine the etiology of the swelling. Some common causes of painless foot and ankle swelling include prolonged standing, heavy exercise, and hot weather. Painless swelling also may be the result of more serious conditions associated with reduced oncotic pressure (as with nephrotic syndrome, cirrhosis, and malnutrition) or elevated hydrostatic pressure within the blood vessels (as with congestive heart failure, and cirrhosis). In contrast, painful swelling may represent an inflammatory reaction and subsequent increased vascular permeability that results from trauma, such as an ankle sprain. Swelling also may occur with increased vascular permeability to proteins (as in allergic edema), inappropriate renal retention of sodium and water (as in nephrotic syndrome) or renal failure, and obstruction of lymphatic flow resulting in lymphedema.

KEY POINTS IN THE HISTORY

- Swelling that occurs suddenly, within hours to days, is often associated with trauma. In contrast, swelling that worsens over a period of weeks to months may suggest a more serious, underlying systemic cause.

- Unilateral swelling often suggests an isolated cause such as trauma or an insect bite to the affected foot, whereas bilateral swelling more likely results from a systemic condition.

- Ankle ligament sprains are the most common cause of sudden, painful foot swelling. The lateral ligament is most commonly affected in foot inversion injuries.

- Systemic diseases such as nephrotic syndrome, congestive heart failure, liver pathology, and malnutrition are commonly associated with progressive, painless foot swelling.

- Cyclic swelling in females may be seen in association with the menstrual cycle.

- Oral contraceptives, ACE inhibitors, tricyclic antidepressants, and antipsychotics such as olanzapine may cause painless, bilateral, foot swelling.

KEY POINTS IN THE PHYSICAL EXAMINATION

- Swelling associated with bruising, a bony deformity, and the inability to bear weight are highly suggestive of a fracture.

- Decreased or absent peripheral pulses and decreased sensation following trauma suggest a compartment syndrome.

- Crepitus in the subcutaneous tissue suggests a fracture.

- Swelling over a bony area indicates either a fracture or a tumor; swelling around a ligament may suggest a sprain.

- Signs of congestive heart failure, such as pulmonary rales and hepatomegaly, may be seen in association with bilateral, painless edema.

- Periorbital edema is often seen in children with nephrotic syndrome.

- Abdominal pain with ascites and jaundice may be seen in children with hepatic cirrhosis.

- Weight loss may suggest malnutrition; congestive heart failure may result in weight gain.

PHOTOGRAPHS OF SELECTED DIAGNOSES

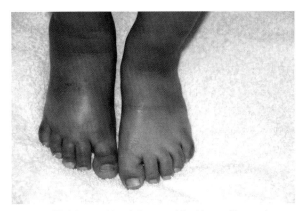

Figure 47-1 Insect bite. A 2-year-old with swelling and erythema of the right foot and ankle because of an insect bite. A pustule and vesicles are noted over the dorsum of the foot. (Courtesy of Julie A. Boom, MD.)

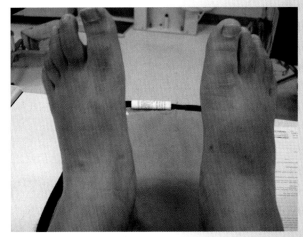

Figure 47-2 Traumatic foot swelling. This 9-year-old boy presents with swelling, bruising, and pain in the right foot 30 minutes after falling during a basketball game at school. This picture shows a comparison of the injured right foot with the normal left foot. Bruising and swelling are visible on the dorsum of the right foot. (Courtesy of Aida Z. Khanum, MD.)

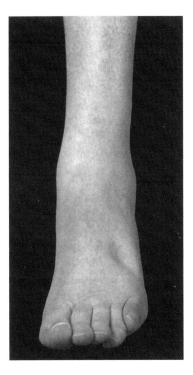

Figure 47-3 Pitting edema of foot. An edematous foot with evidence of pitting following firm pressure. (Used with permission from Bickley LS, Szilagyi P, eds. *Bates' guide to physical examination and history taking.* 8th ed. Philadelphia: Lippincott Williams & Wilkins; 2003:455.)

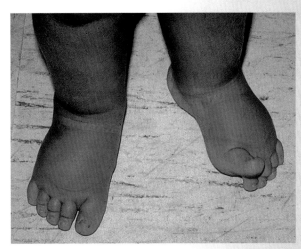

Figure 47-4 Lower extremity and foot edema. Clinical picture of lower extremities showing marked edema. (Used with permission from Gold DH, Weingeist TA. *Color atlas of the eye in systemic disease.* Baltimore: Lippincott Williams & Wilkins; 2001:643.)

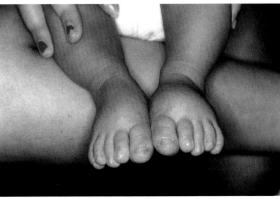

Figure 47-5 Congenital Lymphedema. Bilateral foot swelling noted by the mother of a newborn, 4 days following hospital discharge. (Courtesy of Jan E. Drutz, MD.)

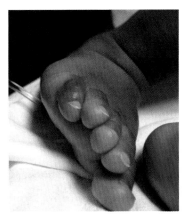

Figure 47-6 Foot edema and erythema in a child with Kawasaki disease. (Courtesy of Esther K. Chung, MD.)

DIFFERENTIAL DIAGNOSIS

DIAGNOSIS	ICD-9	DISTINGUISHING CHARACTERISTICS	DISTRIBUTION	DURATION/ CHRONICITY
Insect Bite	919.4	Pruritus Erythema Central punctum	May be anywhere on body	Swelling may be noted on the day following the actual bite
Ankle Sprain	845.0	Sudden onset Mild to moderate pain	Localized unilateral swelling	Swelling subsides within 48 hours Bear weight without pain 7–10 days for mild sprains; 3–6 weeks for severe sprains
Ankle Fracture	824.8 (closed) 824.9 (open)	Sudden onset Intense pain	Diffuse, unilateral swelling	Until fracture has healed, usually within 6 weeks
Orthostatic Edema	782.3	Painless Pitting on palpation	Bilateral	Duration variable Swelling subsides with sodium restriction and leg elevation
Idiopathic Cyclic Edema	782.3	Painless Cyclic swelling Pitting on palpation	Bilateral	Onset 7–10 days into the menstrual cycle and resolves following menses
Congestive Heart Failure	428.0	Painless, progressive swelling Pitting on palpation	Bilateral	Duration variable Swelling subsides with salt and fluid restriction and diuretic medication
Nephrotic Syndrome	581.9	Painless, progressive swelling Pitting on palpation More common among males aged 2 to 6 years	Bilateral	Duration variable Swelling subsides with start of antihypertensive or diuretic medications

ASSOCIATED FINDINGS	COMPLICATIONS	PREDISPOSING FACTORS
Bites elsewhere	Cellulitis	Warm weather Moist environment
Point tenderness Bruising Difficulty bearing weight Reduced ankle mobility	Joint instability Chronic pain Stiffness Recurrent swelling in 10% to 30% of cases	Sports or recreational injury Inversion more common than eversion injury
Bruising Loss of function of affected limb Numbness and tingling distal to fracture site Bony deformity	Compartment syndrome Arthritis Gait instability Nonunion Infection	Fall from a height Motor vehicle accidents Sports injury Child abuse
None	Leg ulcer	Prolonged standing or sitting
Weight gain of 1.5–2.5 kg on days of edema	None	Premenstrual syndrome
Weight gain Dyspnea Orthopnea Fatigue Hepatomegaly Nocturia	Pulmonary edema Arrhythmias Circulatory collapse	Infection Beta blocker Anemia Arrhythmias Hyperthyroidism
Facial swelling Weight gain Hypertension Protein in urine (foamy appearance) Low serum protein and high triglyceride	Atherosclerosis Congestive heart failure Renal vein thrombosis Renal failure Pneumococcal infections Malnutrition	Infection Drug exposure Malignancy Diabetes Systemic lupus erythematosus (SLE) Multiple myeloma Amyloidosis

OTHER
DIAGNOSES TO
CONSIDER

- Glomerulonephritis

- Pregnancy

- Lymphedema

- Dactylitis

- Kawasaki disease

SUGGESTED READINGS

Artman M, Graham T. Cardiac therapeutics: heart failure. In: Nelson WE, ed. *Nelson textbook of pediatrics.* 16th ed. Philadelphia: WB Saunders; 2000:1440–1445.

Bibbo C, Lin SS. Acute traumatic compartment syndrome of the foot in children. *Pediatr Emerg Care.* 2000;16(4):244–248.

Bickley LS, Szilagyi P, eds. *Bates' guide to physical examination and history taking.* 8th ed. Philadelphia: Lippincott Williams & Wilkins; 2003:455.

Cohn JN. The management of chronic heart failure. *N Engl J Med.* 1996;335:490–498.

Erler K, Oguz E, Komurcu M, et al. Ankle swelling in a 6-year-old boy with unusual presentation: report of a rare case. *J Foot Ankle Surg.* 2003;42(4):235–239.

Gold DH, Weingeist TA. *Color atlas of the eye in systemic disease.* Baltimore: Lippincott Williams & Wilkins; 2001:643.

Mankin KP, Zimbler S. Foot and ankle injuries: solving the diagnostic dilemmas. *Contemp Pediatr.* 1996;13(3):25–45.

Murphy JR, Woodhead JC. Edema. In: Dershewitz R, ed. *Ambulatory pediatric care.* Philadelphia: Lippincott Williams & Wilkins; 1988:697–701.

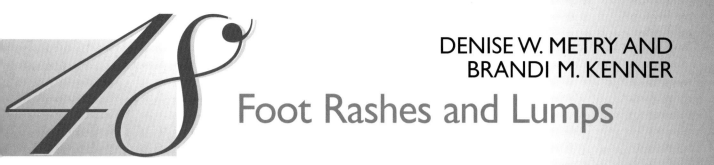

DENISE W. METRY AND
BRANDI M. KENNER

Foot Rashes and Lumps

APPROACH TO THE PROBLEM

Dermatologic conditions of the feet are common and often result from the extreme amount of stress and trauma constantly inflicted by everyday footwear and activities. Some conditions are related to the weight-bearing function of the feet, while others are associated with the warm, moist environment of the shoe-enclosed foot. Feet are also a site of several common dermatologic conditions. Because the feet are so heavily depended on, correct diagnosis and successful treatment of such ailments are important.

KEY POINTS IN THE HISTORY

- Tinea pedis and dyshidrotic eczema are more common in the warm summer months, while juvenile plantar dermatosis is more common during fall and winter months.

- A correlation with new footwear may support the diagnosis of a corn or callus.

- The use of communal showers, baths, and pools has been associated with infections, including tinea pedis and plantar warts.

- Tinea pedis and plantar warts are more common in adolescents, while juvenile plantar dermatosis is more common among prepubertal children.

- Tinea pedis is less common in children younger than 10 years old, but it may occur particularly when other family members are affected.

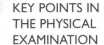 KEY POINTS IN
THE PHYSICAL
EXAMINATION

- After paring, plantar warts will often show pinpoint black dots, which are thrombosed capillaries. Calluses will have a smooth, glassy, homogenous surface.

- Plantar corns are more sensitive to direct pressure, whereas plantar warts are more sensitive to lateral compression (pinching).

- The diagnosis of a scaly, pruritic foot dermatitis may be determined based on the distribution, and juvenile plantar dermatosis tends to affect the balls of the feet bilaterally with a shiny, smooth, "glazed doughnut" appearance. Involvement of the interdigital spaces is seen in tinea pedis, allergic contact dermatitis usually affects the dorsum of the feet sparing the toe webs and soles, and dyshidrotic eczema tends to favor the lateral fingers and toes, palms, and soles.

- Plantar warts usually disrupt skin lines, while skin lines usually are maintained in calluses.

DIFFERENTIAL DIAGNOSIS

DIAGNOSIS	ICD-9	DISTINGUISHING CHARACTERISTICS	DISTRIBUTION	ASSOCIATED FINDINGS	PREDISPOSING FACTORS
Corn or Callus	726.91 (bone)	Corn: • Hard—well-circumscribed, hyperkeratotic lesion with central conical core and a glassy, homogenous surface after paring • Soft—macerated appearance of hyperkeratosis after absorbing an extreme amount of moisture from perspiration Callus: • Broad-based hyperkeratotic plaque of relatively even thickness; skin lines usually maintained; may be painful	Corn: • Hard type—most common on dorsum of fifth toe, but any toe may be affected • Soft type—generally occurs between toes, most commonly between fourth and fifth Callus: • Usually found on the ball of the foot and margins of the heel, under metatarsal heads	Corn: • Hammer toe deformity	High levels of activity/friction, irritation, and pressure, or abnormal foot mechanics Mechanical stress—intrinsic, including bony prominences, or extrinsic, including tight shoes
Plantar Wart	078.19	Round, firm, often callused papule, nodule, or plaque with rough surface; disrupts skin lines and often occurs in multiples Often has "black dot" pattern because of thrombosed capillaries Common in both younger children and adolescents	Especially common over weight-bearing areas of soles	May be painful, especially with application of lateral pressure	Direct contact from person to person or autoinoculation, or indirect by contact with contaminated surfaces or objects (barefoot activities) Trauma may facilitate spread through minor skin abrasions
Tinea Pedis	110.4	Interdigital (most common)—peeling, maceration, and fissuring with erythema Moccasin—dry, fine scaly patches or hyperkeratotic papules with mild erythema, more chronic Vesicular—vesicles and pustules Uncommon before puberty Common in adolescents (M>F)	Generally affects toe webs and soles on one or both feet Often, sharp border between involved and uninvolved skin Interdigital pattern involves web spaces (especially fourth digit space), may spread to dorsal foot and undersurface of toes Moccasin pattern is diffuse and involves plantar and lateral foot surfaces Vesicular usually involves instep	Onychomycosis and tinea manuum ("one hand, two feet")	Use of communal showers, pools Activities that cause feet to sweat; occlusive and/or damp shoes (including not allowing athletic shoes to dry in between activities) Warm weather Household members with tinea pedis
Dyshidrotic Eczema (Pompholyx)	705.81	Two stages: • Vesicular stage—multiple deep-set, tiny, clear vesicles (may coalesce to form bullae) with intense pruritus lasting a few days to weeks, which progresses to the next stage • Dry, desquamating stage—skin peels, cracks, or crusts over 2–3 weeks Recurrent episodes with disease-free periods Uncommon before school-age Most common in ages 20–40 years (F>M)	Along lateral edges of fingers, toes, palms, and soles Usually bilateral and symmetric	N/A	Often associated with hyperhidrosis and exacerbated by warm weather, intense emotions Possible association with primary irritants (excessive washing, detergents, chemicals), nickel allergy, or as an "id" reaction to tinea or candida
Juvenile Plantar Dermatosis	694.2 (dermatosis juvenile)	Chapped, fissured feet with shiny/smooth "glazed doughnut" appearance, erythema, and scaling Pruritus Pain associated with fissuring Mainly in prepubertal children	Bilateral and symmetrical, favors the anterior third of the soles, heels, and toes (especially great toes), with sparing of interdigital spaces	N/A	Associated with hyperhidrosis and exacerbated by occlusive, synthetic footwear (especially tennis shoes), rapid drying without moisturizing Worse in atopic persons during the winter months

PHOTOGRAPHS OF SELECTED DIAGNOSES

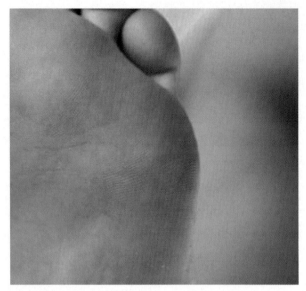

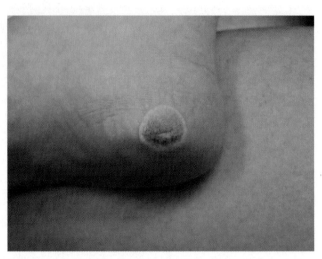

Figure 48-2 Plantar wart on the medial surface of the heel. (Courtesy of Denise W. Metry, MD.)

Figure 48-1 Callus. The skin over the head of the fifth metatarsal is thickened and slightly yellow. Skin lines are maintained. (Courtesy of Julie A. Boom, MD.)

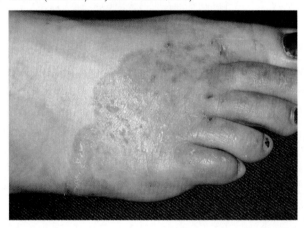

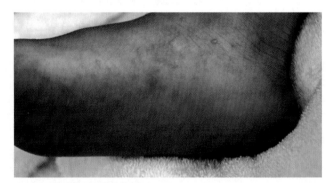

Figure 48-4 Dyshidrotic eczema. A 7-year-old boy with multiple deep-set, clear vesicles over the medical surface of his right foot. (Courtesy of Julie A. Boom, MD.)

Figure 48-3 Tinea pedis. The interdigital pattern of tinea pedis is common. Note the spread onto the dorsum of the foot. (Courtesy of Denise W. Metry, MD.)

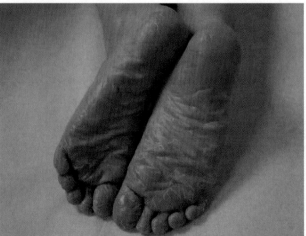

Figure 48-5 Juvenile plantar dermatosis. The skin on the soles has a smooth, shiny appearance with multiple fissures and cracks. (Courtesy of Denise W. Metry, MD.)

OTHER
DIAGNOSES TO
CONSIDER

- Allergic contact dermatitis

- Pustular psoriasis

- Black heel

- Pitted keratolysis

SUGGESTED READINGS

Buescher ES. Infections associated with pediatric sport participation. *Pediatr Clin North Am.* 2002;49(4):743–751.

Freeman DB. Corns and calluses resulting from mechanical hyperkeratosis. *Am Fam Physician.* 2002;65(11):2277–2280.

Guenst BJ. Common pediatric foot dermatoses. *J Pediatr Health Care.* 1999;13(2):68–71.

Omura EF, Rye B. Dermatologic disorders of the foot. *Clin Sports Med.* 1994;13(4):825–841.

TWELVE

Genital and Perineal Region

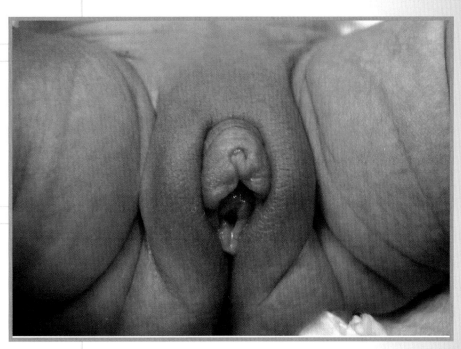

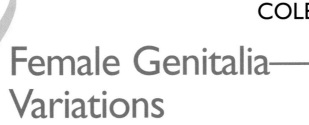

Female Genitalia—Variations

APPROACH TO THE PROBLEM

Variations in the physical appearance of female genitalia encompass findings within the spectrum of normal, ambiguous genitalia, and abnormalities—congenital or acquired. Although most represent isolated external findings, some are associated with variations in the structure and/or function of other organ systems. Identifying such variations depends on the physical characteristics, the stage of the child's genital development, the presence of associated symptoms, ongoing parental involvement in the child's genital care, and the primary care provider's consistent inclusion of a careful genital examination at every health maintenance visit. Early detection may be imperative (ambiguous genitalia), preferred (imperforate hymen), or inconsequential (normal hymenal variants). In addition, any complaints of abdominal pain, urinary symptoms, perineal/vaginal symptoms, change in bowel habits, and/or sexual maltreatment should prompt the clinician to carefully examine the perineum.

KEY POINTS IN THE HISTORY

- A patient's age and Tanner stage are key to establishing whether a particular external genital finding is within the limits of normal.

- Imperforate hymen or a vaginal web may present with complaints of abdominal or lower back pain, pain with defecation, diarrhea, extremity pain, urinary retention, and nausea and vomiting.

- There may be a genetic predisposition to imperforate hymen.

- CAH occurs with higher frequency in Ashkenazi Jewish, Hispanic, Slavic, and Italian populations.

- A family history of neonatal death may represent a missed diagnosis of CAH.

- A family history of ambiguous genitalia, consanguinity, infertility, or amenorrhea suggests a genetic basis for ambiguous genitalia.

- Maternal history of certain ovarian tumors, drug ingestion or teratogen exposure during pregnancy may contribute to the development of ambiguous genitalia.

- Labial adhesions are common and may result from vulvar exposure to irritants, such as residual feces between the labia, bubble baths, or harsh soaps or detergents, or trauma, accidental such as vigorous cleanings, or non-accidental such as sexual maltreatment.

KEY POINTS IN THE PHYSICAL EXAMINATION

- The physiologic red coloring of the prepubertal child's genital mucosae may be mistaken for child maltreatment.

- In a newborn with ambiguous genitalia, gonadal material palpable in the inguinal canal or labioscrotal folds is most commonly testicular material and rarely a herniated ovary or ovotestis in a hermaphrodite; its presence eliminates the diagnoses of Turner syndrome and pure gonadal dysgenesis.

- Varying degrees of labial adhesion typically create a fused segment (posterior to anterior).

- Imperforate hymen may be detected when yellow/white (mucohydrocolpos) or red/blue tissue (hematocolpos) is seen protruding from a child's vagina upon straining or crying.

PHOTOGRAPHS OF SELECTED DIAGNOSES

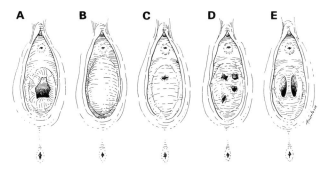

Figure 49-1 Types of hymens: (A) normal, (B) imperforate, (C) microperforate, (D) cribriform, and (E) septate. (Used with permission from Emans SJ, Laufer MR, Goldstein DP, eds. *Pediatric and adolescent gynecology*. 5th ed. Philadelphia: Lippincott Williams & Wilkins; 2005:10.)

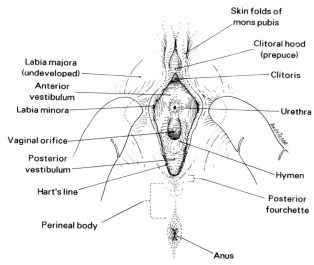

Figure 49-2 Prepubertal child genitalia. (Used with permission from Emans SJ, Laufer MR, Goldstein DP, eds. *Pediatric and adolescent gynecology*. 5th ed. Philadelphia: Lippincott Williams & Wilkins; 2005:3.)

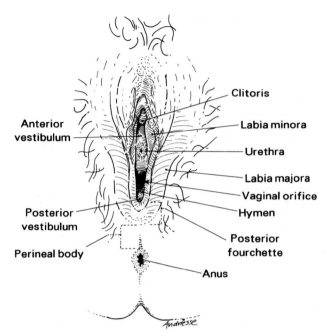

Figure 49-3 Pubertal child genitalia. (Used with permission from Emans SJ, Laufer MR, Goldstein DP, eds. *Pediatric and adolescent gynecology.* 5th ed. Philadelphia: Lippincott Williams & Wilkins; 2005:28.)

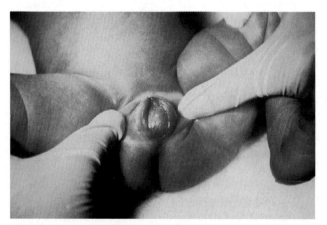

Figure 49-4 Imperforate hymen. (Used with permission from Emans SJ, Laufer MR, Goldstein DP, eds. *Pediatric and adolescent gynecology.* 5th ed. Philadelphia: Lippincott Williams & Wilkins; 2005:plate 21.)

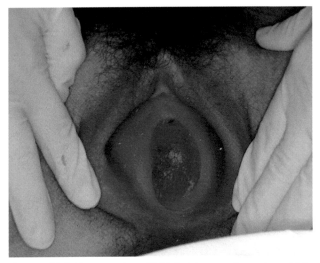

Figure 49-5 Hematocolpos. Bluish bulging membrane in a child with primary amenorrhea and lower abdominal pain. (Used with permission from Fleisher GR, Ludwig S, Baskin MN, eds. *Atlas of pediatric emergency medicine*. Philadelphia: Lippincott Williams & Wilkins; 2004:145.)

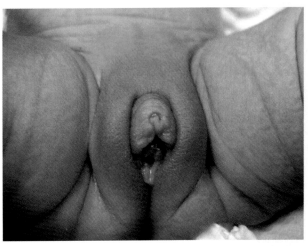

Figure 49-6 Ambiguous genitalia in a child with congenital adrenal hyperplasia. (Courtesy of Philip Siu, MD.)

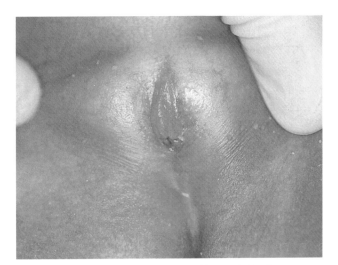

Figure 49-7 Labial adhesions. (Used with permission from Fleisher GR, Ludwig S, Baskin MN, eds. *Atlas of pediatric emergency medicine*. Philadelphia: Lippincott Williams & Wilkins; 2004:146.)

DIFFERENTIAL DIAGNOSIS

DIAGNOSIS	ICD-9	DISTINGUISHING CHARACTERISTICS	DURATION/ CHRONICITY	ASSOCIATED FINDINGS
Normal Genitalia	V65.5 Newborn genitalia	Findings are related to maternal estrogen effects: • Prominent labia majora • Thick labia minora • Pale pink and moist mucosa • Annular or redundant hymen May see variations (septate, microperforate, cribiform hymen)	Continuum between newborn and prepubertal periods	Physiologic leukorrhea Pseudomenses
	Prepubertal genitalia	Larger labia Labia minora exposed Crescentic or posterior rim hymen is common Mucosa pink-red, less moist Redundant or fimbriated hymen and annular hymen can be seen		N/A
	Pubertal genitalia	Labia larger Hymen thick, elastic, and redundant Mucosa pale pink and moist	Puberty	Physiologic leukorrhea Onset of menses
Imperforate Hymen	752.42	Shiny membrane between labia Membrane red/blue or white/yellow and bulging	May present in the newborn period Less commonly detected in early infancy as hydrocolpos, mucocolpos, or hematocolpos Often detected in adolescents with menarche as hematocolpos	Primary amenorrhea Lower abdominal mass Soft, tender, fluctuant mass on rectal exam Abdominal distension
Ambiguous Genitalia	752.7 Female pseudohermaphroditism	Variable virilization Ranges from mild clitoral gland enlargement to "male" phallus and scrotum	Diagnosed at birth	Salt loss Salt retention/hypertension Testicular and ovarian tissue present: true hermaphroditism
	752.7 Ambiguous genitalia Male Pseudohermaphroditism	Inadequate virilization Microphallus, variable hypospadias, chordee, bilateral cryptorchidism, female external genitalia		Salt loss Salt retention, hypertension Hypokalemia
Labial Adhesions	752.49	Pale, smooth, avascular line of fusion between labia minora	3 mos–6 yrs	N/A

COMPLICATIONS	PREDISPOSING FACTORS
N/A	N/A
N/A	Onset of puberty with unopposed estrogen production
Urinary retention Constipation Hydronephrosis	N/A
Vascular collapse and death from salt-wasting nephropathy Gender misassignment	N/A
Variable genitourinary outflow obstruction Urinary tract infections	Vulvar inflammation or irritation

SUGGESTED READINGS

American Professional Society on the Abuse of Children. *Glossary of terms and the interpretations of findings for child sexual abuse evidentiary examinations.* Chicago, IL: APSAC; 1998.

Dickson CA, Saad S, Tesar JD. Imperforate hymen with hematocolpos. *Ann Emerg Med.* 1985;14:467–469.

Emans SJ, Laufer MR, Goldstein DP, eds. *Pediatric and adolescent gynecology.* 5th ed. Philadelphia: Lippincott Williams & Wilkins; 2005:3,10,28.

Fleisher GR, Ludwig S, Baskin MN, eds. *Atlas of pediatric emergency medicine.* Philadelphia: Lippincott Williams & Wilkins; 2004:145,146.

Murray PJ, Davis HW. Pediatric and adolescent gynecology. In: Zitelli BJ, Davis HW, eds. *Atlas of pediatric physical diagnosis.* 4th ed. Philadelphia: Mosby; 2002:609–648.

Styne DM, Glaser NS. Endocrinology. In: Behrman RE, Kliegman RM, eds. *Nelson essentials of pediatrics.* 4th ed. Philadelphia: WB Saunders; 2002:711–766.

Sultan C, Paris F, Jeandel C, et al. Ambiguous genitalia in the newborn: diagnosis, etiology, and sex assignment. *Endocr Dev.* 2004;7:23–38.

Wall EM, Stone B, Klein BL. Imperforate hymen: a not-so-hidden diagnosis. *Am J Emerg Med.* 2003;21:249–250.

T. ERNESTO FIGUEROA
AND ILIA ZELTSER

Penile Abnormalities

APPROACH TO THE PROBLEM

Penile abnormalities occur frequently, and recognition and accurate identification of these conditions are important because some carry significant consequences for the patient and his family. Genital anomalies are often isolated problems, although they may occur as part of a congenital syndrome, such as Noonan, Opitz, Prader Willi, Robinow, or Trisomy 18.

Evaluation for genital anomalies begins in the neonatal period. Palpation of the scrotum, or inguinal area, to assess for two testes in the male, as well as for corporal integrity of the penis, are important diagnostic maneuvers. Systematically, the examination of the genitalia should describe the appearance of the prepuce (normal or incomplete), the location of the urethral meatus (if visible), the size and appearance of the penis, the presence of penile chordee or torsion, the appearance of the scrotum, and the location and size of the testes.

KEY POINTS IN THE HISTORY

- Phimosis is a condition in which the prepuce cannot be retracted. A normal condition in infancy and childhood, it is often referred to as physiologic phimosis. The timing for natural retraction of the prepuce varies, but most uncircumcised boys have a retractile prepuce by 5 years of age.

- Penile adhesions are extremely common. They are universally present in uncircumcised boys and present in about 60% of circumcised boys at some point. The adhesions occur between the glans and the adjacent inner mucosal surface of the prepuce. With time, adhesions separate naturally. Two processes aid in the natural separation of adhesions: erections and formation of smegma between the inner mucosal surface of the prepuce and the glans.

- Hidden penis is a penis that does not protrude beyond the surface of the abdominal wall, mainly because of displacement of the penile skin away from the shaft by subcutaneous fat. In contrast, a concealed penis is buried by a cicatrix of the prepuce that occurs following neonatal circumcision in males who have limited penile skin or when an excessive amount of penile skin is removed during the circumcision. If the glans falls behind the healing preputial scar, then the scar will contract and bury the penis. Concealed penis can be managed nonsurgically by the application of topical corticosteroids, though many procedures will require a surgical release with revision of the circumcision.

- Hypospadias is a frequent anomaly, occurring in 1/300 live male births. Elements of hypospadias include a hooded prepuce, a ventral meatus, and chordee. The severity is variable, with most boys (75%) having a distal abnormality (glanular, coronal, distal shaft). In more severe cases, profound androgenic failure may be evident, with the findings of a microphallus, bifid scrotum, and penoscrotal transposition.

- Chordee, present with or without a hypospadias, is ventral curvature of the penis. Most patients with hypospadias have chordee, partially because of the asymmetry between the normal dorsal penile skin and the hypoplastic ventral penile skin. This is referred to as cutaneous chordee. In more severe cases, as with fibrous chordee, the curvature may involve the ventral surface of the penis (corpus spongiosum and corpora cavernosa) in addition to the cutaneous abnormality.

- Penile torsion is lateral rotation of the penis in reference to the midline penoscrotal raphe. In approximately 5% to 10 % of boys, the raphe may be directed laterally, causing the lateral rotation of the penile shaft.

- A micropenis is a phallus smaller than two standard deviations below the mean for expected age. These are often visually abnormal penises, appearing small in context to the rest of the body habitus of the child. The prepuce is normally formed. If the testes also are abnormally small, or if other findings suggest an endocrine disorder, the patient should be evaluated by an endocrinologist.

- Ambiguous genitalia refers to incomplete or abnormal genital development, preventing accurate definition of gender based on the appearance of the genitalia. These children may suffer from extremely variable conditions, from excessive androgen production in the female with congenital adrenal hyperplasia and virilization of the genitalia to the underdevelopment of the male genitalia in a male patient with 5-alpha reductase insufficiency. This condition is truly a wide spectrum, and awareness of the possibility of sexual and genital ambiguity is critical to its recognition.

KEY POINTS IN THE PHYSICAL EXAMINATION

- Phimosis refers to a conical protrusion of prepuce that cannot be retracted proximally. Contrast this with a secondary phimosis, a cicatrix in a flat distal prepuce that prevents retraction of the prepuce.

- Penile adhesions are soft attachments between inner (mucosal) prepuce and any part of the glans. These will separate in time. Contrast this with skin bridging, a band of skin that has become fused to the corona or glans following circumcision. This will need surgical separation.

- Paraphimosis refers to the condition in which a phimotic prepuce is retracted behind the corona of the glans. Because of the constricting effect of the phimosis, edema and swelling of the glans occur distally to the preputial orifice.

- Hidden penis refers to the appearance of a small penile shaft and excess penile skin. Retracting the prepubic fat pad usually reveals a normal-sized and circumcised penis. Contrast this with concealed penis and micropenis.

- Hypospadias refers to a hooded prepuce; ventral meatus in the area of the corona, shaft, or scrotum; and chordee.

- Chordee refers to abnormal ventral curvature, producing a curved penis.

- Penile torsion refers to clockwise or counterclockwise rotation of the penile shaft and meatus with a laterally displaced penile raphe.

- Micropenis refers to a normally formed penis, although small.

- Ambiguous genitalia refers to the appearance of phallus (penis or clitoris), bifid scrotum or labia, or ventral orifice that could represent hypospadias or urogenital sinus.

DIFFERENTIAL DIAGNOSIS

DIAGNOSIS	ICD-9	DISTINGUISHING CHARACTERISTICS	DISTRIBUTION	DURATION/ CHRONICITY
Phimosis	605	Nonretractile prepuce	Universal at birth	Resolves by 5 years of age
Penile Adhesion	605A	Retractile prepuce with mucosal attachments Distinct from skin bridging	60% of circumcised infants	Resolves by 5 years of age
Paraphimosis	605R	Edema of glans and prepuce	Rare	Acute event
Hidden Penis	752.65	Apparently small size, abundant prepubic fat Distinct from concealed penis	Very common in infancy	Resolves by 2 to 3 years of life
Hypospadias	752.61	Ventral meatus, hooded prepuce	1/300 live male births	Lifelong consequences in more severe cases
Chordee	607.89c	Bent penis, or penile curvature because of abnormal skin (cutaneous chordee) Abnormal corporal bodies (fibrous chordee)	Similar to hypospadias	Correctable in most cases
Penile torsion	607.89	Abnormal axis of meatus and lateral rotation of shaft Most are rotated counterclockwise	15% of boys	Correctable in most cases
Micorpenis	752.64	Abnormally small penis	Rare	May be lifelong condition
Ambiguous Genitalia	752.7 (indeterminate sex)	Abnormal genitalia of uncertain gender	Uncommon	Lifelong condition

ASSOCIATED FINDINGS	COMPLICATIONS	PREDISPOSING FACTORS
Normal penis	Inability to retract prepuce, poor hygiene, urinary tract infection (UTI)	Congenital, normal Secondary to injury to preputial annulus either by circumcision or by forceful retraction of prepuce
Normal penis, either circumcised or uncircumcised	Tearing, penile deviation	—
Tight proximal preputial ring	Glanular ischemia	Tight preputial annulus, retracting the prepuce proximally without returning the prepuce to its normal position
Prepubic fat pad	Skin irritation secondary to urine pooling in the area	Obesity, small penis, excessive or incomplete circumcision
Chordee, micropenis	If meatus is stenotic, difficulty urinating Abnormal penile appearance	Abnormal production/timing of androgens in utero Genetic predisposition
Hypoplastic ventral penile surface Possible hypospadias	May interfere with quality of sexual intercourse	Abnormal corpus spongiosum
Abnormal symmetry of penile skin	Deviated urine stream	—
Hypogonadism	Endocrinopathy Sexual intercourse may be difficult	Endocrinopathy
—	Related to etiology Multiple complications, including need for surgery Psychological adjustment	Depends on underlying etiology

PHOTOGRAPHS OF SELECTED DIAGNOSES

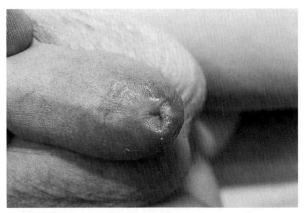

Figure 50-1 Phimosis. (Courtesy of T. Ernesto Figueroa)

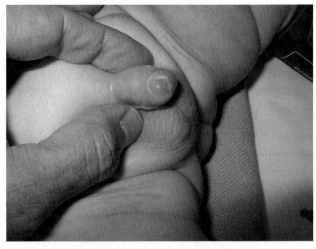

Figure 50-2 Penile adhesion. (Courtesy of T. Ernesto Figueroa)

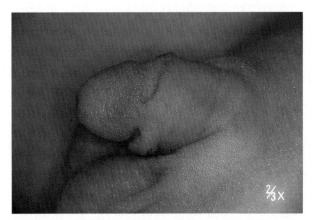

Figure 50-3 Skin bridging. (Courtesy of T. Ernesto Figueroa)

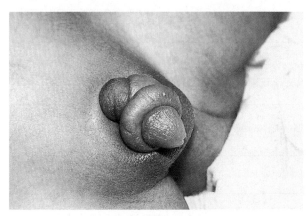

Figure 50-4 Paraphimosis. (Courtesy of T. Ernesto Figueroa)

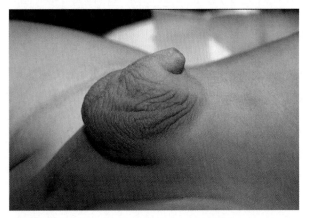

Figure 50-5 Concealed penis. (Courtesy of T. Ernesto Figueroa)

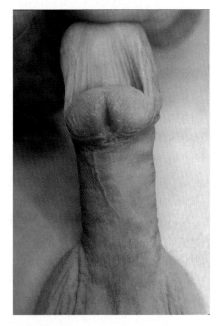

Figure 50-6 Coronal hypospadias. Note the associated hooded prepuce. (Courtesy of T. Ernesto Figueroa)

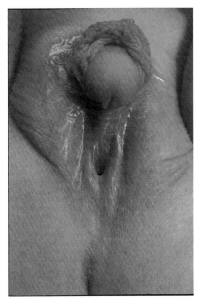

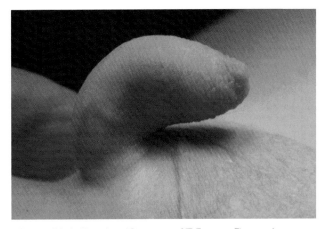

Figure 50-8 Chordee. (Courtesy of T. Ernesto Figueroa)

Figure 50-7 Perineal hypospadias. (Courtesy of T. Ernesto Figueroa)

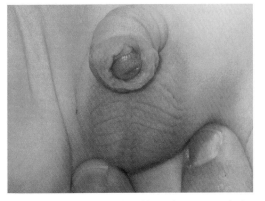

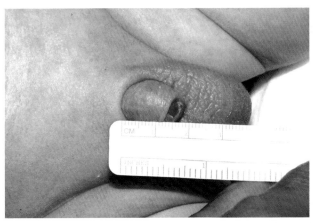

Figure 50-9 Penile torsion. Note the counterclockwise rotation of the penile meatus and shaft. (Courtesy of T. Ernesto Figueroa)

Figure 50-10 Micropenis. (Courtesy of T. Ernesto Figueroa)

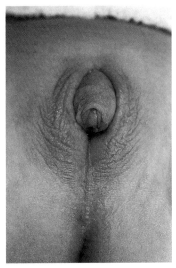

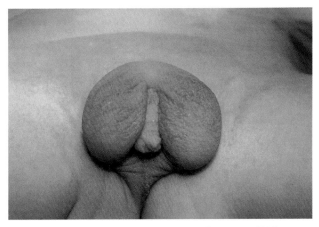

Figure 50-12 Penoscrotal transposition. (Courtesy of T. Ernesto Figueroa)

Figure 50-11 Ambiguous genitalia. (Courtesy of T. Ernesto Figueroa)

OTHER DIAGNOSES TO CONSIDER

- Secondary phimosis

- Concealed penis

- Penile skin bridging

- Idiopathic penile edema

- Epispadias

SUGGESTED READINGS

Elder JS. Abnormalities of the genitalia in boys and their surgical management. In: Walsh, ed. *Campbell's urology.* 8th ed. Philadelphia: WB Saunders; 2002.

Figueroa TE. Congenital adrenal hyperplasia. In: Siedmon EJ, Hanno PM, Kaufman JJ, eds. *Current urological therapy.* 3rd ed. Philadelphia: WB Saunders; 1994.

Figueroa TE, Casale P. Circumcision. In: Mattei, ed. *Surgical directives: pediatric surgery.* New York: Lippincott Williams & Wilkins; 2002.

Kennedy AP, Figueroa TE. Common urological problems in the fetus and neonate. In: Spitzer A, ed. *Intensive care of the neonate and fetus.* 2nd ed. Philadelphia: Hanley & Belfus Press; 2003.

Perovic S. *Atlas of congenital anomalies of the external genitalia.* Yugoslavia: Refot-Arka; 1999.

51

T. ERNESTO FIGUEROA AND ILIA ZELTSER

Penile Swelling

Penile swelling, or edema, is often a sudden, alarming departure from the normal appearance of the genitalia in boys. The penile skin and prepuce are unique tissues in their ability to stretch and tolerate trauma. The penile skin can respond to trauma or inflammation with the development of significant tissue edema. The normal penile skin has a very subtle, rugated appearance, and edema produces a full and tight appearance. Erythema often accompanies penile edema, and this combination implies an acute inflammatory condition. Proximal extension of penile erythema into the prepubic skin or scrotum suggests tissue infection or cellulitis.

Penile edema may be a primary or secondary process, and it may occur in the presence or absence of the prepuce. In the uncircumcised penis, primary penile conditions include posthitis (preputial inflammation) and balanoposthitis (acute glanular inflammation). In the circumcised penis, primary penile conditions include idiopathic penile edema and edema related to accidental or postsurgical trauma. Congenital genital lymphedema is recognized in infancy by the thickened and leathery appearance of the penile skin and scrotum, distended appearance of the penile and scrotal raphe, and lack of erythema or acute inflammation. These patients with lymphedema precox usually have coexisting lower extremity edema. Secondary penile edema is seen in association with systemic conditions that result in decreased oncotic pressure, including conditions associated with hypoalbuminemia, or other causes of generalized or dependent edema. On rare occasions, penile edema may be the first sign of an allergic reaction to certain medications. In these patients, the term *angioedema* is used to describe diffuse swelling of the loose subcutaneous tissues in addition to the dermis. This reaction can be seen with and without urticaria.

In the presence of diffuse dermatitis, penile edema represents a secondary process.

KEY POINTS IN THE HISTORY	• Posthitis, or acute inflammation of the prepuce, presents with sudden onset and rapid progression (for example, several hours) of redness, swelling, and penile pain.

• Balanoposthitis, or inflammation of the glans and prepuce because of bacteria in the preputial space, presents with redness, preputial swelling, penile pain, and suppuration of the glans, with urination difficulty.

• Penile trauma generally presents with a history of trauma. Patients will complain of penile swelling, bruising, broken skin margins, and bleeding.

• Allergic penile edema, also referred to as angioedema, may present with a history of exposure to medications, including antibiotics or topical products.

KEY POINTS IN THE PHYSICAL EXAMINATION

• In assessing a patient with acute penile edema, it is important to determine whether the glans is involved or evidence of vascular compromise exists.

• An important component of the physical examination is the determination of a distended bladder representing urinary retention because of pain or difficulty with urination related to the penile condition.

• Posthitis refers to florid redness, tight-appearing swelling, and tenderness of the penile skin and prepuce. It is often seen in association with phimosis. Suppuration of the glans is generally not present.

• Balanoposthitis: similar to posthitis; however, suppuration of the glans and significant difficulty with urination are present. A palpable bladder may be evident because of urinary retention.

• Penile trauma refers to edema that generally is localized to the area of trauma, with adjacent ecchymotic areas, lacerated skin, and bleeding. Old blood may be evident in the underwear.

• Congenital genital lymphedema, a lymphatic disorder affecting the genitalia and lower extremities, produces a nontender, nonerythematous, chronic, leathery, thickened edematous appearance, with common involvement of the lower extremities.

• Dependent edema, or pitting, non-tender edema, is seen in postsurgical or posttrauma patients who remain recumbent.

• With allergic penile edema, the glans appears normal but there is a bulbous-appearing, edematous mucosal skirt of the distal penile skin and mucosal edema. The transition to the normal penile skin from the edematous mucosal skirt is smooth. One must differentiate this condition from paraphimosis, in which a constricting band is present.

• Penile edema with mild erythema may occur with generalized conditions that are associated with penile cutanenous lesions, such as varicella.

PHOTOGRAPHS OF SELECTED DIAGNOSES

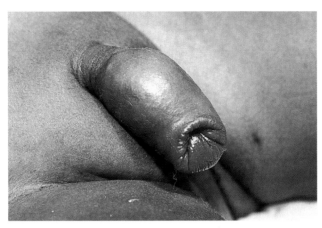

Figure 51-1 Penile edema after reduction of paraphimosis. (Courtesy of T. Ernesto Figueroa, MD.)

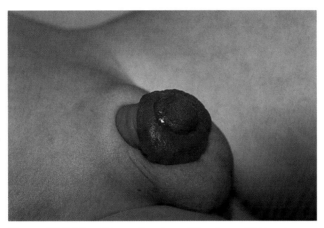

Figure 51-2 Idiopathic penile edema. (Courtesy of T. Ernesto Figueroa, MD.)

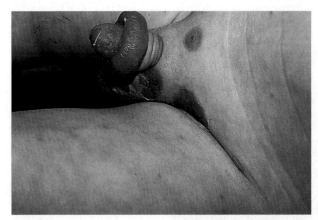

Figure 51-3 Penile edema in association with varicella. (Courtesy of T. Ernesto Figueroa, MD.)

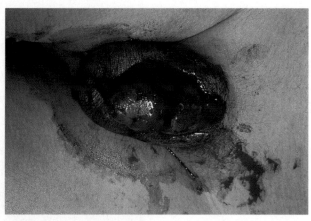

Figure 51-4 Penile trauma. (Courtesy of T. Ernesto Figueroa, MD.)

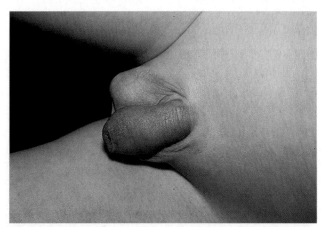

Figure 51-5 Balanoposthitis. (Courtesy of T. Ernesto Figueroa, MD.)

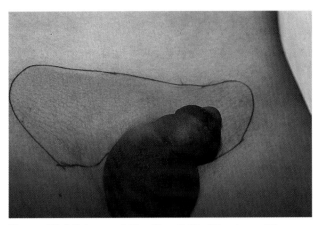

Figure 51-6 Balanoposthitis with cellulitis. (Courtesy of T. Ernesto Figueroa, MD.)

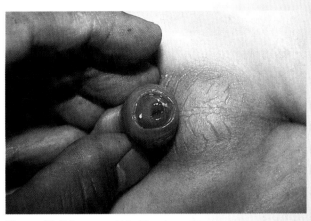

Figure 51-7 Acute posthitis. (Courtesy of T. Ernesto Figueroa, MD.)

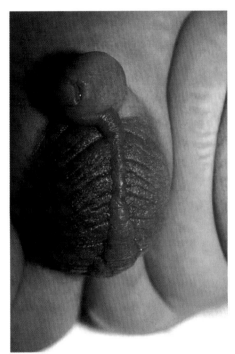

Figure 51-8 Lymphedema. (Courtesy of T. Ernesto Figueroa, MD.)

DIFFERENTIAL DIAGNOSIS

DIAGNOSIS	ICD-9	DISTINGUISHING CHARACTERISTICS	DURATION/ CHRONICITY	ASSOCIATED FINDINGS
Penile Edema	607.93	Diffuse edema of penis • May occur as dependent edema in association with anasarca • May occur as angioedema or an allergic response to medications • May be seen as a local response to penile cutaneous lesions seen with generalized rashes, such as varicella	Acute condition, except in congenital lymphedema	Balanoposthitis Erythema and associated physical findings will distinguish primary edema from secondary causes Secondary edema may be pitting
Penile Trauma	911.8G	History of trauma Ecchymoses Broken skin Bleeding Localized edema	Acute condition	Ecchymoses Bleeding
Balanoposthitis	607.1B	Inflammation of glans Penile edema, phimosis, and suppuration from glans and preputial space	Acute condition	Erythema Diffuse edema Pain and tenderness Suppuration Phimosis
Posthitis	.607.1	Diffuse inflammation of prepuce and penile skin Less severe than balonoposthitis	Acute condition	Diffuse and florid erythema and edema Phimosis Glans not visible
Congenital Lymphedema	607.93	Leathery, thickened penile skin	Chronic condition	Lower extremity edema

COMPLICATIONS	PREDISPOSING FACTORS
Difficulty urinating	Phimosis Fluid overload Hypoalbuminemia Severe anemia
Pain Difficulty urinating Cosmetic deficits Loss of penile skin Scar formation	Clamp circumcision Sexual abuse
Injury to glans because of inflammation Secondary phimosis Progression to cellulitis	Phimosis Separation of prepuce from glans
Worsening of phimosis Difficulty urinating Progression to cellulitis	Phimosis
Difficulty with urination Mass effect of genitalia Difficulty with sexual activity	Abnormal lymphatic channels Hypoplasia of lymphatic channels

SUGGESTED READINGS

Bloom DA, Wan J, Key DW. Disorders of the male external genitalia and inguinal canal. In: Kelalis, King, Belman, eds. *Pediatric urology*. 3rd ed. Philadelphia: WB Saunders; 1992.

Elder JS. Abnormalities of the genitalia in boys and their surgical management. In: Walsh, ed. *Campbell's urology*. 8th ed. Philadelphia: WB Saunders; 2002.

Figueroa TE, Casale P. Circumcision. In: Mattei P, ed. *Surgical directives: pediatric surgery*. New York: Lippincott Williams & Wilkins; 2002.

Lakshmaran Y, Pakulkar BG. Edema-external genitalia. In: Gomella, ed. *The 5-minute urology consult*. Philadelphia: Lippincott, Williams & Wilkins; 2000.

Netter F. *The Ciba collection of medical illustrations (vol 2)—Reproductive system*. New York: Ciba; 1965.

Perineal Red Rashes

APPROACH TO THE PROBLEM

Diaper dermatoses, some of the most common skin disorders in infants and toddlers, peak at age 9 to 12 months. The term encompasses a variety of acute inflammatory skin reactions in the diaper area. Contact diaper dermatitis is the most frequent cause of diaper rash. Older children and adolescents with groin rashes present with lesions predominantly caused by fungal infections, such as vulvovaginitis and tinea cruris. In most cases, frequent diaper changes and application of topical barrier agents are the mainstay of therapy. Groin rashes that indicate the presence of infection require topical antifungal or antibiotic agents. It is crucial to perform an entire body exam when evaluating rashes in the groin area.

KEY POINTS IN THE HISTORY

- A history of a rash elsewhere on the skin suggests the possibility of seborrhea; psoriasis; or less likely, histiocytosis X.

- A history of recent antibiotic use often precedes a *Candida albicans* diaper rash or vulvovaginitis in an adolescent female.

- Extremes of moisture or heat in the groin area may lead to contact dermatitis, candida diaper dermatitis, or tinea cruris.

- Seborrheic, atopic, and contact dermatitis disrupt the integrity of the skin and place the host at risk for infection with *Candida albicans*.

- Overall, disposable diapers are more effective than cloth diapers in preventing and resolving contact diaper dermatitis.

- Persistent diarrhea may contribute to contact diaper dermatitis.

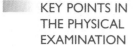 KEY POINTS IN
THE PHYSICAL
EXAMINATION

- Seborrhea, psoriasis, and histiocytosis X are associated with rashes outside of the diaper region.

- The distribution of the diaper rash provide clues to the diagnosis: a red rash in the intertriginous areas indicates seborrhea, *Candida albicans*, or tinea cruris, while a rash on the exposed convex surfaces is suggestive of contact dermatitis.

- Evaluation of the margins of the rash assists in making the diagnosis. Satellite lesions are seen with candidal dermatitis, and sharp borders are seen with tinea curtis.

- The color may help to distinguish one rash from another. Red beefy lesions indicate candidal diaper dermatitis, salmon yellow lesions suggest seborrhea, silvery scales overlying red bases indicate psoriasis, and yellow to reddish brown papules may suggest histiocytosis X.

PHOTOGRAPHS OF SELECTED DIAGNOSES

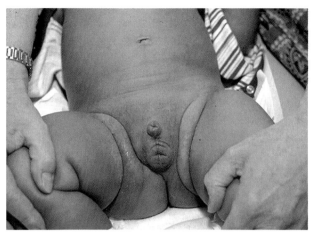

Figure 52-1 Contact dermatitis. Erythematous diaper dermatitis distributed primarily on convex surfaces with sparing of the intertriginous folds in an infant. (Courtesy of George A. Datto, III, MD.)

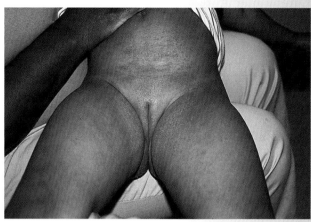

Figure 52-2 Contact dermatitis. Older child with contact dermatitis from a bathing suit. (Courtesy of George A. Datto, III, MD.)

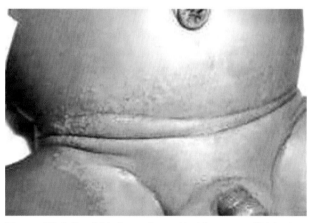

Figure 52-3 Candidal diaper dermatitis. (Courtesy of Moise L. Levy, MD.)

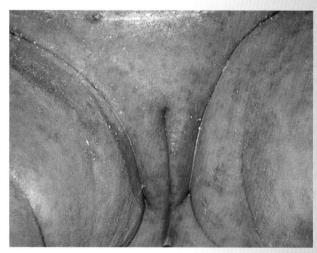

Figure 52-4 Seborrhea greasy intertriginous dermatitis with yellowish scale. (Used with permission from the Benjamin Barankin Dermatology Collection.)

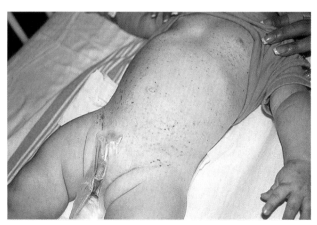

Figure 52-5 Histiocytosis. Clusters of hemorrhagic papules in groin and on abdomen. (Courtesy of George A. Datto, III, MD.)

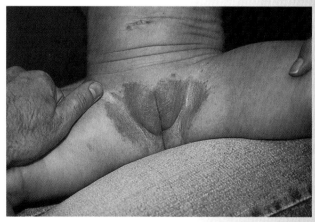

Figure 52-6 Psoriasis. Erythematous plaque with scale in diaper area; also note smaller lesions on abdomen. (Courtesy of George A. Datto, III, MD.)

DIFFERENTIAL DIAGNOSIS

DIAGNOSIS	ICD-9	DISTINGUISHING CHARACTERISTICS	DISTRIBUTION	ASSOCIATED FINDINGS
Contact Dermatitis	692.9	Spares intertriginous areas Located on convex surfaces Erosions occur occasionally	Buttocks Perineum Lower abdomen Upper thighs	N/A
Candidal Infection	112.2	Vivid beefy red color Raised edges with sharp margination White scales at the border Pinpoint satellite lesions	Buttocks Lower abdomen Inner thighs Intertriginous areas Occasionally generalized with an "id" reaction	Oral thrush
Seborrhea	690.12	Salmon-colored, greasy lesions—yellowish scale	Intertriginous areas Spares convex areas	Involvement of the scalp, face, neck, postauricular areas, and flexural areas
Tinea Cruris	110.3	Symmetrical, scaly, erythematous plaque Sharply demarcated Most common in male adolescents	Intertriginous folds near the scrotum and upper inner thighs Occasionally on buttocks, perineum Spares penis	Leukorrhea Itching Burning Painful urination
Cutaneous Candidiasis (Adolescent Female)	112.1	Redness and swelling White patches on red bases on mucosal surfaces Cheesy exudate	Labia Perineum Perianal area Gluteal folds	Pruritus
Histiocytosis X	202.56	Clusters of yellow-to-reddish brown papules with hemorrhagic qualities Hemorrhagic, seborrhea-like eruption	Groin Axilla Retroauricular areas	Bone lesions, particularly skull Premature tooth eruption Draining ears Lymphadenopathy Exophthalmos
Psoriasis	696.1	Erythematous plaques with a scaling eruption Remissions and exacerbations typical Fails to respond to usual diaper dermatitis therapies	Girls—clitoral hood to upper gluteal cleft Boys—base of penis, inner thighs, gluteal cleft	Dark red plaques with silvery scales on the trunk, face, scalp Nail involvement

COMPLICATIONS	PREDISPOSING FACTORS
Bacterial superinfection	Contact with proteolytic enzymes and irritant chemicals Alkaline pH Excessive heat and moisture Moderate to severe diarrhea Infrequent diaper changes
None	Systemic antibiotic therapy Warm, moist, occluded skin
None	N/A
Bacterial superinfection	*Epidermophyton floccosum* *Tinea rubrum* Hot, humid weather Vigorous exercise Tight-fitting clothing
None	Antibiotics Diabetes mellitus Pregnancy Oral contraceptives
Varies with extent of disease	Abnormal proliferation/accumulation of cells of the monocyte-macrophage system
None	Genetic predisposition

OTHER
DIAGNOSES TO
CONSIDER

- Acrodermatitis enteropathica

- Kawasaki disease

- Scarlet fever

SUGGESTED READINGS

Diaper dermatitis. In: Hurwitz. *Clinical pediatric dermatology.* 2nd ed. Philadelphia: WB Saunders; 1993:34–38.

Boiko S. Making rash decisions in the diaper area. *Pediatr Ann.* 2000;29:50–56.

Hansen RC, Krafchik BR, Lane AT, et al. Dealing with diaper dermatitis. *Contemp Pediatr.* 1998;(Suppl):5–14.

Ward DB, Fleischer AB Jr, Feldman SR, et al. Characterization of diaper dermatitis in the United States. *Arch Pediatr Adoles Med.* 2000;154:943–946.

Zsolway K, Harrison A, Honig P. Diaper rash in a young infant. *Pediatr Case Rev.* 2002;2(4):220–225.

53

Perineal Sores and Lesions

ALLAN R. DE JONG

APPROACH TO THE PROBLEM

The most common cause of genital irritation and bleeding in a prepubertal girl beyond the neonatal period is vulvovaginitis, and hygiene-related problems are often implicated. Other causes of postneonatal genital bleeding include genital warts, trauma, vaginal foreign body, hemangioma, tumors, and urethral prolapse. Dermatologic conditions—psoriasis; lichen sclerosis; impetigo; and seborrheic, contact, and atopic dermatitis—commonly cause rashes, pain, itching, bleeding, and fissures in the anogenital area. The distribution of the individual lesions is important for differentiating a generalized dermatitis from localized infections, trauma, and congenital lesions. The differential diagnosis of perineal sores and lesions includes child sexual abuse, which must be addressed by an experienced clinician.

KEY POINTS IN THE HISTORY

- When approaching child sexual abuse, most of the medical history, review of systems, and context and content of the child's disclosure can be obtained from adults who accompany the child without the child present. The child should be interviewed without the caretakers present, if necessary for medical management. Questioning should be nonleading, open-ended, and carefully documented.

- The key to diagnosis of sexual abuse is the clear history of sexual contact provided by the child, while the diagnosis of straddle injury is supported by a clear history of blunt genital impact particularly during a fall onto an object.

- Midline fusion defects and hemangiomas should be recognized within the first few months of life if not detected at birth.

- The history of painful oral plus genital lesions suggests herpes or Behçet's syndrome.

- The history of dermatological or allergic conditions involving other body sites should be considered because the anogenital rash, itching, pain, bleeding, or lesions may be the result of the same generalized condition.

- A history of maternal, congenital, or acquired syphilis with inadequate treatment precedes the condyloma lata of secondary syphilis.

- Genital itching typically accompanies candidal dermatitis and/or vaginitis, lichen sclerosis, and genital warts.

- Pain typically accompanies trauma (which may result from rubbing or itching), lesions from viral infections (including herpes, varicella, Epstein-Barr, coxsackie, or influenza), and Behçet's syndrome.

KEY POINTS IN THE PHYSICAL EXAMINATION

- The evaluation of a child who presents with a chief complaint of sexual abuse is often done best at a local or regional sexual abuse center. Clinicians should explain the examination in advance to the child who should be reassured that examination of the genital area by a physician is all right and that it will not be painful. A gentle, deliberate manner is appropriate, and physical force should not be used.

- The most common physical findings in cases of sexual abuse are normal or nonspecific anogenital examinations. When sexual abuse injuries are found, they are typically near the posterior midline within the vaginal vestibule and involve the hymen.

- Injuries from straddle trauma are typically unilateral or asymmetrical and anterior or anterolateral in location.

- Lesions associated with bleeding include acute straddle or sexual abuse injuries, hemangiomas, lichen sclerosis, and genital warts. Unlike most of the other lesions, hemangiomas and failure of midline fusion should be completely unchanged when reexamined 2 to 4 weeks later.

- Oral ulcerations with genital ulcerations suggest herpes virus or Behçet's syndrome.

- Lesions in nongenital areas may be found in some individuals with perineal hemangiomas, genital warts, or both.

- Molluscum contagiosum does not involve mucous membranes or palms and soles, but a rash of the palms and soles may accompany condyloma lata.

- Bilateral, diffuse labial redness usually is from vulvovaginitis, but it may also accompany lichen sclerosis.

- Hemangiomas typically blanch with pressure, but most other lesions do not.

PHOTOGRAPHS OF SELECTED DIAGNOSES

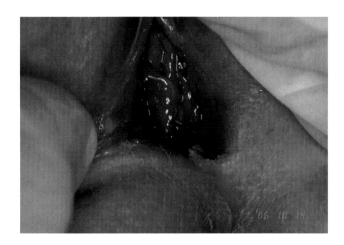

Figure 53-1 Sexual abuse, acute. Tissue edema and hemorrhage in a 19-month-old girl 4 days after penile vaginal penetration. Prominent lacerations to the vaginal wall, hymenal membrane and posterior commissure are present. (Used with permission from De Jong AR, Finkel MA. Medical findings in child sexual abuse. In: Reece R, Ludwig S, eds. *Child abuse: medical diagnosis and management.* 2nd ed. Philadelphia: Lippincott Williams & Wilkins; 2001:248.)

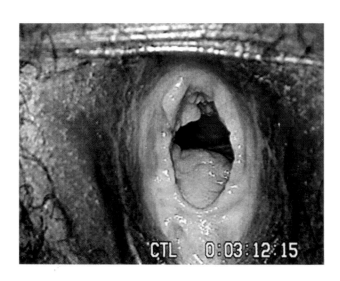

Figure 53-2 Sexual abuse, nonacute. Deep, wide posterior midline hymenal cleft extending to the vaginal wall. Cleft represents healed complete hymenal tear or transection in a 15-year-old who disclosed multiple acts of penile vaginal penetration. (Courtesy of Allan R. De Jong, MD.)

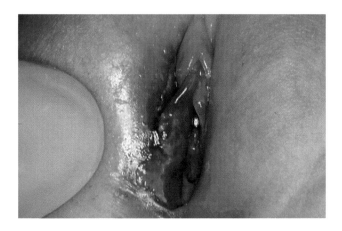

Figure 53-3 Straddle injury. Crush injury to the right labia minor and labia major in a 6-year-old who provided a clear history of a fall onto a metal bar of a jungle gym. (Used with permission from De Jong AR, Finkel MA. Medical findings in child sexual abuse. In: Reece R, Ludwig S, eds. *Child abuse: medical diagnosis and management.* 2nd ed. Philadelphia: Lippincott Williams & Wilkins; 2001:249.)

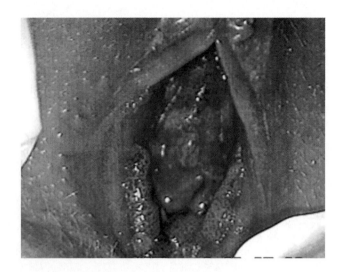

Figure 53-4 Genital warts. Multiple genital warts are seen in vaginal vestibule of 6-year-old who disclosed only digital penetration. Blood vessels in the irregular masses create the red stippling of the wart surface. (Courtesy of Allan R. De Jong, MD.)

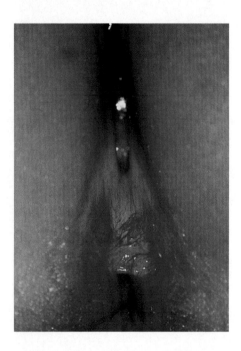

Figure 53-5 Failure of midline fusion. Midline, pale indented defect with prominent vascularity and the appearance of mucosa that was initially mistaken for trauma. (Used with permission from Bays J. Conditions mistaken for child sexual abuse. In: Reece R, Ludwig S, eds. *Child abuse: medical diagnosis and management.* 2nd ed. Philadelphia: Lippincott Williams & Wilkins; 2001:292.)

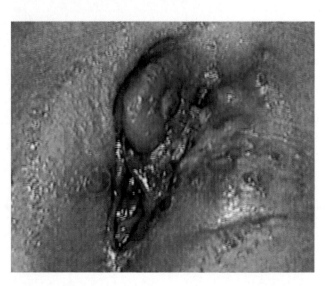

Figure 53-6 Herpes simplex virus. Multiple, painful, erythematous ulcerations on the labia of a 4-year-old girl who reported penile genital contact with an adult relative. Culture was positive for herpes simplex virus type II. (Courtesy of Allan R. De Jong, MD.)

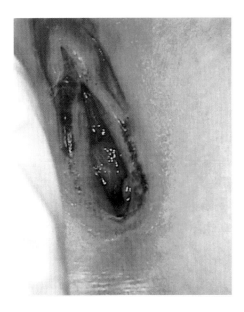

Figure 53-7 Lichen sclerosus et atrophicus. Characteristic subepidermal hemorrhages in a 4-year-old with a 3 week history of genital itching and intermittent dysuria. Lesions showed only slight improvement at follow-up weeks later. (Courtesy of Allan R. De Jong, MD.)

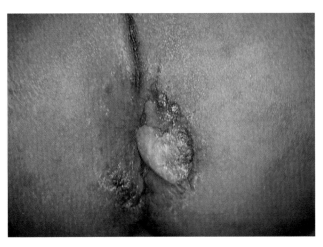

Figure 53-8 Condyloma lata. Pale hypertrophic plaque of condyloma lata in a 2-year old with previously untreated primary syphilis. (Used with permission from De Jong AR, Finkel MA. Medical findings in child sexual abuse. In: Reece R, Ludwig S, eds. *Child abuse: medical diagnosis and management.* 2nd ed. Philadelphia: Lippincott Williams & Wilkins; 2001:259.)

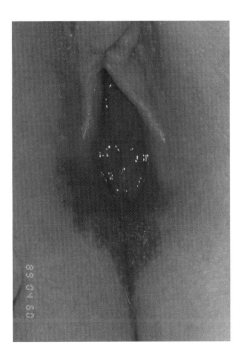

Figure 53-9 Hemangioma. Superficial, red capillary hemangioma of the posterior commissure and perineal body. Initially mistaken as an abrasion, it blanched with pressure. (Used with permission from Bays J. Conditions mistaken for child sexual abuse. In: Reece R, Ludwig S, eds. *Child abuse: medical diagnosis and management.* 2nd ed. Philadelphia: Lippincott Williams & Wilkins; 2001:290.)

DIFFERENTIAL DIAGNOSIS

DIAGNOSIS	ICD-9	DISTINGUISHING CHARACTERISTICS	DISTRIBUTION	DURATION/ CHRONICITY
Sexual Abuse	995.53	Acute—laceration or bruising of hymen Nonacute—hymenal transection or healed tear (cleft) extending to the base of hymen or vaginal wall	Injuries when present typically involve posterior one third of hymen and vestibule	Acute or nonacute Single episode or multiple episodes (chronic)
Straddle Injury	926.0	Asymmetrical bruising, swelling, or laceration accompanied by acute pain Has clear history of blunt impact or straddle event	Typically involves anterior two thirds of vulva especially the labia, periclitoral folds, or folds between labia majora and labia minora	Acute onset Resolving completely in days to weeks
Genital Warts	078.11	On mucosal surfaces, flesh-colored to pink, raised lesions with red stippling On moist skin surfaces usually multiple irregular papules, filiform, and multidigited lesions	Usually multifocal Can involve skin and mucosal surfaces	Variable duration, can grow very slowly and spontaneously Regress after months or years
Molluscum Contagiosum	078.0	Dome-shaped, skin-colored papules on nonerythematous base Often umbilicated with white center	Any body surface except palms and soles	Chronic, variable duration
Herpes Simplex Virus	054.1	Multiple vesicular and ulcerative lesions Associated with pain and erythema	Often involves both skin and mucosa May be clustered or scattered individual lesions	Acute lesions resolve within 2–3 weeks Can be recurrent
Lichen Sclerosus et Atrophicus	701.0	White, wrinkled plaques with fissures producing "parchment-like" skin Subepidermal bruising or bullae and bleeding with minor trauma	Sharp demarcation from normal skin Symmetrical "figure 8" or "hour glass" depigmentation and involvement of vulva and perianal area	Chronic but variable course; many cases improve with puberty
Hemangioma	228.0	Reddish-to-bluish flat or elevated lesions that often blanch with pressure Appearance depends on type and size of blood vessels	Often asymmetrical Single or multiple lesions	Chronic, with typically unchanging appearance
Failure of Midline Fusion	759.9 (congenital anomaly) NOS	Painless indented midline lesion Pale tissue centrally at base of lesion with normal vascularity and smooth edges bordering lesion	Midline and symmetrical lesion extending posteriorly from posterior commissure	Chronic (congenital)
Condyloma Lata	091.3	Large, moist, pale, hypertrophic plaques	Moist, warm areas including labia and perianal tissues	Chronic
Behçet's Syndrome	136.1	Painful, persisting ulcerations of vagina, vulva, and cervix associated with simultaneous oral ulcers	Genital area but not involving genitocrural folds or interlabial sulci	Chronic, relapsing pattern

ASSOCIATED FINDINGS	PREDISPOSING FACTORS
Sexually transmitted disease occasionally present Most victims show no specific injuries or infections	Multiple psychosocial risk factors, such as poor parental attachment, nonbiologically related males in household, parental drug/alcohol abuse, child with unmet emotional needs, adolescent risk taking
Rarely involves injury to hymen	Activities involving boys' bicycles, monkey bars, balance beams, and falls onto other objects or being kicked in genital area
Occasionally, warts present on hands or feet or around lips	Sexual contact Autoinnoculation Perinatal transmission Vertical transmission
Can appear inflamed or pustular when resolving	Exposure to individual infected with viral agent (5% of all children infected)
Primary infection often associated with fever and inguinal adenopathy Pain may precede rash	Caretaker or child with oral herpes (cold sores) Perinatal transmission Primary herpes gingivostomatitis Sexual contact
Peak at 6–8 years of age Itching and burning are frequent symptoms	Predilection for areas of mechanical or thermal skin injury
Can ulcerate and bleed or change slowly with involution Other nongenital lesions common	None (congenital)
Mucosal appearance Often associated with anterior placement of anal opening	None (congenital)
Secondary syphilis lesions including maculopapular or papulosquamous rash, especially on palms, soles	Untreated congenital syphilis or primary syphilis
Triad of recurrent oral ulcers, genital ulcers, and eye lesions Skin lesions and positive pathergy test (induration and erythema produced at the site of a sterile needle stick)	None

- Poor hygiene

- Seborrheic, psoriatic, atopic, or contact dermatitis

- Impetigo, streptococcal vulvovaginitis

- Labial adhesions or agglutination

- Ulcerations from varicella, herpes zoster, influenza, Epstein-Barr, or coxsackie viruses

- Stevens-Johnson syndrome

- Crohn disease

SUGGESTED READINGS

Baldwin DD, Landa HM. Common problems in pediatric gynecology. *Urol Clin North Am.* 1995;22:161–176.

Bays J. Conditions mistaken for child sexual abuse. In: Reece R, Ludwig S, eds. *Child abuse: medical diagnosis and management.* 2nd ed. Philadelphia: Lippincott Williams & Wilkins; 2001:287–306.

De Jong AR, Finkel MA. Medical findings in child sexual abuse. In: Reece R, Ludwig S, eds. *Child abuse: medical diagnosis and management.* 2nd ed. Philadelphia: Lippincott Williams & Wilkins; 2001:207–286.

Emans SJH, Laufer MR, Goldstein DP, eds. *Pediatric and adolescent gynecology.* 5th ed. Philadelphia: Lippincott–Raven Publishers; 2005:565–684, 939–975, 1024–1036.

Quint EH, Smith YR. Vulvar disorders in adolescent patients. *Pediatr Clin North Am.* 1999;46:593–606.

54

ALLAN R. DE JONG
Vulvar Swelling and Masses

Swelling and masses found in the female external genitalia include acquired and congenital lesions. Acquired lesions typically present with symptoms including masses, pain, urinary symptoms, and/or bleeding but may be found as incidental findings on examination. Congenital lesions often are recognized as masses in the perinatal period, but they may go unrecognized until later childhood. The presence or absence of symptoms and the location of the mass are essential pieces of information when considering the differential diagnosis. Some benign lesions may require surgical intervention. Malignant tumors are rare in childhood.

**KEY POINTS IN
THE HISTORY**

- Neonatal onset of swelling is common in paraurethral duct cysts, mucocolpos or hematocolpos, and inguinal hernias, but these lesions can also appear later in life. Other masses rarely present in the neonatal period.

- Painless genital bleeding or spotting is the presenting symptom in most cases of urethral prolapse and in some cases of genital tumors.

- Labial abscesses, incarcerated or strangulated hernias, or secondarily infected cysts are accompanied by acute pain, while other genital masses usually are not.

- Typically, a history of urinary tract infections, incontinence, or voiding difficulties accompanies prolapsed ureteroceles, and occasionally accompanies Gartner duct cysts and urethral prolapse. They are rarely associated with other genital masses.

- A history of intermittent swelling, particularly increasing with crying or Valsalva maneuvers, is only typical for masses caused by hernias.

- Abdominal pain, lower abdominal mass or increasing abdominal girth, and amenorrhea are common symptoms of hematocolpos or hematometrocolpos.

- A positive family history is present in 10% of children with hernias.

KEY POINTS IN THE PHYSICAL EXAMINATION

- Masses that originate or are present in the midline include urethral caruncle, urethral prolapse, prolapsed ureterocele, sarcoma botryoides, mucocolpos, and hematocolpos.

- Asymmetrical or nonmidline masses include most inguinal hernias; labial abscesses; and Bartholin, Gartner, and paraurethral duct cysts.

- Paraurethral duct cysts usually displace the urethral opening from the midline; whereas, all other common genital masses do not.

- Urethral prolapse is the only vulvar or urogenital lesion producing a circular mass surrounding the urethral opening.

- Most urogenital masses are nontender to palpation except for labial abscesses, incarcerated or strangulated hernias, or secondarily infected cysts.

- If painful, enlarged inguinal nodes accompany the mass, the mass is either a labial abscess or secondarily infected cyst.

- The presence of blood with the mass is most indicative of a urethral prolapse, but occasionally blood will accompany a sarcoma botryoides.

- Lower abdominal masses may accompany mucocolpos and hematocolpos because retained mucus and/or blood causes distention of the uterus.

DIFFERENTIAL DIAGNOSIS

DIAGNOSIS	ICD-9	DISTINGUISHING CHARACTERISTICS	ASSOCIATED FINDINGS	PREDISPOSING FACTORS
Labial Hypertrophy	624.3	Painless enlargement of labia minora in adolescents Usually bilateral, about 10% unilateral	Labia minora measure more than 4 cm in span from medial to most lateral point	None known
Inguinal Hernia	550.90 (unilateral) 550.92 (bilateral)	Bulge or lump in mons pubis or labia majora, usually unilateral Often intermittent, increases with crying or Valsalva maneuver	May include ovary, fallopian tube in hernia Only 2% to 3% have testes (testicular feminization) and rarely ovotestes (true hermaphroditism) in sac Discoloration, pain with incarceration/strangulation	Family history in 10% Male:female 8:1 Bilateral hernias in girls associated with high risk of testicular feminization
Urethral Prolapse	599.5	Circular, doughnut-shaped bright red, purple-to-blue protrusion of the urethral meatus Anterior to hymenal orifice; has urethral meatus in center Usually nontender	Typically presents with painless bleeding or spotting, but may be associated with dysuria or frequency (<25%) May present with urinary retention Predominantly in prepubertal (5- to 8-year-old) black girls (<10% white)	Hereditary disposition Urinary tract infections (UTI) Increased abdominal pressure Constipation Chronic cough Trauma Lack of estrogen
Labial Abscess	616.4	Acute, painful swelling with overlying redness or discoloration	Enlarged, tender, inguinal lymph nodes common	Trauma, obesity, excessive shaving, poor hygiene, diabetes, folliculitis, or infected cyst
Paraurethral Duct Cyst	599.84	Glistening, tense, bulging, yellowish-white mass Urethral meatus is usually displaced laterally	May cause dysuria or obstruction May cause deflected urinary stream	Most often noted in neonatal period because of congenital obstruction May be result of acquired obstruction from infection
Gartner Duct Cyst	752.11	Visible, palpable, nontender, unilateral perihymenal or perivaginal mass, in anterolateral wall of vaginal vestibule Often translucent with retained, pearly white secretions under surface	Usually asymptomatic Visible, normal vaginal and urethral openings Abnormal ureters or kidneys may be present	Congenital Vestigial remnants of mesonephric ducts
Bartholin Duct Cyst	616.2	Visible, palpable, nontender, unilateral mass, medial to labia minora, in posterior part of vaginal vestibule (5 o'clock and 7 o'clock locations) Visible, normal vaginal and urethral openings	Often asymptomatic Infected cysts are accompanied by severe pain and increased swelling	None with cysts Recurrent infection or abscess of cysts sometimes associated with STDs
Prolapsed Ureterocele	753.23	Soft, smooth cystic mass with whitish glistening surface protruding from urethral meatus Commonly presents in infancy or early childhood as urinary tract infection (UTI)	No evidence of bleeding Incontinence, voiding dysfunction common May have significant upper tract abnormalities and bladder outlet obstruction	Mostly associated with abnormal insertion of the ureter, duplicating collection system, and obstructed upper pole
Hematocolpos	626.8	Presents in neonates as mucocolpos or hydrocolpos with shiny, pearly grey-to-blue midline mass with hymen stretched over it Presents in adolescents as bulging blue-to-red midline mass covered by hymen	Urethra is superior to mass and hymenal opening is absent Can present as abdominal pain, lower abdominal mass, or amenorrhea May have other genitourinary (GU) tract anomalies	Results from imperforate hymen, transverse hymenal septum, or atretic vagina
Sarcoma Botryoides	171.6	Lobulated mass protruding or prolapsing through hymenal opening Moist, grape-like clusters	May present as spotting of blood or vaginal discharge A type of rhabdomyosarcoma	Peak incidence <2 years, 90% before 5 years of age
Urethral Caruncle	599.3	Thin, reddish polypoid mass or membrane protruding from a portion of urethral opening Usually asymptomatic	Occasionally associated with dysuria, frequency, urgency, or recurrent UTI	Cause unknown

■ PHOTOGRAPHS OF SELECTED DIAGNOSES

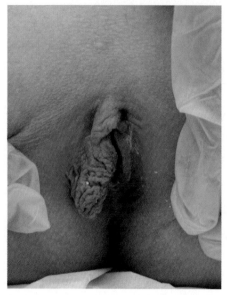

Figure 54-1 Labial hypertrophy. Unilateral hypertrophy of the right labia minor in an 8-year-old girl with Down syndrome. (Courtesy of Joyce Adams, MD.)

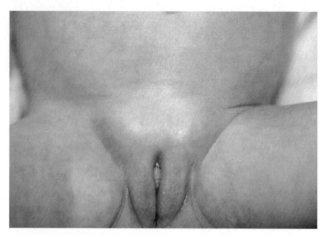

Figure 54-2 Inguinal hernia. One-month-old girl with bilateral inguinal hernias. Normal ovaries were found in the hernia sacs. (Courtesy of Allan R. De Jong, MD.)

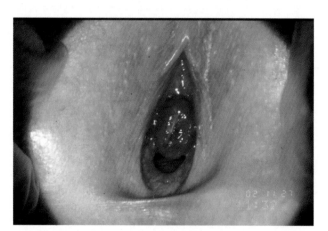

Figure 54-3 Urethral prolapse. Circular, reddish mass in the anterior midline, with the urethral opening in the center of the mass and a portion of the crescentic hymen and hymenal opening seen inferior to the mass. This 4-year-old girl presented with painless genital bleeding. (Courtesy of Tony Olsen, MD.)

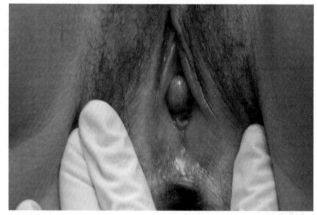

Figure 54-4 Paraurethral duct cyst. Yellowish, smooth mass in a 12-year-old with dysuria. Urethral opening is obscured, but hymenal opening is clearly visible below mass. (Courtesy of Joyce Adams, MD.)

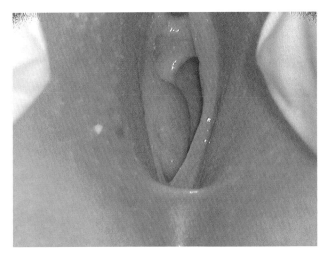

Figure 54-5 Gartner duct cyst. Cystic perihymenal mass in anterolateral wall of vaginal vestibule. Incidental finding in asymptomatic 8-year-old girl evaluated for suspected sexual abuse. (Courtesy of Jayme Coffman, MD.)

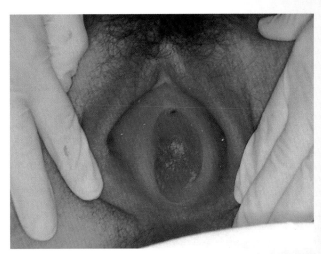

Figure 54-6 Hematocolpos. Bulging midline mass in a 14-year-old girl with imperforate hymen resulting in hematocolpos. Girl presented with amenorrhea and lower abdominal mass. (Used with permission from Fleisher GR, Ludwig S, Baskin MN, eds. *Atlas of pediatric emergency medicine.* Philadelphia: Lippincott, Williams & Wilkins; 2004:145.)

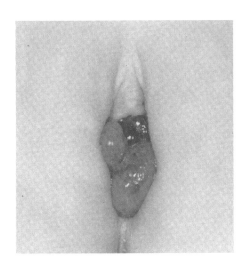

Figure 54-7 Sarcoma botryoides. Grape-like cluster of tissue protruding between the labia of a prepubertal girl. (Used with permission from Emans SJH, Laufer MR, Goldstein DP, eds. *Pediatric and adolescent gynecology.* 5th ed. Phildelphia: Lippincott–Raven Publishers; 2005:446–447.)

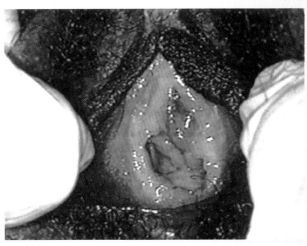

Figure 54-8 Urethral caruncle. Red polypoid mass is seen protruding from a portion of the urethral opening. Incidental finding in an asymptomatic 16-year-old girl who reported being raped 4 months earlier. (Courtesy of Allan R. De Jong, MD.)

OTHER
DIAGNOSES TO
CONSIDER

- Labial hematoma

- Lipoma

- Lymphangioma

- Henoch-Schönlein purpura

- Urethral polyps

- Hymenal cysts

- Epithelial inclusion cysts

SUGGESTED READINGS

Baldwin DD, Landa HM. Common problems in pediatric gynecology. *Urol Clin North Am.* 1995;22:161–176.

Bays J. Conditions mistaken for child sexual abuse. In: Reece R, Ludwig S, eds. *Child abuse: medical diagnosis and management.* 2nd ed. Philadelphia: Lippincott Williams & Wilkins; 2001:287–306.

Brown MR, Cartwright PC, Snow BW. Common office problems in pediatric urology and gynecology. *Pediatr Clin North Am.* 1997;44:1091–1106.

De Jong AR, Finkel MA. Medical findings in child sexual abuse. In: Reece R, Ludwig S, eds. *Child abuse: medical diagnosis and management.* 2nd ed. Philadelphia: Lippincott Williams & Wilkins; 2001:207–286.

Eilber KS, Raz S. Benign cystic lesions of the vagina: a literature review. *J Urol.* 2003;170:717–722.

Emans SJH, Laufer MR, Goldstein DP, eds. *Pediatric and adolescent gynecology.* 4th ed. Philadelphia: Lippincott–Raven Publishers; 1998:446–447.

Fleisher GR, Ludwig S, Baskin MN, eds. *Atlas of pediatric emergency medicine.* Philadelphia: Lippincott, Williams & Wilkins; 2004:145

Quint EH, Smith YR. Vulvar disorders in adolescent patients. *Pediatr Clin North Am.* 1999;46:593–606.

Scrotal Swelling

WILLIAM R. GRAESSLE

APPROACH TO THE PROBLEM

Common causes of scrotal swelling vary by age. Inguinal hernia is a common cause of scrotal swelling at any age. Spermatocele, varicocele, and primary testicular tumors are seen predominantly during adolescence. An acute scrotum may be caused by epididymitis, testicular torsion, or torsion of the testicular appendage (appendix testis torsion). At any age, generalized edema or edema in reaction to local trauma or inflammation may cause scrotal swelling that can be quite significant. Rapid diagnosis and intervention is essential when testicular torsion is suspected to prevent ischemic damage and the need for removal of the testicle.

KEY POINTS IN THE HISTORY

- A swelling present since birth suggests a hydrocele or hydrocele of the spermatic cord, while the acute onset of scrotal swelling would be more suggestive of a reactive hydrocele, testicular torsion, or epididymis.

- Fluctuation of the swelling size with physical activity or Valsalva maneuvers may be seen with a communicating hydrocele or inguinal hernia.

- A history of sexual activity, urethral discharge, or both may be present in patients with epididymitis.

- Pain, especially acute, raises the concern for testicular torsion.

- A history of nausea, vomiting, or abdominal distension in a patient with a suspected inguinal hernia suggests incarceration.

- Recurrent epididymis may be seen in patients with dysfunctional voiding.

KEY POINTS IN THE PHYSICAL EXAMINATION

- The scrotum of an adolescent male should be examined in the standing position. Varicoceles may be missed when the patient is recumbent.

- Scrotal swelling with fullness at the inguinal ring is consistent with an inguinal hernia or hydrocele of the spermatic cord.

- A smooth mass that transilluminates when a light source is applied directly to the scrotum suggests a hydrocele.

- In testicular torsion, the affected testes may appear to sit higher than the contralateral testes.

- Redness limited to the upper pole of the testis is consistent with torsion of the appendix testis.

- The testicular surface should be smooth; an irregular surface should raise suspicion for a testicular tumor.

- The presence of tenderness, firmness, or discoloration suggests incarceration or strangulation of an inguinal hernia.

- Reduction of an apparent hydrocele is consistent with a communicating hydrocele or an inguinal hernia.

- Edema affecting both sides of the scrotum may occur in patients with generalized edema (for example, in patients with hypoalbuminemia) and in patients with local trauma, including blunt trauma to the perineal area or severe perineal dermatitis.

DIFFERENTIAL DIAGNOSIS

DIAGNOSIS	ICD-9	DISTINGUISHING CHARACTERISTICS	AGE	ASSOCIATED FINDINGS	PREDISPOSING FACTORS
Varicocele	456.4	Swelling in upper part of scrotum Feels like a "bag of worms" Usually left-sided	10% to 15% of postpubertal boys	More pronounced with standing	Acute varicocele may be caused by intra-abdominal venous obstruction
Hydrocele	603.9	Swelling around testicle Normal cord palpated above the mass	Common in newborns	Transilluminates If reducible, hernia should be suspected	Congenital May be reactive to a torsion of an appendix testis
Hydrocele of the Spermatic Cord	603.9	Inguinal fluid mass not in communication with peritoneum or scrotum	Infancy	Often associated with hernia and scrotal hydrocele	Congenital
Inguinal Hernia	550.90 B/L 550.92	Reducible swelling in inguinal area	Any	Inguinal swelling may be accompanied by scrotal mass Swelling may be fixed when incarcerated	Increased intra-abdominal pressure Ventriculoperitoneal shunt or dialysis catheter (The extra fluid may make an underlying hernia apparent)
Testicular Torsion	608.2	Enlarged testicle Painful Does not transilluminate	Peak in neonates and adolescents Can occur at any age	High-riding testicle Nodular cord swelling superior to testicle	Some males predisposed because of a high insertion of tunica vaginalis on cord
Appendix Testis Torsion	608.2	Infarcted appendage may be palpated or visible (blue dot sign) at the upper pole of testis	Most commonly at the onset of puberty	Reactive hydrocele may make differentiation from testicular torsion difficult without imaging	Cause unknown
Epididymis	604.90	Enlargement and tenderness of epididymis Scrotum may be painful and swollen Testis should be normal	Adolescents Younger children with urinary tract abnormalities Older children with voiding dysfunction	Urethral discharge may be present Pyuria and bacteriuria	Commonly idiopathic Hematogenous spread of viral disease Sexually transmitted diseases
Spermatocele	608.1	Cystic swelling separate from the testis	After onset of puberty	Transilluminates	N/A
Meconium Sequestration	608.89 (mass scrotum)	Firm, nodular scrotal mass	Any	Usually calcifications on ultrasound	History of meconium peritonitis may be present
Testicular Cancer	186.9	Painless mass	More commonly adolescent or young adult	Secondary hydrocele may be present Abdominal mass, prominent inguinal lymph nodes	N/A

PHOTOGRAPHS OF SELECTED DIAGNOSES

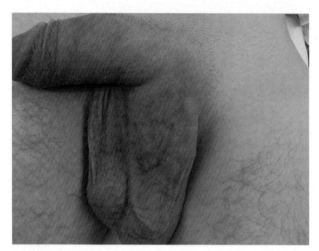

Figure 55-1 Varicocele with "bag of worms" appearance above the testicle. (Courtesy of T. Ernesto Figueroa, MD.)

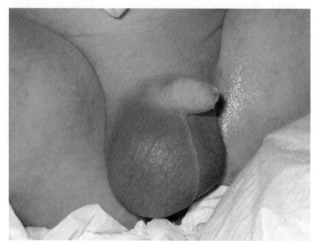

Figure 55-2 Infant with a hydrocele. (Courtesy of T. Ernesto Figueroa, MD.)

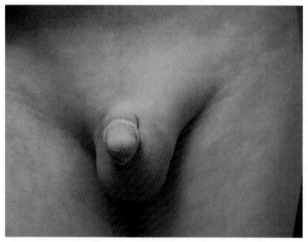

Figure 55-3 Inguinal hernia. Note the fullness near the inguinal ring. (Courtesy of Philip Siu, MD.)

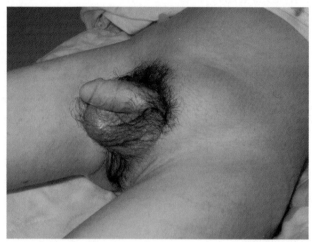

Figure 55-4 Adolescent with testicular torsion. (Courtesy of T. Ernesto Figueroa, MD.)

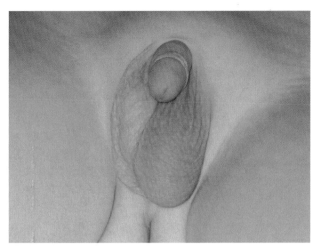

Figure 55-5 Torsion of the appendix testis with reactive hydrocele. (Courtesy of T. Ernesto Figueroa, MD.)

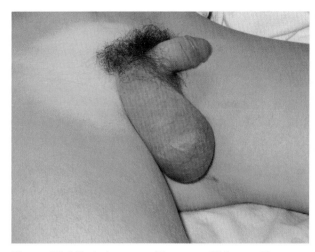

Figure 55-6 Testicular tumor. (Courtesy of T. Ernesto Figueroa, MD.)

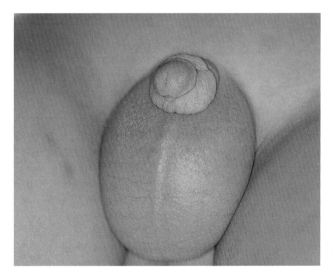

Figure 55-7 Scrotal swelling in a 7-year-old with nephrotic syndrome. (Used with permission from Fleisher GR, Ludwig S, Baskin MN. *Atlas of pediatric emergency medicine.* Philadelphia: Lippincott Williams & Wilkins; 2004:304.)

- Henoch-Schönlein purpura

- Leukemic infiltration

- Intraperitoneal hemorrhage

- Inguinal lymphadenopathy

SUGGESTED READINGS

Fleisher GR, Ludwig S, Baskin MN. *Atlas of pediatric emergency medicine*. Philadelphia: Lippincott Williams & Wilkins; 2004:304.

Kass EJ. Adolescent varicocele. *Pediatr Clin North Am.* 2001;48:1559–1569.

Kass EJ, Lundak B. The acute scrotum. *Pediatr Clin North Am.* 1997;44:1251–1266.

Kapur P, Caty MG, Glick PL. Pediatric hernias and hydroceles. *Pediatr Clin North Am.* 1998;45:773–789.

Katz DA. Evaluation and management of inguinal and umbilical hernias. *Pediatr Ann.* 2001;30:729–735.

Sheldon CA. The pediatric genitourinary examination. *Pediatr Clin North Am.* 2001;48:1339–1380.

Wan J, Bloom DA. Genitourinary problems in adolescent males. *Adolesc Med.* 2003;14:717–731.

THIRTEEN

Perianal Area and Buttocks

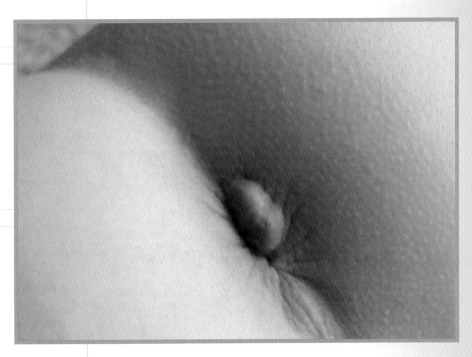

56 Perianal and Buttock Swelling

KARINA IRIZARRY AND MICHAEL J. WILSEY, JR.

APPROACH TO THE PROBLEM

Pediatricians often encounter concerns about symptoms related to the anorectal region. In children, most of these concerns represent benign entities that seldom require surgical intervention. Symptoms may include perianal masses, rectal pain, bleeding, and pruritus. Careful review of the history, with particular attention to bowel movement patterns and associated symptoms, will help guide the physical examination and facilitate identification of the problem.

KEY POINTS IN THE HISTORY

- Perirectal abscesses are more common in infants and children who are less than 1 year of age.

- Inflammatory bowel disease (IBD), human immunodeficiency virus (HIV) infection, diabetes mellitus, and neutrophil dysfunction may predispose children to develop perirectal abscesses.

- Perirectal abscesses present with perianal pruritus, redness, swelling, or a lump near the anus. They are very painful, and the pain worsens with movement, sitting, and defecation (and diaper changing in infants).

- Multiple draining midline sinus tracts that often soil underclothes with cloudy or bloodstained discharge may accompany pilonidal abscesses.

- Skin tags, rectal prolapse, and hemorrhoids in children usually result from functional constipation. A history of large, hard, and painful bowel movements and/or encopresis should be considered.

- A history of bright red, blood-streaked stools, blood dripping into the toilet, or blood seen on the toilet paper after wiping is suggestive of a perianal fissure.

- A fibrotic "sentinel" skin tag may be present over a chronic fissure.

- Large, edematous, shiny perianal skin tags should raise concern about the presence of Crohn disease.

- External hemorrhoids are varicose veins involving the skin surrounding the anus. They rarely cause symptoms.

- Acutely thrombosed external hemorrhoids present as a sudden onset of throbbing, burning pain at the end of defecation associated with a new bulge in the anal region.

- Internal hemorrhoids, which arise from the rectal submucosa, are uncommon in children and should raise concern for portal hypertension.

- Anogenital warts are often asymptomatic and found incidentally by parents or physicians.

- Anogenital warts in children may be acquired vertically during birth or by autoinoculation from common hand warts.

KEY POINTS IN THE PHYSICAL EXAMINATION

- A localized tender, well-defined, fluctuant mass may be palpated on the anal verge or on digital examination whenever there is a perirectal abscess.

- Ischiorectal abscesses are often large and visible on the surface of the buttock.

- Pilonidal abscesses occur at the site of an ingrown hair follicle and present as a midline sacral boil approximately 1 to 2 cm above the anus. If the boil spontaneously drains, it may be associated with a fistulous tract.

- A hard, painful bluish lump may be seen in the anal opening whenever there is a thrombosed, external hemorrhoid.

- Ninety percent of anal fissures are located at the six o'clock position (midposterior region), with the 12 o'clock position (midanterior region) being the next most common. Anal fissures in unusual locations should raise concern about inflammatory bowel disease (IBD), occult abscesses, and infections such as herpes or syphilis.

- Anogenital warts will turn white when soaked in 3% to 5% acetic acid (vinegar).

- Rectal prolapse may involve only the mucosa or all layers of the rectum (most commonly). In complete prolapse, concentric rings of rectal mucosal are seen herniating through the anus on examination.

- After reduction of rectal prolapse, the anal tone may be absent or decreased during rectal examination. The normal tone will return after several hours.

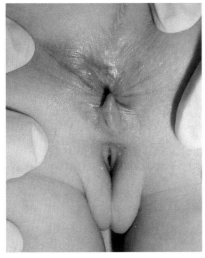

Figure 56-1 Perianal skin tag. A "sentinel" perianal skin tag seen in a female infant. (Courtesy of Mary L. Brandt, MD.)

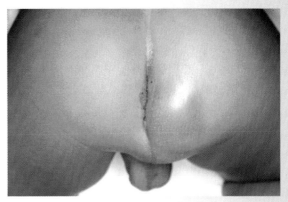

Figure 56-2 Perirectal abscess. A 12-month-old male presenting with a perirectal mass. (Courtesy of Mark A. Ward, MD.)

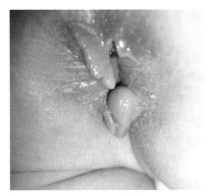

Figure 56-3 Perianal Crohn disease in a child with multiple large, edematous skin tags and a perianal fissure at the 7-o'clock position. (Courtesy of Martin Fried, MD.)

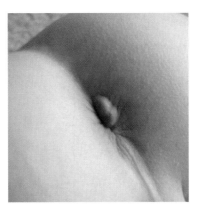

Figure 56-4 External hemorrhoid in a 2-year-old male with recurrent straining because of chronic constipation. (Courtesy of Michael J. Wilsey, Jr., MD.)

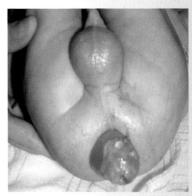

Figure 56-5 Rectal prolapse seen in a male infant. (Courtesy of Mary L. Brandt, MD.)

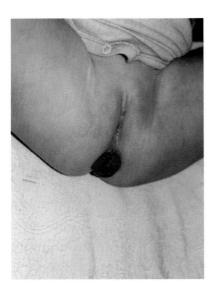

Figure 56-6 Rectal prolapse. Concentric rings of rectal mucosa (all the layers of the rectum) are seen herniating through the anus, indicating a complete prolapse. (Courtesy of Fernando L. Heinen, MD.)

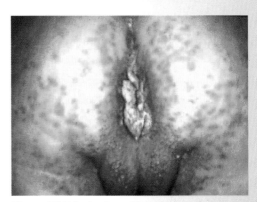

Figure 56-7 Perianal condylomata seen following sexual abuse. (Courtesy of Fernando L. Heinen, MD.)

DIFFERENTIAL DIAGNOSIS

DIAGNOSIS	ICD-9	DISTINGUISHING CHARACTERISTICS	DISTRIBUTION	DURATION/ CHRONICITY
Perirectal Skin Tag	455.9	Painless, shapeless lumps or flaps of skin or flesh Painful defecation when associated with anal fissure	Anal verge Sentinel tags form above chronic anal fissures	Chronic
Perirectal Abscess	566	Tender, fluctuant mass near anus or upon digital exam Pilonidal abscess—midline boil +/- fistula	Perianal (60%) Ischiorectal Intersphincteric Supralevator	Present until it drains spontaneously or surgically
Hemorrhoids	455.6	Firm bulge at anal verge, may have bluish discoloration Usually asymptomatic Can be acutely painful when thrombosed (external)	External (below dentate line)—most common Internal (above dentate line)—rare in pediatrics	Acute pain lasts hours to 1–2 weeks (until spontaneously or surgically corrected)
Rectal Prolapse	569.1	Painless, bright-red tissue protruding from anus In mucosal prolapse, radial folds seen at junction with anal skin In complete rectal prolapse, circular folds seen at junction with anal skin Highest incidence in the first year of life	Anal herniation of rectal mucosa	May become chronic, occurring with most bowel movements (weeks to months)
Anogenital Warts	078.19	Four types: • Condyloma acuminatum-cauliflower-like lesions • Flat-macular • Papular • Keratotic-thick, crusty Usually multiple	May be found as discrete lesions or may coalesce to form plaques	N/A

ASSOCIATED FINDINGS	COMPLICATIONS	PREDISPOSING FACTORS
Anal pruritus Rectal bleeding	Hygiene-related problems (may impair cleaning of perineum when wiping)	Constipation Fissures Fistulas Injury from rectal surgery Hemorrhoids
Fever Perianal pruritus Pain worse with defecation	Fistula Recurrence Stricture Incontinence	Infancy More common in immunosuppressed patients and patients with diabetes mellitus
Painless rectal bleeding Occasional discomfort with defecation Anal pruritus	Thrombosis Prolapse Strangulation	Constipation often precedes external hemorrhoids Portal hypertension may precede internal hemorrhoids
Pruritus Bleeding Urgency	Edema and necrosis of prolapsed tissue Fecal incontinence	Constipation Acute or chronic diarrhea Chronic lung disease Cystic fibrosis Pelvic floor weakness because of myelomeningocele, postanal surgery, or Ehlers Danlos syndrome Parasitic infestations, especially with *Trichuriasis* (whipworm) Hirschsprung disease Malnutrition Congenital hypothyroidism
Can be friable, pruritic, and painful	Cancer (very rarely)	Human papillomavirus (HPV) infection (low risk types: 6,11) Sexual abuse Autoinoculation from hand wart

<table>
<tr><td>

OTHER
DIAGNOSES TO
CONSIDER

</td><td>

- Protruding colonic polyp

- Protruding ileocecal intussusception

- Chronic solitary ulcer

</td></tr>
</table>

SUGGESTED READINGS

Blumberg D, Wald A. Other diseases of the colon and rectum. In: Feldman , Friedman, Sleisenger, eds. *Sleisenger and Fordtran's gastrointestinal and liver disease.* 7th ed. Philadelphia: WB Saunders; 2000:2294–2296.

Budayr M, Ankney RN, Moore RA. Condyloma acuminata in infants and children. A survey of colon and rectal surgeons. *Dis Colon Rectum.* 1996;39(10):1112–1115.

Johnson S, Jaksic T. Benign perianal lesions. In: Walker WA, Goulet O, Kleinman RE, et al., eds. *Pediatric gastrointestinal disease: pathophysiology, diagnosis, management.* 4th ed, vol 1. Hamilton, Ontario: BC Decker; 2004:598–601.

Pfenninger JL, Zainea GG. Common anorectal conditions: Part II. Lesions. *Am Fam Physician.* 2001;64(1):77–88.

Raimer SS. Family violence, child abuse, and anogenital warts. *Arch Dermatol.* 1992;128:842–844.

Siafakas C, Vottler TP, Andersen JM. Rectal prolapse in pediatrics. *Clin Pediatr.* 1999;38(2):63–72.

57 Perianal and Buttock Redness

APPROACH TO THE PROBLEM

Friction and exposure to excessive moisture are often the predisposing factors in many diseases that cause redness in the buttock and perianal area. The specific location of redness, whether found over convex surfaces, in the gluteal fold, in the perianal area, or in other intertriginous areas, will help to determine the specific etiology of the problem. Redness over convex surfaces may result from primary irritant diaper dermatitis or folliculitis. Perianal redness may result from several problems, including streptococcal dermatitis, pinworm infestation, candidiasis, psoriasis, and seborrheic dermatitis. Redness in intertriginous areas is often caused by candidiasis, seborrheic dermatitis, and, more rarely, psoriasis. The presence or absence of rash in other areas of the body will also assist in making an accurate diagnosis.

KEY POINTS IN THE HISTORY

- Fifty percent of infants develop primary irritant diaper dermatitis usually between 9 and 12 months of age.

- Perianal streptococcal dermatitis may present with perianal itching and rash. Rectal pain may occur with defecation, and there may be a history of bloody stools.

- Perianal streptococcal colonization may occur concomitantly with streptococcal pharyngitis.

- Streptococcal dermatitis typically is seen between the ages of 7 months to 12 years. It is more common in males.

- Pinworm infestation may present with severe nocturnal and early morning itching, enuresis, changes in bowel habits, insomnia, restlessness, anorexia, weight loss, and abdominal cramping.

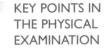 **KEY POINTS IN THE PHYSICAL EXAMINATION**

- Shiny erythematous macules and papules over convex surfaces with sparing of the creases suggest primary irritant diaper dermatitis.

- Erythema in the inguinal and other creases is suggestive of candidal diaper dermatitis.

- The presence of satellite lesions is a hallmark of candidal diaper dermatitis.

- Streptococcal dermatitis often presents as a bright red, well-demarcated, superficial, confluent redness, sometimes with associated swelling, exudate, pustules, and bleeding.

- There may be a paucity of physical findings with pinworm infestation, but excoriation may be present because of intense itching.

- Perianal erythema and desquamation may be seen in toxin-mediated disease resulting from staphylococcal or streptococcal infection, and these may be seen in Kawasaki disease.

- Psoriasis in the diaper area of an infant or toddler may not have the classic thick-silvery scale that is seen in psoriatic lesions in drier areas of the skin.

DIFFERENTIAL DIAGNOSIS

DIAGNOSIS	ICD-9	DISTINGUISHING CHARACTERISTICS	DISTRIBUTION	ASSOCIATED FINDINGS	COMPLICATIONS
Primary Irritant Diaper Dermatitis	691.0	Erythematous shiny or glazed-appearing areas with possible areas of erosion	Convex surfaces of the perineum that are maximally exposed to moisture, stool, and friction	Skin erosion with bleeding if untreated	Persistence after 48–72 hours of treatment may suggest secondary candidal or bacterial infection
Candidiasis	691.0	Confluent papular erythema with erythematous satellite papules in intertriginous areas	Groin and diaper area	Adverse effect of oral antibiotic treatment Persistently moist perirectal area Thrush in infants	Focal areas of skin erosion with possible bleeding if left untreated
Streptococcal Dermatitis	041.0	No itching Bright red, well-defined erythema	Perianal	Streptococcal pharyngitis	None
Folliculitis	704.8	Erythema surrounding the hair follicle with a small, central, yellow pustule Multiple lesions may occur	Buttocks in infants and toddlers wearing diapers	May also occur in other areas where hair follicles are present	May progress to a furuncle, a deeper infection with a larger area of erythema with a central cavity of pus May persist or spread if left untreated
Pinworm	127.4	Intense nocturnal itching Excoriations	Perianal	Restlessness Insomnia Urinary tract infection in girls	Perianal abscess Appendicitis Salpingitis

PHOTOGRAPHS OF SELECTED DIAGNOSES

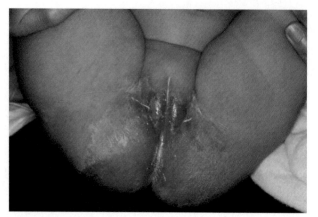

Figure 57-1 Primary irritant diaper dermatitis. Confluent areas of shiny erythema over labia majora and buttocks. (Courtesy of Jan E. Drutz, MD.)

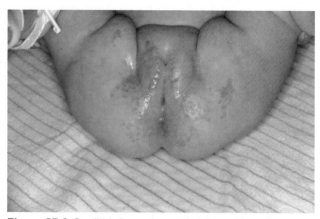

Figure 57-2 Candidal diaper dermatitis. Infant with erythematous rash with satellite lesions in the groin. (Courtesy of Jan E. Drutz, MD.)

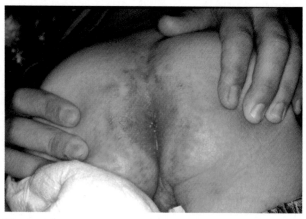

Figure 57-3 Perianal group A beta-hemolytic streptococcus (GABHS). Intense erythema is noted in the immediate perianal area of this toddler. (Courtesy of Jan E. Drutz, MD.)

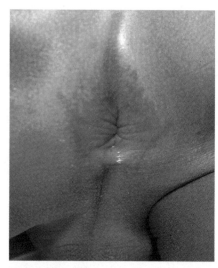

Figure 57-4 Perianal group A beta-hemolytic streptococcal infection (GABHS). Perianal streptococcal disease in an African American child. (Courtesy of George A. Datto, III, MD.)

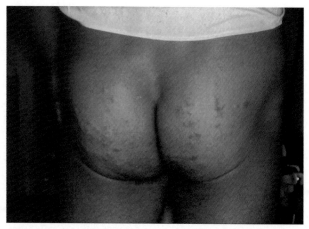

Figure 57-5 Buttock folliculitis. A child with erythematous papules over the posterior buttocks consistent with folliculitis. (Courtesy of Jan E. Drutz, MD.)

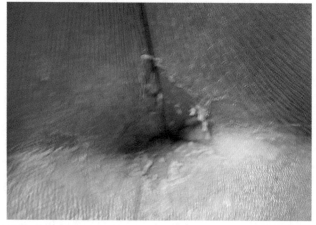

Figure 57-6 Perianal erythema and desquamation in a patient with Kawasaki disease. (Courtesy of Esther K. Chung, MD.)

OTHER
DIAGNOSES TO
CONSIDER

- Acrodermatitis enteropathica (zinc deficiency)

- Histiocytosis X

- Seborrheic dermatitis

- Granuloma gluteale infantum

- Inflammatory bowel disease (IBD)

- Sexual abuse

SUGGESTED READINGS
Brilliant LC. Perianal streptococcal dermatitis. *Am Fam Physician.* 2000;61:391–397.
Bugatti L. Filosa G. Ciattaglia G. Perianal dermatitis in a child. Perianal streptococcal dermatitis (PSD). *Arch Dermatol.* 1998;134(9):1147–1150.
Elston DM. What's eating you? Enterobius vermicularis (pinworms, threadworms). *Cutis* 2003;71(4):268–270.
Friedlander SF. Contact dermatitis. *Pediatr Rev.* 1998;(19):166–171.
Jones JE. Pinworms. *Am Fam Physician.* 1998;38(3):159–164.
Shwayder T. Five common skin problems—and a string of pearls for managing them. *Contemp Pediatr.* 2003;20(7):34–54.

58 Imperforate Anus

APPROACH TO THE PROBLEM

The imperforate anus, also termed *anorectal malformation*, is a congenital anomaly that occurs with an incidence of 1 to 4 cases/5,000 live births. Most of these anomalies are evident at birth and result from faulty development in utero of the anus, lower rectum, and urogenital tract. The imperforate anus can be classified into three main categories based on the position of the rectum relative to the puborectalis muscle. The rectum ends above the puborectalis muscle in high anomalies. Intermediate malformations develop at the same level or just below the puborectalis muscle. The low anomalies terminate below the level of the puborectalis muscle. The classification of these malformations is significant because the high anomalies are more often associated with other congenital anomalies compared to the low lesions. There is a higher incidence of both genitourinary and lower spinal abnormalities in patients with imperforate anus.

KEY POINTS IN THE HISTORY

- When evaluating an infant during the neonatal period, it is important to check the delivery record to note whether meconium was passed by the infant or was present in the amniotic fluid.

- Infants often present with delayed passage of meconium in the neonatal period (beyond 24 hours of life).

- Severe anorectal anomalies usually present with signs and symptoms of intestinal obstruction, such as abdominal distension, within 72 hours of birth.

- Diagnosis beyond the neonatal period may occur in low anorectal malformations and can present as chronic constipation (usually prior to 12 months of age) and overflow incontinence.

KEY POINTS IN THE PHYSICAL EXAMINATION

- Fistulas can present with discharge of meconium from the perineum, scrotum, vagina, or urethra. The presence of stool in the diaper does not rule out imperforate anus.

- A prominent midline groove and anal dimple indicate a low level anomaly; whereas, the absence of a midline groove and anal dimple in association with a flat perineum are seen with a high level anomaly.

- Higher defects may present with a poorly formed or absent sacrum.

- Cloaca, the most complex type of imperforate anus, is a high level anomaly with the vagina, urethra, and rectum sharing a single perineal opening.

- It is important to detect the presence of other congenital anomalies, such as musculoskeletal anomalies, cardiovascular anomalies, and dysmorphic features.

DIFFERENTIAL DIAGNOSIS

DIAGNOSIS	ICD-9	DISTINGUISHING CHARACTERISTICS	ASSOCIATED FINDINGS	COMPLICATIONS
Perineal Fistula	565.1	Small orifice in the perineum, anterior to the external sphincter	"Bucket-handle" or "black ribbon" structure, which is a subepithelial fistula filled with meconium	Associated defects are rare
Rectovestibular Fistula	619.1	Rectum opens through the vestibule, outside the hymenal orifice	Meconium is passed through the vagina	Urologic defects
Rectourethral Fistula	619.1	Rectum opens through the lower urethra (bulbar) or upper urethra (prostatic)	Meconium is passed through the urethra	Urologic defects
Rectovesical Fistula	596.1	Rectum opens through the bladder neck	Meconium is passed through the urethra	Urologic defects
Rectal Atresia	751.2	Externally normal appearing anus	Failure to pass meconium	Associated defects are rare
Cloaca	751.5	Single orifice behind the clitoris for the rectum, vagina, and urethra	Abnormally large vagina filled with mucous secretions	Urologic defects

PHOTOGRAPHS OF SELECTED DIAGNOSES

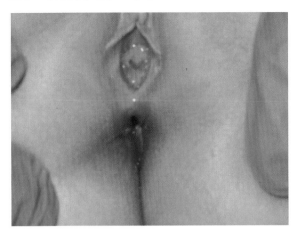

Figure 58-1 Perineal fistula opening into the perineum just posterior to the fourchette. (Courtesy of Christine Finck, MD.)

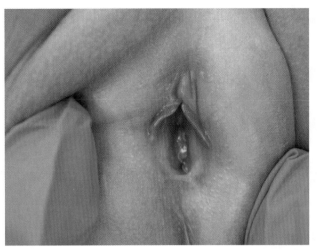

Figure 58-2 Rectovestibular fistula. While there may be a normal appearing vagina and urethra, the rectum opens through the vestibule and causes meconium to pass through the vagina. There is no visible anal orifice. (Courtesy of Mary L. Brandt, MD.)

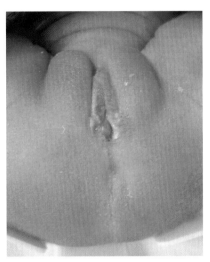

Figure 58-3 Rectovestibular fistula. The rectum opens through the posterior fourchette, and there is no visible anal orifice. (Courtesy of Mary L. Brandt, MD.)

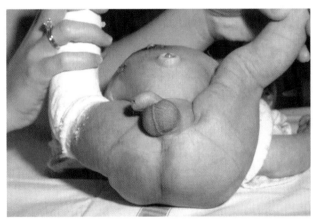

Figure 58-4 Rectourethral fistula. Meconium is passed through a fistula opening into the urethra, and there is no visible anal orifice. (Courtesy of Kevin P. Lally, MD.)

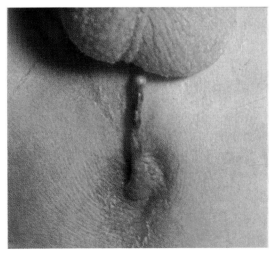

Figure 58-5 Imperforate anus without fistula. The visible meconium streak along the raphe is consistent with a low imperforate anus. (Courtesy of Kevin P. Lally, MD.)

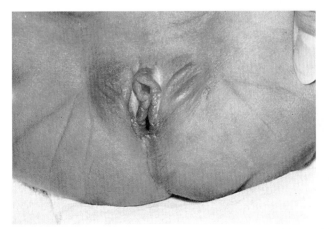

Figure 58-6 Cloaca is a high level anomaly with the vagina, urethra, and rectum sharing a single perineal opening. (Courtesy of Kevin P. Lally, MD.)

OTHER
DIAGNOSES TO
CONSIDER

- VATER—vertebral defects, anal atresia, tracheoesophageal fistula with esophageal atresia, radial and renal dysplasia

- VACTERL—above anomalies as well as additional cardiac and limb anomalies

- Sacral agenesis

SUGGESTED READINGS

Behrman RE, Kliegman RM, Arvin AM, eds. *Nelson textbook of pediatrics.* 15th ed. Philadelphia: WB Saunders; 1996:1075–1078.

Cho S, Moore SP, Fangman T. One hundred three consecutive patients with anorectal malformations and their associated anomalies. *Arch Pediatr Adolesc Med.* 2001;155:587–591.

Cuschieri A. Anorectal anomalies associated with or as part of other anomalies. *Am J Med Genet.* 2002;110:122-130.

Da Silva GM, Jorge JM, Belin B, et al. New surgical options for fecal incontinence in patients with imperforate anus. *Dis Colon Rectum.* 2004;47:204–209.

Di Lorenzo C, Benninga MA. Pathophysiology of pediatric fecal incontinence. *Gastroenterology.* 2004;126:S33–S40.

Kim HL, Gow KW, Penner JG, et al. Presentation of low anorectal malformations beyond the neonatal period. *Pediatrics.* 2000;105:E68.

Zitelli BJ, Davis HW. *Atlas of pediatric physical diagnosis.* 4th ed. Philadelphia: Mosby; 2002:606–608.

Skin

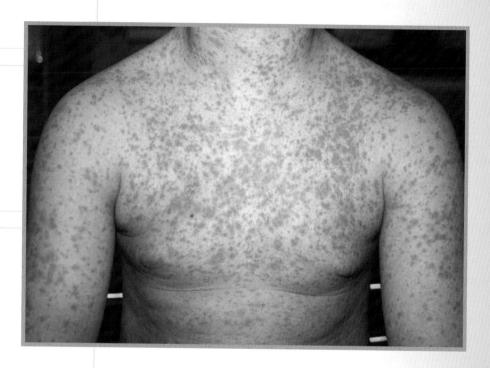

DENISE A. SALERNO

Newborn Physical Findings: Skin Abnormalities

APPROACH TO THE PROBLEM

A thorough inspection of the skin for rashes and skin abnormalities is an essential part of the newborn examination. Most skin findings are transient and very rarely require treatment, but it is important to distinguish benign skin lesions from cutaneous manifestations of more serious disorders. Knowledge and recognition of common, benign lesions of the newborn is also important in counseling parents about the natural course of these dermatological lesions.

KEY POINTS IN THE HISTORY

- A maternal history of a primary active genital herpes infection perinatally puts the infant at the highest risk for developing herpes neonatorum. A negative history from mother does not exclude the possibility of this diagnosis.

- A history of cyanosis of the hands and feet is often benign, while cyanosis of the lips and mouth is a sign of hypoxia.

- Physiologic cutis marmorata, a transient rash brought on by exposure to cold or distress, resolves once the baby is warmed. Cutis marmorata telangiectatica is always visible.

- Mongolian spots are present at birth in more than 90% of African Americans, 80% of Asians, and rarely in Caucasians.

- The lesions of epidermolysis bullosa heal slowly, while sucking blisters heal within 48 hours.

KEY POINTS IN
THE PHYSICAL
EXAMINATION

- Mongolian spots are nontender, gray-blue macular lesions primarily located on the lumbosacral area, but may be seen over the entire back and on the shoulders and extremities. Familiarity with these lesions will enable a clinician to distinguish these from ecchymoses.

- Miliaria crystallina are pinpoint vesicles containing clear fluid. The lesions are easily denuded with pressure.

- The lesions of erythema toxicum resemble flea bites.

- Erythema toxicum spares the palms and soles, while pustular melanosis may involve the palms and soles.

- Pustular melanosis may present at birth with small hyperpigmented macular lesions if the pustular phase occurred in utero.

- Milia are white pinhead-sized papules that usually occur on the face.

- Initially, neonatal acne may resemble milia, but the lesions become larger and pustular in the first month of life.

- Acropustulosis of infancy consists of extremely pruritic lesions concentrated on the palms and soles.

- Neonatal seborrhea usually involves the ears, back of neck, and shoulders. Neonatal eczema spares these areas.

- The vesicles of herpes simplex often occur on the presenting body part of the infant during birth.

- Cultures of pustular or vesicular lesions can help distinguish benign cutaneous lesions from those of infectious etiology.

PHOTOGRAPHS OF SELECTED DIAGNOSES

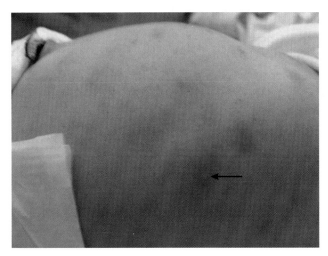

Figure 59-1 Erythema toxicum. Note the central papule with surrounding erythema. (Courtesy of Esther K. Chung, MD.)

Figure 59-2 Mongolian spots. Bluish-gray macular pigmentation on back of neonate. (Courtesy of George A. Datto, III, MD.)

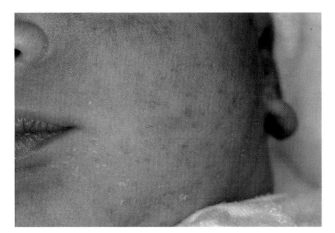

Figure 59-3 Pustular melanosis. Hyperpigmented macules with adherent white scale seen after the pustular lesions have ruptured. (Courtesy of Paul S. Matz, MD.)

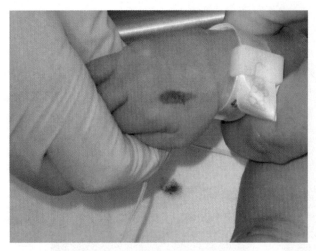

Figure 59-4 Sucking blister. The lesion on the left hand of this newborn is the result of sucking that occurred in utero. (Courtesy of Denise A. Salemo, MD.)

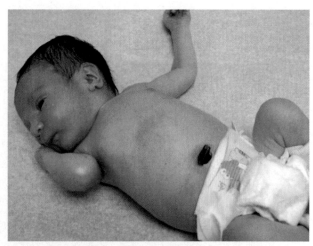

Figure 59-5 Jaundice. Physiologic jaundice. (Courtesy of Denise A. Salemo, MD.)

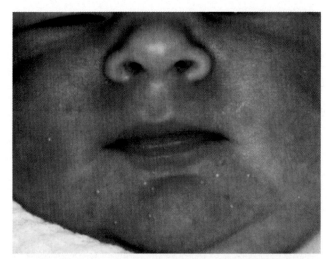

Figure 59-6 Milia. (Used with permission from Fletcher MA. *Physical diagnosis in neonatology.* Philadelphia: Lippincott Williams & Wilkins; 1998:124.)

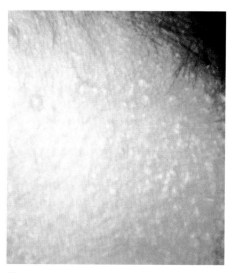

Figure 59-7 Miliaria crystallina alba. (Used with permission from Fletcher MA. *Physical diagnosis in neonatology.* Philadelphia: Lippincott Williams & Wilkins; 1998:124.)

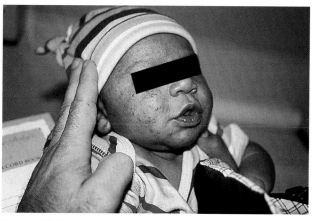

Figure 59-8 Neonatal acne. Erythematous pustular rash on cheeks of a 3-week-old neonate. (Courtesy of George A. Datto, III, MD.)

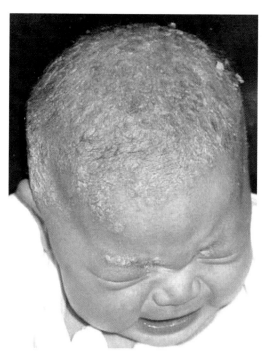

Figure 59-9 Seborrhea. Greasy, scaly lesions of scalp and eyebrows. (Courtesy of the Benjamin Barankin Dermatology Collection.)

DIFFERENTIAL DIAGNOSIS

DIAGNOSIS	ICD-9	DISTINGUISHING CHARACTERISTICS	DISTRIBUTION
Erythema Toxicum	778.8	Small white-yellow papules with surrounding flare of erythema Papules contain eosinophils	Trunk Arms Legs Face Palms and soles spared Few to several hundred
Mongolian Spots	757.33	Bluish-gray macular lesions Varying size Resulting from accumulation of melanocytes Incidence varies with ethnicity No risk of malignancy	Lumbosacral area Extensor surfaces Spares face, palms, and soles Single or multiple
Pustular Melanosis	782.1	Pustules present in utero or at birth Pustules unroof leaving brown macules surrounded by scale Pustules contain neutrophils	Chin Face Lower back Nape of neck
Sucking Blister	959.09	Bullous lesion or erosion	Finger Hand Wrist Lip
Neonatal Jaundice (Physiologic)	774.6	Usually noted at 48–72 hours Yellow discoloration of skin Spreads cephalocaudally as the bilirubin level increases	Skin Mucous membranes Sclera
Cutis Marmorata (Physiologic)	782.61	Reticulated mottling of skin Disappears with rewarming	Arms Legs Torso
Milia (Epidermal Inclusion Cyst)	706.2	Results from retention of keratin and sebaceous material within sebaceous glands Grouped whitish pin-head-sized papules Not denuded by pressure	Forehead Chin Cheeks Nose
Miliaria	705.1	Crystallina • Clear pinpoint vesicles • Appear as early as first day of life Rubra • Erythematous papules or vesicles • Appear after first week	Around hairline Face Nape of neck Upper trunk Intertriginous areas Occluded areas
Acne Neonatal	706.1	Comedones	Cheeks Forehead
Seborrhea	706.3 Infantile -690.12 Dermatitis -690.10	Greasy Red scaling Yellow crusting Nonpruritic	Scalp Diaper area Face Postauricular area Shoulder
Acropustulosis of Infancy	696.1	Pruritic papulopustules or vesiculopustules Appear in crops Recur every few weeks Topical steroids and antihistamines relieve itch	Hands Feet Wrists Ankles

DURATION/ CHRONICITY	DIFFERENTIAL DIAGNOSIS	PREDISPOSING FACTORS
Self-limited Few days to few weeks	Herpes simplex neonatorum Congenital candidiasis Miliaria rubra Staphylococcal skin infection	More common in full-term infants
Fade during childhood Seldom last into adulthood	Bruises Blue nevus	N/A
Pustular phase—24 to 48 hours Melanosis stage—Few weeks to few months	Staphylococcal skin infection Candidal skin infection	N/A
Resolve in 24–48 hours	Bullous impetigo Epidermolysis bullosa Herpes neonatorum	Results from vigorous sucking on affected part of the body in utero
Depends on severity Resolution can be accelerated by phototherapy	Gram-negative infection Biliary atresia Choledochal cyst	ABO or Rh incompatibility Excessive bruising Breastfeeding
Lasts until 6 months of life	Cutis marmorata telangiectatica congenita (CMTC) Vascular diseases Homocystinuria Down syndrome Cornelia de Lange syndrome	Physiologic response to chilling
Few weeks to few months	Hereditary trichodysplasia Orofacial-digital syndrome type I	N/A
Resolves with elimination of excessive heat	Erythema toxicum	Hot, humid weather Over-bundled infants
Resolves spontaneously over a few months	Milia	Placental transfer of maternal androgens
Scalp-improves with antiseborrheic shampoos Responds to topical steriods	Infantile atopic dermatitis Leiner's disease Histiocytosis X Psoriasis of scalp Candidal skin infection	N/A
Crops last 2–3 weeks Disorder resolves by 2 years of age	Scabies Dyshidrosis	N/A

SUGGESTED READINGS

Devillers AC, de Waard-van der Spek FB, Oranje AP. Cutis marmorata telangiectatica congenital: clinical features in 35 cases. *Arch Dermatol.* 1999;135(1):34–38.

Esterly NB, Solomen. Neonatal dermatology. III. Pigmentary lesions and hemangiomas. *J Pediatr.* 1972;81(5):1003–1013.

Fletcher MA. *Physical diagnosis in neonatology.* Philadelphia: Lippincott Williams & Wilkins; 1998:124.

Hodgman JE, Freeman RI, Levan NE. Neonatal dermatology. *Pediatr Clin North Am.* 1971;18(3):713–756.

Hurwitz S. Clinical pediatric dermatology. 2nd ed. Philadelphia: WB Saunders; 1993:7–9, 12–18, 116–117, 215–216.

Solomon LM, Esterly NB. Neonatal dermatology. I. The newborn skin. *J Pediatr.* 1970;77(5):888–894.

Treadwell PA. Dermatoses in newborns. *Am Fam Physician.* 1997;56(2):443–450.

60

Facial Rashes

GARY A. EMMETT

APPROACH TO THE PROBLEM

Facial rashes may be local processes or signs of systemic illness. The distribution (rash follows a dermatome, is asymmetric or symmetric, is a well-defined shape), the anatomical location of the rash within the skin (superficial versus subcutaneous), the classification of the rash (vesicle, papule, plaque), and the color of the rash are all potential clues to their etiology. Acne is the most common chronic facial rash seen in adolescents. The psychological consequences of all facial rashes must be considered when counseling families and addressing their treatment.

KEY POINTS IN THE HISTORY

- Acne is often the first sign of adrenal gland activation associated with the onset of puberty.

- The facial lesions of tuberous sclerosis often are misdiagnosed as acne.

- With impetigo, the gradual spread of golden-crusted, inflamed sores from the nares across the face is caused by bacterial spread from scratching.

- A family history of eczema, allergies, or asthma is almost always found in children with significant eczema.

- Facial rashes associated with skin dryness, including eczema, pityriasis alba, and lip-licking dermatitis, are often worse in the winter when there is relatively low humidity.

KEY POINTS IN THE PHYSICAL EXAMINATION

- Impetigo or tinea corporis usually presents with focal facial rashes.

- Skin lesions resulting from acute infectious systemic illnesses, such as erythema infectiosum or scarlet fever, usually are symmetric.

- Acne can present with the following types of lesions: open and closed comedones, papules, pustules, and nodulocystic lesions.

- Contact dermatitis occurs in areas exposed to the offending agent, such as under nickel-containing jewelry.

- Vesicles are seen with herpes infections, contact dermatitis, and eczema.

- Vesicular lesions that are grouped or that follow a dermatome are classic for herpes infections.

- Many forms of papules are associated with specific diseases such as the very hard, subcutaneous papules seen in tuberous sclerosis; comedones seen in acne; the small, rough papules of scarlet fever; and the polished, pearl-like lesions of molluscum contagiosum.

- Eczema, seborrhea, psoriasis, and pityriasis alba are scaly facial rashes that can be found elsewhere on the body.

- Pityriasis alba can be differentiated from tinea infections by performing a KOH examination of the scale.

- Seborrhea has a predilection for areas in which there is hair, including the scalp, eyebrows, eyelashes, and beard, but it is also found just under and behind the earlobes.

- Chronic facial rashes associated with signs of inflammation, including fever and arthritis, raise concerns for and should prompt further evaluation for autoimmune diseases.

PHOTOGRAPHS OF SELECTED DIAGNOSES

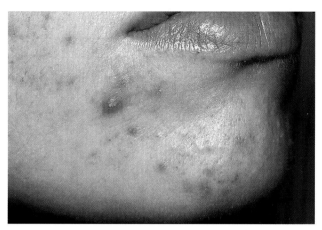

Figure 60-1 Inflammatory acne. Erythematous papules and pustules on chin. (Used with permission from Goodheart HP. *Goodheart's photoguide to common skin disorders.* 2nd ed. Philadelphia: Lippincott Williams & Wilkins; 2003:14.)

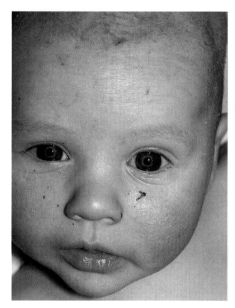

Figure 60-2 Eczema. Symmetric bilateral scaly rash on cheeks. (Used with permission from Goodheart HP. *Goodheart's photoguide to common skin disorders.* 2nd ed. Philadelphia: Lippincott Williams & Wilkins; 2003:46.)

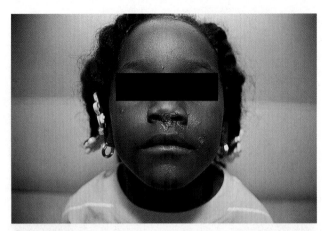

Figure 60-3 Impetigo. Honey-crusted lesions at base of nares that are self-inoculated onto other parts of the face. (Courtesy of George A. Datto III, MD.)

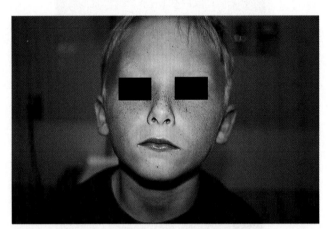

Figure 60-4 Erythema infectiosum. Bilateral erythematous macular rash on cheeks—"slapped cheeks." (Courtesy of George A. Datto, III, MD.)

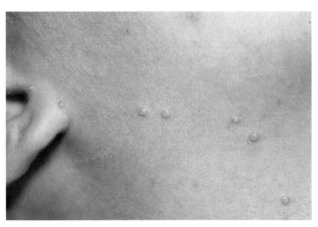

Figure 60-5 Molluscum contagiosum. Umbilicated papules on face of child. (Used with permission from Goodheart HP. *Goodheart's photoguide to common skin disorders*. 2nd ed. Philadelphia: Lippincott Williams & Wilkins; 2003:138.)

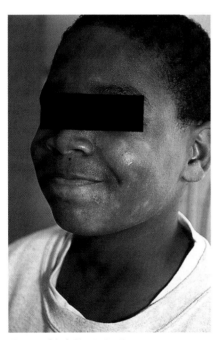

Figure 60-6 Pityriasis alba. Hypopigmented scaly macules on cheeks. (Courtesy of George A. Datto, III, MD.)

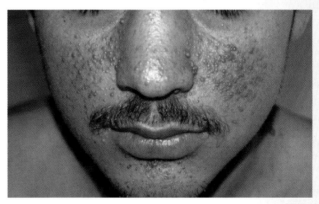

Figure 60-7 Tuberous sclerosis. Adenoma sebaceum (angiofibroma). (Used with permission from Goodheart HP. *Goodheart's photoguide to common skin disorders*. 2nd ed. Philadelphia: Lippincott Williams & Wilkins; 2003:388.)

DIFFERENTIAL DIAGNOSIS

DIAGNOSIS	ICD-9	DISTINGUISHING CHARACTERISTICS	DISTRIBUTION	ASSOCIATED FINDINGS
Acne	706.1	Open comedones—blackhead Closed comedones—whitehead Papules Nodules in dermis	Forehead Chest and back in males	N/A
Eczema	691.8	Scaly Erythema, exudation, microvesicles (acute) Lichenification (chronic)	Symmetric Cheeks, chin, forehead	Extremity lesions Pruritus Asthma Allergic symptoms
Impetigo	684.0	Golden-crusted lesions	Nares	May spread to other parts of body by self-inoculation
Seborrhea	706.3	Greasy, scaly, papules	Scalp Retroauricular Eyebrows Blepharitis External ear canal	Pruritus
Scarlet Fever	034.1	Small "sandpaper" papules	Diffuse	Pharyngitis Strawberry tongue Fever Circumoral pallor
Erythema infectiosum	057.0	Erythematous "slapped cheeks"	Cheeks Trunk Proximal extremities	Prodrome of fever, headache, symptoms of upper respiratory tract infection (URI)
Molluscum Contagiosum	078.0	Firm, pearly papules Central umbilication	Eyelids Cheeks	N/A
Pityriasis Alba	696.5	Hypopigmented Oval shaped Fine scale	Cheeks	Lesions may also be on trunk and upper arms
Adenoma Sebaceum (see with Tuberous Sclerosis)	759.5 (tuberous sclerosis)	Pink firm papules	Nasolabial folds Cheeks	Ash leaf spots Shagreen patch

COMPLICATIONS	PREDISPOSING FACTORS
Scarring Emotional impact	Adolescent Increased sebum production *Propionibacterium acnes*
Superinfection	Family history of atopic disease
Cellulitis Poststrep glomerulonephritis	Skin trauma *Staphylococcus aureus* Group A beta-hemolytic streptococci (GABHS)
Loss of hair	Infants Adolescents
Glomerulonephritis Rheumatic fever	Pyrogenic exotoxins GABHS
Arthritis Arthralgias Aplastic crisis	Parvovirus B19
Conjunctivitis Genital involvement—sexual abuse	Poxvirus
N/A	Skin dryness
Seizure Cardiac rhabdomyoma CNS tubers	Chromosome 9q34 and 16q13.3 mutations Autosomal dominant 50% new mutation

OTHER
DIAGNOSES TO
CONSIDER

- Hemangiomas

- Lipomas

- Purpura

- Dermatomyositis

SUGGESTED READINGS

Barron RP. Kainulainen VT. Forrest CR. Tuberous sclerosis: clinicopathologic features and review of the literature. *J Craniomaxillofac Surg.* 2002;30:361–366.

Goodheart HP. *Goodheart's photoguide to common skin disorders.* 2nd ed. Philadelphia: Lippincott Williams & Wilkins; 2003:14,46,138,388.

Gupta AK, Bluhm R, Cooper EA, et al. Seborrheic dermatitis. *Dermatol Clin.* 2003;21(3):401–412.

Hurwitz S. *Clinical pediatric dermatology.* 2nd ed. Philadelphia: WB Saunders; 1993:45–59,62,66,136–149,279–281,319–321,338–339,357,379–381,629–632.

Illi S, von Mutius E, Lau S, et al. The natural course of atopic dermatitis from birth to age 7 years and the association with asthma. *J Allergy Clin Immunol.* 2004;113(5):925–931.

Krowchuk DP. Managing acne in adolescents. *Pediatr Clin North Am.* 2000;47:841–857.

Silverberg N. Pediatric molluscum contagiosum: optimal treatment strategies. *Paediatr Drugs.* 2003;5:505–512.

Smolinski KN, Yan AC. Acne update: 2004. *Curr Opin Pediatr.* 2004;16:385–391.

SUSANNE KOST

Diffuse Red Rashes

61

APPROACH TO THE PROBLEM

A diffuse erythematous rash may range in significance from a minor cosmetic annoyance to a life-threatening problem. Diffuse erythema may result from toxins found in the environment, such as sunlight or certain medications, or from toxins produced by infectious organisms, such as staphylococci.

KEY POINTS IN THE HISTORY

- Typical sunburn causes erythema and pain after 30 minutes to 4 hours of sun exposure, depending on the skin type and intensity of the ultraviolet (UV) radiation.

- Photosensitizing agents, including doxycycline, sulfonamides, oral contraceptives, griseofulvin, phenothiazines, NSAIDs, some diuretics, and phytotoxins, accelerate UV toxicity; significant erythema may occur after only minutes of sun exposure.

- Patients complain of skin burning or itching with photodermatitis.

- Drug-related erythema is most often related to antibiotics, anti-epileptics, and anti-inflammatory and anti-anxiety medications and is most common within 1 to 3 weeks of starting the medication.

- Rapid intravenous infusion of vancomycin may cause the "Red Man syndrome," characterized by sudden hypotension, erythematous rash (most prominent over the upper body), urticaria, and/or respiratory distress.

- A prodrome of conjunctivitis or sore throat often precedes staphylococcal scalded skin syndrome (SSSS).

- In addition to diffuse macular erythroderma, a diagnosis of toxic shock syndrome requires four of five of the following:

  - Fever $\geq 38.9^\circ$C

  - Desquamation 1 to 2 weeks postonset

  - Hypotension

- Multisystem organ involvement of three systems—gastrointestinal (vomiting or diarrhea), muscle (severe myalgia or elevated CPK), and mucosal, renal, hepatic, hematologic or central nervous system

- Negative test results for other infections

- Nasal packing and tampon use are associated with one form of toxic shock syndrome.

KEY POINTS IN THE PHYSICAL EXAMINATION

- Erythema may be easier to detect in light-skinned individuals.

- Drug rashes usually progress proximally to distally. Although they are difficult to distinguish from viral exanthems, they are generally more intensely erythematous, confluent, and pruritic.

- Prominence in sun-exposed areas, such as nose, cheeks, and extensor surfaces, and sharp demarcations at clothing borders strongly suggest photomediated erythema.

- A staphylococcal source, such as a wound, conjunctivitis, sinusitis, pneumonia, or abscess, is often apparent in toxin-mediated infectious erythema.

- SSSS progresses from diffuse erythema to formation of large bullae characterized by a positive Nikolsky's sign.

- The rash from scarlet fever is often diffuse with intensified erythema in the groin area.

PHOTOGRAPHS OF SELECTED DIAGNOSES

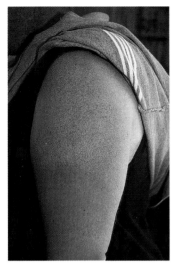

Figure 61-1 Sunburn. Diffuse erythema on lateral aspect of arm. (Courtesy of George A. Datto, III, MD.)

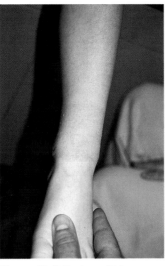

Figure 61-2 Photosensitivity. Edematous and erythematous sharp-bordered lesion that developed on ankle after sun exposure. (Courtesy of George A. Datto, III, MD.)

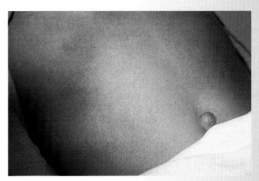

Figure 61-3 Drug rash. Erythroderma with fine morbilliform rash that developed after antibiotic exposure. (Courtesy of George A. Datto, III, MD.)

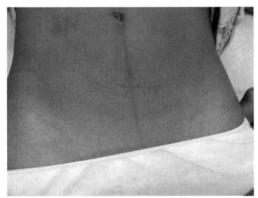

Figure 61-4 Rash seen with scarlet fever. Note the diffuse distribution of this rash that is more intense in the lower abdomen and groin. (Courtesy of Esther K. Chung, MD.)

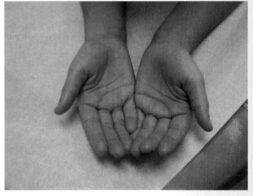

Figure 61-5 Palmar erythema. Note the intense palmer redness seen in a child with Scarlet fever. (Courtesy of Esther K. Chung, MD.)

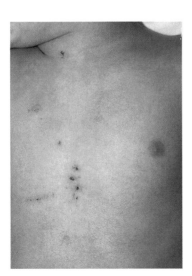

Figure 61-6 Staphylococcal scalded skin syndrome. Erythroderma and desquamation that appears on the chest secondary to impetigo caused by *S. aureus*. (Used with permission from Fleisher GR. *Atlas of pediatric emergency medicine.* Philadelphia: Lippincott Williams & Wilkins; 2004:90.)

DIFFERENTIAL DIAGNOSIS

DIAGNOSIS	ICD-9	DISTINGUISHING CHARACTERISTICS	DISTRIBUTION	ASSOCIATED FINDINGS
Sunburn	692.71	Diffuse erythema and warmth	Sun-exposed areas; sharp borders at clothing margins	Vesicles, bullae generally peaking on the second day; later desquamation
Photosensitivity	692.72	Exaggerated sunburn, sometimes associated with edema or urticaria	Sun-exposed areas; sharp borders at clothing margins	Skin burning
Drug Rash	693.0	May develop rapidly as erythroderma or evolve from coalescent macular or morbilliform rash	Generalized; mucosal surfaces usually spared	Scaling, pruritus
Scarlet Fever	034.1	Generally described as a fine, sandpapery rash. May be pruritic	May be limited to the upper torso, head, and neck or may be more diffuse. Enhanced erythema in the groin	Pruritus Desquamation Petechiae Sore throat Fever Strawberry tongue
Toxic Shock Syndrome (TSS)	040.89	Diffuse scarlatiniform erythroderma that desquamates, mucosal and conjunctival hyperemia, swelling of hands and feet	Generalized; may be more prominent in groin and axillae	High fever, myalgia, hypotension, vomiting, diarrhea, lethargy
Staphylococcal Scalded Skin Syndrome (SSSS)	695.1	Most common in 5-year olds; begins as faint macular erythema progressing in 1–2 days to tender scarlatiniform rash, then large flaccid bullae that rupture to reveal bright red "scalded" appearing skin	May be patchy or generalized	Prodrome of sore throat or conjunctivitis; fever, malaise, irritability

COMPLICATIONS	PREDISPOSING FACTORS
Fever/chills, nausea, headache, malaise if burn is extensive Potential malignant risk with blistering sunburns	Sunbathing No sunscreen use Inadequate protective clothing and hats
Inflammation may lead to chronic hyperpigmentation (sometimes in odd patterns)	Photosensitizing substance exposure (medications, plants, perfumes)
Fever, malaise, hepatosplenomegaly, jaundice, alopecia, lymphadenopathy in severe cases	Drug exposure 1–3 weeks prior to rash
Rheumatic fever Glomerulonephritis	Infection with Group A beta hemolytic streptococci
Severe prolonged shock, death (3–5% mortality)	Staphylococcal infection Tampon use
Low mortality with appropriate treatment unless immunosuppressed; heals without scarring	Staphylococcal infection

OTHER
DIAGNOSES TO
CONSIDER

- Systemic lupus erythematosus (SLE)

- Erythrodermic psoriasis

SUGGESTED READINGS

Fleisher GR. *Atlas of pediatric emergency medicine*. Philadelphia: Lippincott Williams & Wilkins; 2004:90.

Millikan LE. Feldman M. Pediatric drug allergy. *Clin Dermatol*. 2002;20:29–35.

Patel GK. Finlay AY. Staphylococcal scalded skin syndrome: diagnosis and management. *Am J Clin Dermatol*. 2003;4:165–175.

Roelandts R. The diagnosis of photosensitivity. *Arch Dermatol*. 2000;136:1152–1157.

62 Red Patches and Swellings

APPROACH TO THE PROBLEM

Common causes of skin redness or swelling include infections, vascular malformations, and autoimmune and toxin reactions. Infectious causes may be serious and need immediate treatment to prevent complications. Pain and warmth at the site of the swelling is suspicious for an infectious cause. Differentiating between infectious and allergic/toxin-mediated rashes is often based clinically on the presence or absence of pain and pruritus since both rashes tend to be erythematous and warm.

KEY POINTS IN THE HISTORY

- Redness preceded by a break or abnormality in the skin such as a wound, a bite (animal or human), or an area of eczema suggests infection.

- In the case of infection, the patient may complain of pain, swelling, fevers, chills, or worsening symptoms.

- Erythema nodosum is most commonly associated with infections, including strep infections, cat scratch disease, Epstein-Barr virus infection, tularemia, tuberculosis, and fungal infections. It may also occur with drug exposure, leukemia, lymphoma, or inflammatory bowel disease (IBD).

- In Lyme disease, erythma (chronicum) migrans appears at the site of a tick bite 7 to 14 days after tick exposure; however, only 25% of patients recall having had the tick bite.

- The only symptom that is specific for Lyme disease is the rash of erythema migrans. A variety of systemic complaints, such as fever, headache, malaise, and myalgia—although associated with early and late disease—may have other causative etiologies.

- Hemangiomas often increase in diameter, elevation, and redness over the first year of life before regressing and involuting.

- Following a spider bite, patients may feel a pinprick (black widow bite) or a sharp sting with itching and burning (brown recluse bite) at the site of redness.

- The presence of pruritus with elevated erythema suggests an allergic process.

KEY POINTS IN THE PHYSICAL EXAMINATION

- The erythema in erysipelas is circumscribed and well-demarcated with elevation above the skin.

- Cellulitic lesions appear to involve the dermis as well as subcutaneous tissues, and patches are poorly defined.

- Hemangiomas may appear in the superficial dermis as raised, lobulated, and intensely red and will appear bluer in the deep dermis. As they involute, the color becomes pearl to gray.

- Erythema nodosum lesions, painful to palpation, are classically red-to-blue, raised nodules found in the deep dermis and subcutaneous tissues in the pretibial area.

- The target lesion of erythema (chronicum) migrans should be at least 5 cm in size to make the diagnosis.

- Spider bites can be associated with severe systemic findings that may mimic acute abdomen or sepsis.

PHOTOGRAPHS OF SELECTED DIAGNOSES

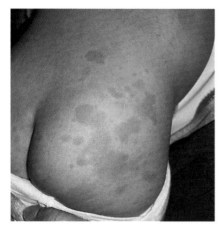

Figure 62-1 Urticaria. Erythematous wheals on buttocks of child. (Courtesy of George A. Datto, III, MD.)

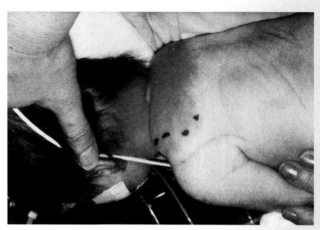

Figure 62-4 Erysipelas. Very erythematous rash on neck with sharply demarcated borders. (Courtesy of George A. Datto, III, MD.)

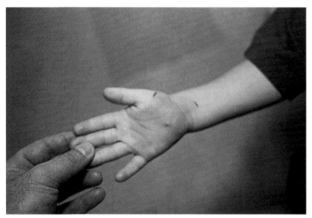

Figure 62-2 Cellulitis. Poorly defined erythematous lesion on hand that developed after skin abrasion. (Courtesy of George A. Datto, III, MD.)

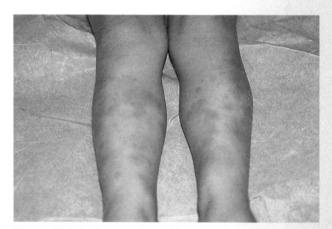

Figure 62-5 Erythema nodosum. Tender erythematous nodules on extensor aspects of lower legs. (Courtesy of George A. Datto, III, MD.)

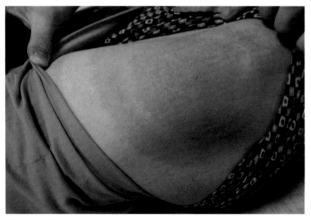

Figure 62-3 Erythema (chronicum) migrans. Note the central punctum following a tick bite and the ring-like appearance. (Courtesy of Paul S. Matz, MD.)

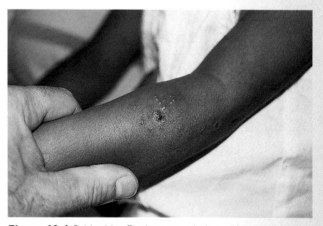

Figure 62-6 Spider bite. Erythematous lesion with central eschar following a spider bite. (Courtesy of George A. Datto, III, MD.)

DIAGNOSIS	ICD-9	DISTINGUISHING CHARACTERISTICS	DISTRIBUTION
Insect Bite	919.4	Raised, warm symmetrical lesion with central punctum	Exposed skin
Urticaria	708.9	Well-circumscribed erythematous wheals	Diffuse
Cellulitis	528.3	Poorly defined raised, warm, painful erythematous lesion	Involvement of the dermis and subcutaneous tissues 85% of cases involve the legs and feet
Hemangioma	228.0	Superficial lesions appear bright red and lobulated while deeper lesions have a bluish hue	60% head and neck 25% trunk 15% extremities
Erythema Migrans	088.81	Flat, red, uniform, circular lesion with central clearing in 40% of cases (bull's eye) and/or expanding ring lesion	Depends on the initial site of tick exposure Disseminated Lyme disease; multiple sites
Erysipelas	035	Red, warm, raised lesion with well-demarcated borders	Similar in distribution to cellulitic lesions
Erythema Nodosum	695.2	Red-to-blue, circular, raised, extremely tender nodules	Pretibial area in the deep dermis and subcutaneous tissues Other common sites include the face and arms
Spider Bites	E905.1	Black widow bites—two red punctae with local swelling Recluse spider bite—painful, red, then it blisters and becomes hemorrhagic	Distribution depends on area bitten by spider Common sites include extremities
Cutaneous Anthrax	022.0	Painless papule that enlarges into a vesicle or bulla in the first day Surrounded by redness and edema Becomes hemorrhagic, ulcerates, and is covered by a 1–5 cm black eschar	Distribution depends on the area exposed to the spore, but most commonly occurs on the upper extremities

ASSOCIATED FINDINGS	COMPLICATIONS	PREDISPOSING FACTORS
Pruritus	None	Hypersensitivity to insect venom
Pruritus Angioedema	None	Food Drugs Infections Physical factors
Fever, malaise, chills, pain.	Superinfection with gram negative or anaerobic bacteria	Preceded by breaks in the skin for any reason including abrasions, wounds, punctures, ulcerations, etc
May be associated with visceral, airway, or neurologic symptoms depending on distribution	Can be compressive in the airway or spinal cord Congestive heart failure (CHF) in large liver lesions Scarring and ulceration near mucosa surfaces	Sporadic presentation because of various defects in angiogenesis
Lesion may be itchy or painful; systemic features include fever, myalgia, headache, malaise, joint pain	Early or late disseminated Lyme disease Sequelae include meningitis, cranial neuropathies, carditis, cardiac conduction abnormalities, synovitis, and arthritis	*Borrelia burgdorferi* spirochete from the bite of the *Ixodes* (deer) tick
Fever, malaise, chills, pain	Superinfection with gram negative or anaerobic bacteria	Erysipelas is not always preceded by breech of skin integrity Prodrome of flu-like symptoms Streptococcal pharyngitis Respiratory infection
Fever Corresponding infectious or autoimmune diseases will have various associated symptoms	Self-limited	Streptococcal, yersinia, mycobacterial, or fungal infections Autoimmune causes include IBD, sarcoidosis, and spondyloarthropathies Drugs as causes include Phenytoin (Dilantin), sulfa drugs, and oral contraceptives
Black widow bites: • Severe muscle cramps • Chest pain • HTN • Tachycardia • Acetylcholinergic overload • Symptoms of uncontrolled salivation, lacrimation, urination, and defecation Brown recluse bites: • Fever • Nausea • Vomiting • Pain • Headache	Life-threatening hypertension Recluse bites—thrombocytopenia, hemolysis, and renal failure that may progress to disseminated intravascular coagulation (DIC), shock, and death	Symptoms preceded by the offending arachnid bite
Fever, headache, lethargy, impressive regional lymphadenopathy	Superinfection, overwhelming sepsis, malignant edema of the head and neck leading to SVC-type syndrome	Exposure to anthrax spores in farming, veterinary trade, laboratory exposure, or terrorist attacks

SUGGESTED READINGS

Bisno A. Current concepts: streptococcal infections of the skin and soft tissues. *N Engl J Med.* 1996;334(4):240–245.

Diekema DS, Reuter DG. Environmental emergencies. *Clin Pediatr Emerg Med.* 2001;2(3)155–167.

Edlow JA. Tick-borne diseases. *Med Clin North Am.* 2002;86(2)239–260.

Kakourou T. Erythema nodosum in children: a prospective study. *J Am Acad Dermatol.* 2001;44(1)17–21.

Sadick N. Current aspects of bacterial infections in the skin. *Dermatol Clin.* 1997;15(2)341–349.

Wenner KA, Kenner JR. Anthrax. *Dermatol Clin.* 2004;22(3)247–256.

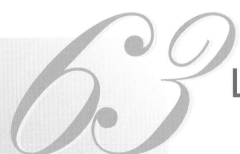

Linear Red Rashes

APPROACH TO THE PROBLEM

Linear red rashes may result from numerous causes, including congenital diseases, infectious processes, environmental exposures, or inflammatory conditions. These rashes may be isolated or may be associated with more systemic conditions. The linear nature of rashes may be subtle and missed during a cursory physical exam.

KEY POINTS IN THE HISTORY

- Age, gender, and ethnic background are important to consider because certain skin disorders show a predilection for certain populations. Girls are two to three times more likely to be affected by lichen striatus.

- Lichen striatus often starts as a small patch of papules on an extremity that expands linearly over a few months.

- Environmental exposures including clothing, outdoor activity, or occupational hazards often provide etiologic sources of linear rashes.

- The presence of pruritus is intense in scabies and rhus dermatitis.

- Scabies often causes other family members to itch.

- Recent travel to a tropical beach potentially exposes feet to parasitic eggs.

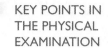

KEY POINTS IN THE PHYSICAL EXAMINATION

- Rhus dermatitis is often only present on exposed skin that is not covered by clothing.

- The presence of excoriations on the lesions suggests that the rash is pruritic.

- Lichen striatus appears hypopigmented in dark-skinned individuals.

- A pruritic rash is at risk for bacterial superinfection, which may make it difficult to diagnose the primary dermatologic condition.

- The distribution of scabies depends on the age of the child.

- The presence of linear burrows in the webbed spaces of the parent's fingers may confirm the diagnosis of scabies in their child.

- Rhus dermatitis will often demonstrate the Koebner phenomenon.

- Linear erythema without overlying epidermal changes is seen with cutaneous larva migrans and in lymphangitis.

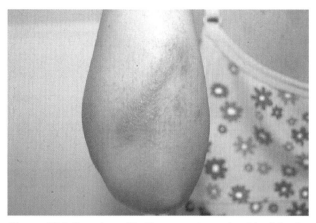

Figure 63-1 Rhus dermatitis. Linear papules and vesicles following exposure to poison ivy. (Courtesy of George A. Datto, III, MD.)

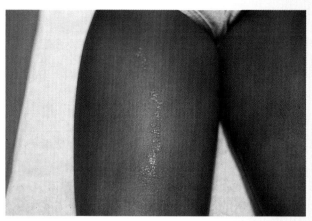

Figure 63-2 Lichen striatus. Small, shiny, hypopigmented papules in a linear distribution on the posterior thigh. (Courtesy of George A. Datto, III, MD.)

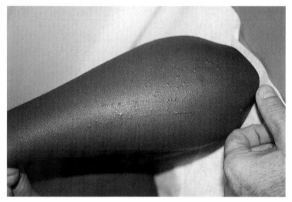

Figure 63-3 Koebner phenomenon. Papulovesicular eruption in a linear distribution on the forearm of a child with an id reaction (autosensitization dermatitis) associated with tinea capitis. (Courtesy of George A. Datto, III, MD.)

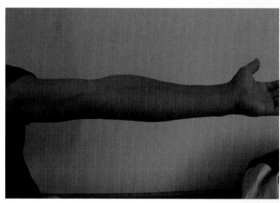

Figure 63-4 Lymphangitis. Linear red streak proximal to skin infection. (Courtesy of Paul S. Matz, MD.)

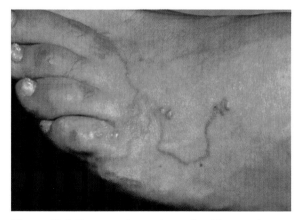

Figure 63-5 Cutaneous larva migrans. Serpiginous red streaks on sole of foot. (Used with permission from Goodheart HP. *Goodheart's photoguide of common skin disorders*. 2nd ed. Philadelphia: Lippincott Williams & Wilkins; 2003:315.)

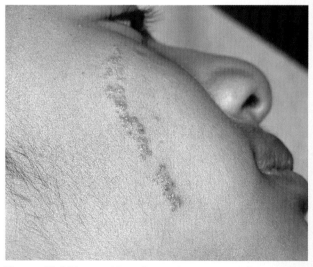

Figure 63-6 Linear epidermal nevus. Warty, linear lesions on face. (Used with permission from Goodheart HP. *Goodheart's photoguide of common skin disorders*. 2nd ed. Philadelphia: Lippincott Williams & Wilkins; 2003:9.)

DIFFERENTIAL DIAGNOSIS

DIAGNOSIS	ICD-9	DISTINGUISHING CHARACTERISTICS	DISTRIBUTION	ASSOCIATED FINDINGS
Rhus Dermatitis	692.6	Pruritic papules, vesicles, or bullae	Exposed surfaces Most commonly on arms and legs Face and groin when scratched	Koebner phenomenon
Lichen Striatus	697.8	Pink-colored papules along Blaschko's lines	Usually extremities Less common on face, trunk, and buttocks	N/A
Scabies	133.0	Linear, thread-like burrows Pruritic papules	Infant—generalized Toddler—axilla and groin Children—webs of fingers and toes	N/A
Koebner Phenomenon	N/A	Isomorphic response along site of injury	Along site of injury	N/A
Lymphangitis	682.3	Tender and warm red streaks	Proximal to the site of skin infection	Regional adenopathy Pain Fever
Cutaneous Larva Migrans	126.8	Erythematous serpiginous tracks Larvae migrate at a rate of 1–2 cm per day	Feet Hands	Regional lymph node enlargement
Linear Epidermal Nevus	216.9	Linear, warty papules	Face Trunk Extremities	N/A

COMPLICATIONS	PREDISPOSING FACTORS
Bacterial superinfection	Sap-like allergen: oleoresin Poison ivy, sumac, and oak
Hypopigmentation	N/A
Eczematous changes Bacterial superinfection	*Sarcoptes scabiei*
N/A	Warts Molluscum contagiosum Rhus dermatitis Psoriasis Lichen planus
Bacteremia Sepsis	Skin infection due to *Staphylococcus aureus* Group A streptococci
N/A	Cutaneous exposure to larval nematodes
N/A	N/A

OTHER
DIAGNOSES TO
CONSIDER

* Striae

* Linear morphea

* Contact dermatitis

SUGGESTED READINGS

Goodheart HP. *Goodheart's photoguide of common skin disorders*. 2nd ed. Philadelphia: Lippincott Williams & Wilkins; 2003:9, 315.

Hanson S, Nigro J. Office dermatology. Part II. *Med Clin North Am*. 1998:82(6):1381–1402.

Hartley A, Rabinowitz L. Advances in clinical research. *Dermatol Clin*. 1997:15(1):111–120.

Hurwitz S. *Clinical pediatric dermatology: a textbook of skin disorders of childhood and adolescence*. Philadelphia: WB Saunders; 1993:3,4,64–65,71–72,218.

Schachner L, Hansen R. *Pediatric dermatology*. New York: Churchill Livingstone; 1995.

64

Focal Red Bumps

APPROACH TO THE PROBLEM

Parents and physicians readily identify red bumps on a child's skin. The redness may be caused by vascular, infectious, or allergic etiologies. Vascular lesions tend to be chronic in nature, while infectious and inflammatory lesions have more acute presentations. Vascular lesions tend to be asymptomatic, infectious lesions are painful, and allergic lesions are generally pruritic.

KEY POINTS IN THE HISTORY

- Hemangiomas grow rapidly during the first year of life, regress, then typically show complete involution by the time the child is 3 years of age.

- Pyogenic granuloma, a vascular lesion, often has a history of bleeding easily with minor trauma.

- Impetigo is contagious and may affect other children in the household.

- An erythematous bump is found at the site of a cat scratch in 50% of patients who present with lymphadenitis caused by cat scratch disease.

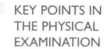

KEY POINTS IN THE PHYSICAL EXAMINATION

- Pyogenic granuloma occurs most often in areas that sustain trauma, such as the face, fingers, and forearms.

- A punctum is found at the center of a red bump because of an insect bite.

- The swelling caused by an insect bite is erythematous, indurated, and warm but not very painful on examination.

- The swelling from an insect bite has very sharp margins as compared to the more diffuse swelling associated with an infectious etiology.

- Impetigo caused by *Staphylococcus aureus* presents as bullous lesions, while impetigo caused by beta-hemolytic streptococcus is more often crusted.

- Purulent, blood-tinged discharge may be expressed from a furuncle when firm pressure is applied around the lesion.

- Strawberry hemangiomas are bright red or purplish red, while cavernous hemangiomas are bluish and have less distinct borders.

PHOTOGRAPHS OF SELECTED DIAGNOSES

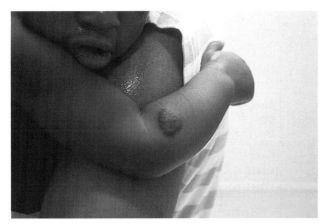

Figure 64-1 Hemangioma on the forearm of an infant with darkly pigmented skin. The lesion appears more purple in color than red. (Courtesy of George A. Datto, III, MD.)

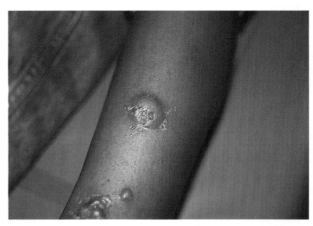

Figure 64-2 Insect bite on extensor surface of lower leg. The patient gets similar lesions every summer. (Courtesy of George A. Datto, III, MD.)

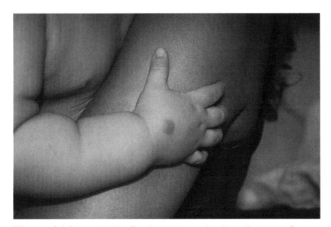

Figure 64-3 Insect bite. Erythematous wheal on dorsum of hand. (Courtesy of George A. Datto, III, MD.)

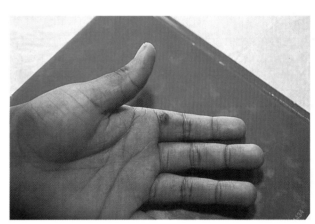

Figure 64-4 Pyogenic granuloma A lobulated vascular nodule on finger. (Courtesy of George A. Datto, III, MD.)

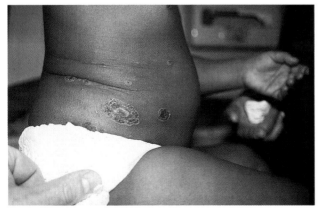

Figure 64-5 Ecthyma. Erythematous papules that develop central-adherent central crust. (Courtesy of George A. Datto, III, MD.)

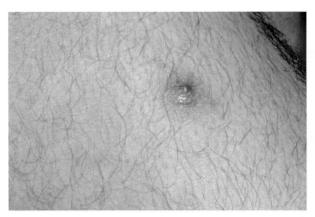

Figure 64-6 Furuncle. Painful, red, tender nodule on thigh. (Used with permission from Goodheart HP. *Goodheart's photoguide of common skin disorders.* 2nd ed. Philadelphia: Lippincott Williams & Wilkins; 2003:126.)

DIFFERENTIAL DIAGNOSIS

DIAGNOSIS	ICD-9	DISTINGUISHING CHARACTERISTICS	DISTRIBUTION	ASSOCIATED FINDINGS
Hemangioma	228.0	Raised, red, lobulated, vascular tumor	Head Neck Trunk	None
Insect Bite	919.4	Urticarial wheal with central punctum	Arms Legs May occur anywhere on the body	None
Pyogenic Granuloma	686.1	Bright red, firm nodule	Face Hands Forearms	None
Impetigo	684.0	Crusted, erythematous papule Bullous lesion	Face Nares Extremities	Pain at site Fever Lymphadenopathy
Ecthyma	686.8	Erythematous papule that progresses to punched out, crusted ulcer	Trunk	None
Cat Scratch Disease	078.3	Small, indurated, erythematous papule at site of cat scratch	Hands Forearm Neck	Regional lymphadenopathy Fever
Furuncle	680.0	Red, tender, nodule Central necrosis Purulent discharge	Hairy skin areas	None

COMPLICATIONS	PREDISPOSING FACTORS
May compromise vital function of eyesight (when on eyelid), breathing (when involving the larynx), Kasabach-Merritt syndrome	Female gender
Superinfection	Exposed skin Brightly colored clothes
May bleed easily with trauma	Trauma to skin
Cellulitis	Beta-hemolytic streptococci *Staphylococcus aureus* Traumatized skin
Scar formation upon healing	Beta-hemolytic streptococci
Prolonged fever Hepatitis Encephalopathy	Scratch by kitten *Bartonella henselae*
Cellulitis	Folliculitis Skin trauma

- Trauma

- Glomus tumor

- Infected cysts

SUGGESTED READINGS

Bhurmba NA, McCullough SG. Skin and subcutaneous infections. *Prim Care.* 2003;30:1–24.

Bruckner AL. Hemangiomas of infancy. *J Am Acad Dermatol.* 2003;48:477–493.

Goodheart HP. *Goodheart's photoguide of common skin disorders.* 2nd ed. Philadelphia: Lippincott Williams & Wilkins; 2003:126.

Weston WI, Lane AT, Morelli JG, eds. *Color textbook of pediatric dermatology.* 3rd ed. St. Louis: Mosby; 2002.

65

KATHLEEN CRONAN

Raised Red Rashes

APPROACH TO THE PROBLEM

Raised red rashes, common in pediatrics, often present a cause for concern among parents and practitioners. The majority of raised red rashes are not indicative of serious illness. Many red rashes have associated symptoms that may be helpful in making a final diagnosis. For example, symptoms of fatigue, fever, and lymphadenopathy suggest infectious mononucleosis. Complications occur in some individuals with certain red rashes. For example, exposure of a pregnant woman to parvovirus may place her fetus at risk. At times, typical eruptions may not follow a predicted pattern—the distribution may be atypical, the season may not fit, or the age may be unusual. These diagnostic challenges emphasize the importance of a detailed history and astute observation.

KEY POINTS IN THE HISTORY

- High fever for 3 to 5 days followed by acute defervescence that precedes the rash eruption is characteristic of roseola.

- Antibiotic exposure is associated with a drug rash and erythema multiforme.

- Individuals acutely affected by infectious mononucleosis are at risk for rash development following exposure to penicillin.

- Pruritus is typical in erythema multiforme, hot tub folliculitis, and scabies.

- Seasonal occurrence can provide clues to the diagnosis: late summer and fall (coxsackie virus); spring and fall (erythema multiforme).

- The location of rash origin is important. For example, a red rash that begins on the scalp and travels downward is characteristic of measles.

- Family members with a similar rash may suggest scabies.

- Classic characteristics in the history aid in the diagnosis. For example, a history of "slapped cheeks" indicates Fifth's disease; the presence of Koplik spots denotes measles.

KEY POINTS IN THE PHYSICAL EXAMINATION

- Erythema may be more apparent in light-skinned children.

- The size and types of papules may support specific diagnoses: fine micropapules indicate scarlet fever; target lesions denote erythema multiforme.

- The color of the lesions aids in the diagnosis of the rash: rose pink lesions are seen in roseola; red maculopapular lesions, in measles; and brownish lesions on the palms and soles, in syphilis.

- Red lesions on the palms and soles are present in syphilis, measles, erythema multiforme, scabies, and Gianotti-Crosti syndrome.

- Symmetric lesions may be noted in erythema multiforme, syphilis, and Gianotti-Crosti syndrome.

- Diffuse mucosal inflammation (urethritis, conjunctivitis, pharyngitis) is seen with Kawasaki disease.

- There are often oral mucous membrane findings in infectious, mononucleosis, erythema multiforme, Kawasaki disease, and measles.

- Conjuctivitis is seen in Kawasaki disease and measles.

- The rash follows lines of skin cleavage in syphilis.

- Periorbital edema is associated with roseola and infectious mononucleosis.

PHOTOGRAPHS OF SELECTED DIAGNOSES

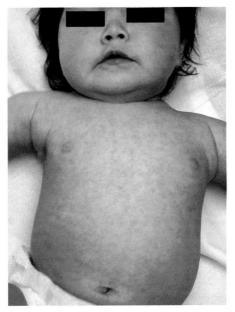

Figure 65-1 Roseola. (Courtesy of John Loiselle, MD.)

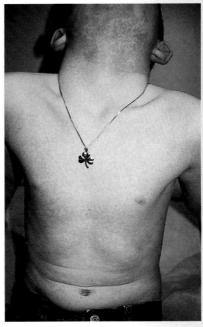

Figure 65-2 Scarlet fever. (Courtesy of George A. Datto, III, MD.)

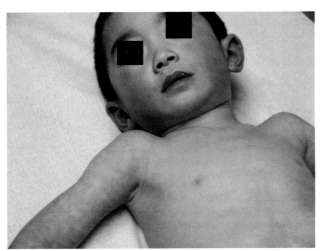

Figure 65-3 Erythema infectiosum. Erythematous "slapped" cheeks along with erythematous rash on extensor surfaces of arms. (Courtesy of Philip Siu, MD.)

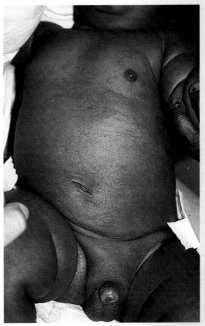

Figure 65-4 Kawasaki disease. Erythematous maculopapular rash that started in groin and spread onto trunk. (Courtesy of George A. Datto, III, MD.)

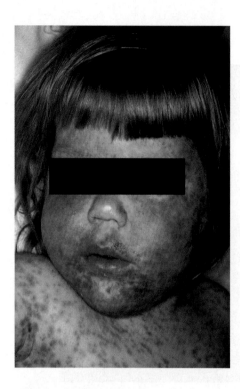

Figure 65-5 Infectious mononucleosis. (Courtesy of Kathleen Cronan, MD.)

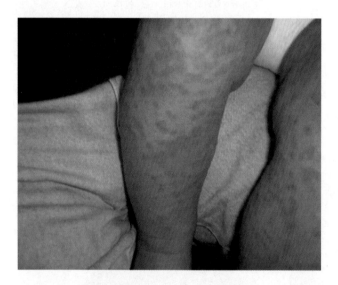

Figure 65-6 Gianotti-Crosti Syndrome. Note the reddish-brown papular lesions on extremities. (Courtesy of John Loiselle, MD.)

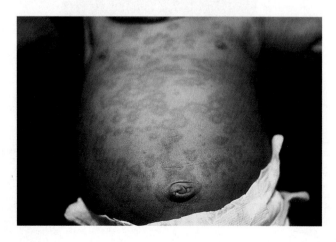

Figure 65-7 Erythema multiforme. (Courtesy of George A. Datto, III, MD.)

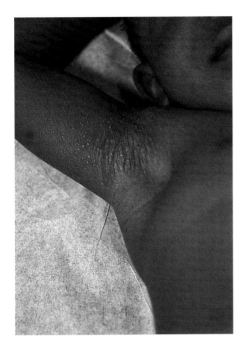

Figure 65-8 Scabies. Note the lesions in the axilla of a child. (Courtesy of George A. Datto, III, MD.)

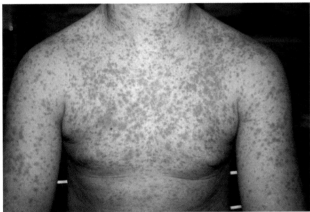

Figure 65-9 Measles. (Courtesy of Kathleen Cronan, MD.)

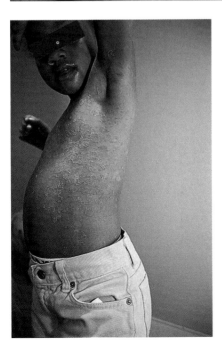

Figure 65-10 Unilateral laterothoracic exanthema. (Courtesy of George A. Datto, III, MD.)

DIFFERENTIAL DIAGNOSIS

DIAGNOSIS	ICD-9	DISTINGUISHING CHARACTERISTICS	DISTRIBUTION
Roseola	057.8	Rose-pink lesions that blanch with pressure Rarely coalesce <2 years of age	Trunk Extremities Neck
Scarlet Fever	034.1	Erythematous punctate rash that blanches with pressure Generalized sandpaper rash School age	Begins in axillae and groin then generalizes Often seen on the face and neck areas
Erythema Infectiosum	079.99	Three stages: • Erythematous malar blush "slapped cheeks" • Erythematous maculopapular eruption on extensor surfaces of the extremities • Lacy reticulated pattern	Face Extremities Trunk Proximal extremities
Kawasaki Disease	446.1	Maculopapular to morbilliform rash <5 years of age	Often starts in groin
Infectious Mononucleosis	075	Macular or maculopapular Morbilliform eruption Exanthem occurs in 10% to 15% of patients Adolescents	Trunk Upper arms Face Forearms Thighs
Gianotti-Crosti Syndrome	782.1	Monomorphous red to red-brown papules 1–6 years of age	Begins on extensor surfaces of legs and arms Buttocks Cheeks Symmetric distribution
Erythema Multiforme (Minor)	695.1	Papules that develop into erythematous ring with dusky center (target lesion)	Trunk, face, neck, palms, soles, dorsal hands and feet; extensor surfaces of arms and legs Oral lesions—buccal mucosa
Scabies	133	Papules, pustules, vesicles Linear burrows	Infants—trunk, palms, soles, neck, face Older children—flexural areas, interdigital spaces, wrists, axillae
Measles	055	Erythematous maculopapular lesions followed by brawny desquamation Enanthem—Koplik spots	Progresses from scalp to hairline to face to neck to upper extremities to trunk to upper and lower extremities to feet
Asymmetric Lateral Exanthem of Childhood (Asymmetric Periflexural Exanthem)	05.78	Pink-red, scaly papules Initial eruption—unilateral palms, soles, and face spared	Axilla Torso
Hot Tub Folliculitis	704.8	Pruritic papules may change to pustules or nodules Occurs 1–2 days after exposure	Torso Hot tub exposed areas

ASSOCIATED FINDINGS	COMPLICATIONS	PREDISPOSING FACTORS
Rash preceded by high fever Periorbital edema Leukopenia	Febrile seizures	Human herpes virus 6
Fever, malaise, sore throat, palatal petechiae, abdominal pain, pharyngo-tonsillitis, strawberry tongue Pastia lines	Glomerulonephritis Rheumatic fever	Group A beta-hemolytic streptococcus (GABHS)
Low-grade fever Aches and pains Mild arthritis Arthralgia Cold symptoms	Red-cell aplasia Nonimmune fetal hydrops	Parvovirus B19
High fever for 5 days Lymphadenopathy Swelling of hands and feet Mucositis	Coronary artery aneurysms	Unknown
Fever Headache Malaise Pharyngitis Lymphadenopathy Periorbital swelling Splenomegaly Hepatomegaly	Splenic rupture Neurological symptoms Hemolytic anemia	Epstein-Barr Virus
Fever Cough Lymphadenopathy Hepatomegaly in hepatitis B–associated cases	None	Viral infections Hepatitis B virus infection
Low-grade fever Arthralgias Malaise	None	Viral infections Recurrent herpes infections Drugs
Intense pruritus	Secondary infection Id reaction Eczematous changes	*Sarcoptes scabiei*
Cough Coryza Fever Conjunctivitis Ill appearance	Pneumonia Encephalitis	Paramyxovirus
Pruritus Localized lymphadenopathy Fever Sore throat Vomiting Diarrhea	None	Unknown
Occasional fever Malaise Headache	Cellulitis	*Pseudomonas aeruginosa*

- Drug eruptions

- Urticaria

- Contact dermatitis

SUGGESTED READINGS
Carder KR. Weston WL. Atypical viral exanthems: new rashes and variations on old themes. *Contemp Pediatr.* 2003;12:111–127.
Cohen BA. A baby, a cutaneous lesion—and an efficient approach to recognition and management. *Contemp Pediatr.* July 2004;28–50.
Hurwitz. *Clinical pediatric dermatology.* Philadelphia: WB Saunders; 1993:347–366.
Mancini AJ. Exanthems in childhood: an update. *Pediatr Ann.* 1998;27:163–170.
Shwayder T. Five common skin problems—and a string of pearls for managing them. *Contemp Pediatr.* 2003;34–54.

66 Vesicular Rashes

SHIRLEY P. KLEIN

APPROACH TO THE PROBLEM

A vesicle is a circumscribed, raised lesion filled with clear fluid and measuring less than 1 cm. A fluid-filled lesion that is 1 cm or greater is a bulla. The etiology of the vesicular rash may be infectious, allergic/contact/reactive, or congenital/inherited. Children with herpetic vesicular rashes have the potential to be quite ill, especially as neonates or when they have an underlying immunodeficiency. Smallpox and chickenpox, which once were common causes of vesicular rashes, have been eliminated (smallpox) or have diminished significantly (chicken pox) with vaccines.

KEY POINTS IN THE HISTORY

- Distinguishing whether the lesions are painful or pruritic can be helpful in differentiating vesicular rashes.

- Season may suggest etiology: varicella is more common in the spring, poison ivy and papular urticaria in the late spring through fall, and hand-foot-and-mouth disease in late summer and early fall.

- A vaccinated child can still acquire varicella because the varicella vaccine is not 100% effective, and milder breakthrough cases occur with increasing frequency over time.

- The incidence of zoster is 30 times lower in children who received vaccine compared to children who had a history of chicken pox.

- Patients with zoster often have a prodrome of pain, tingling, or burning in the affected dermatome.

- Zoster that presents with severe dermatomal disease or organ involvement should raise suspicion of an underlying immunodeficiency syndrome.

- A newborn with a vesicular rash on a presenting part or who appears toxic should be suspected of having herpes even when the mother does not have a history of genital herpes.

- Recurrent herpes simplex may occur at the site of previous infection or more commonly on the nearby lip, because the virus remains latent in the dorsal nerve root ganglia.

- Lesions of papular urticaria result from a delayed hypersensitivity reaction from the bite of cat or dog fleas. Usually, only one person in the family is affected—most commonly a toddler or preschooler.

- The last case of naturally occurring smallpox in the world was in 1977, but the threat of biologic warfare or bioterrorism has increased awareness of this disease.

KEY POINTS IN THE PHYSICAL EXAMINATION

- Children with smallpox are severely ill with lesions appearing primarily on the extremities that are all in the same stage, and these progress from papules to vesicles to pustules to crusts with each stage lasting 1 to 2 days.

- Lesions of chicken pox are predominantly on the trunk, nearly always on the scalp, and in different stages (macules, papules, vesicles) with rapid evolution to crusts, usually within 1 day.

- Zoster can affect any dermatome with the thorax being the most common and the facial dermatomes associated with the highest morbidity. Herpes zoster rarely crosses the midline.

- Vesicles that are present in a newborn or develop within 48 hours suggests intrauterine herpes simplex infection, often resulting in premature birth with other findings of congenital infection, such as microcephaly.

- The lesions of hand-foot-and-mouth disease often are found initially on the medial aspect of the feet as small papules that progress to palmar, plantar, and oral vesicles.

- More severe cases of papular urticaria include vesicles and bullae as well as the typical erythematous papules.

- Linear vesicles suggest a contact dermatitis.

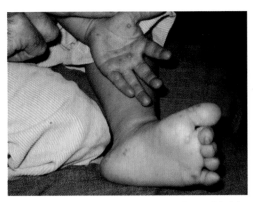

Figure 66-1 Hand-foot-and-mouth disease. Vesicles on palms and soles. (Courtesy of Philip Siu, MD.)

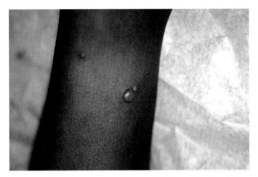

Figure 66-2 Papular urticaria. Vesicular lesion following an insect bite on the lower leg of a child. (Courtesy of Shirley P. Klein, MD.)

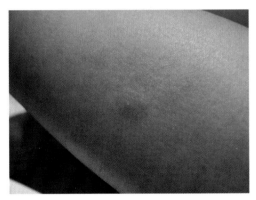

Figure 66-3 Breakthrough varicella. Note the "dew-drop-on-a-rose-petal" appearance of this lesion in a child previously immunized against varicella. (Courtesy of Esther K. Chung, MD.)

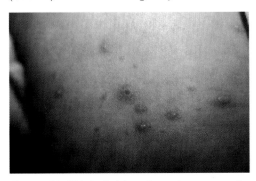

Figure 66-4 Varicella. Note the various stages of the lesions: papular, vesicular, and crusted lesions. (Courtesy of Shirley P. Klein, MD.)

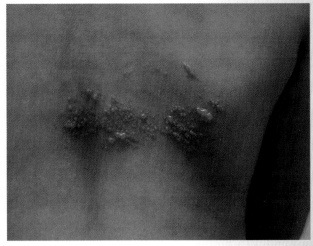

Figure 66-5 Herpes zoster. Grouped vesicles on an erythematous base in a dermatomal distribution. (Courtesy of Hans Kersten, MD.)

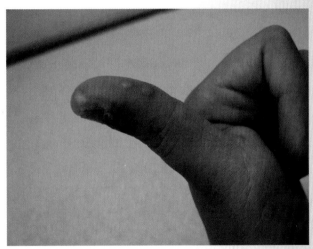

Figure 66-6 Herpetic whitlow. A group of vesicular lesions on the distal phalanx. (Courtesy of Paul S. Matz, MD.)

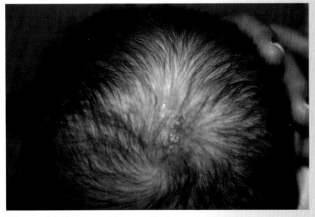

Figure 66-7 Neonatal herpes. Scalp erythema and vesicle at site of scalp electrode. (Courtesy of Shirley P. Klein, MD.)

DIFFERENTIAL DIAGNOSIS

DIAGNOSIS	ICD-9	DISTINGUISHING CHARACTERISTICS	DISTRIBUTION	ASSOCIATED FINDINGS
Hand-Foot-and-Mouth Disease	074.3	Irregular and elongated vesicles	Posterior palate, pharynx, palms, soles, and buttocks	Oral lesions: painful Extremity lesions: asymptomatic
Contact Dermatitis	692.9	Linear vesicles, erythema, oozing	Site of contact with allergen	Pruritus
Papular Urticaria	698.2	Crops of papules with urticarial flare and progress to vesicles	Mainly lower legs, other exposed areas	Pruritus
Chicken pox (varicella)	052.9	Crops of lesions, different stages, "dew-drop-on-a-rose-petal"	Trunk, face, scalp, less on extremities, rarely on palms and soles	Fever (mild) at onset Pruritus All lesions usually crusted by day 6
Herpes Zoster	053.9	Several clusters of vesicles on an erythematous base	Unilateral, 1–3 sensory dermatomes	Localized pain Hyperesthesias Pruritus
Herpetic Whitlow	054.6	Group vesicles on distal phalanx	Distal phalanx	Swelling of distal phalanx Pain
Herpes Simplex	054.9			
Primary	054.9	Mainly oral lesions or inoculated from saliva	Anterior buccal mucosa, gums, and tongue	Fever up to 10 days Submandibular/cervical nodes
Recurrent	054.9	Triggered by physical or mental stress	At or near site of previous lesions	Pain or tingling preceding rash
Neonatal	054.9		Scattered clusters; frequently at site of scalp monitor electrode	
CNS (Central Nervous System)	054.3	Skin lesions may occur late in illness		Fever, irritability Septic neonate
Sepsis	054.5			Multi-organ involvement
Smallpox	050.9	Severely ill Lesions all the same stage	Mainly face and extremities, usually including palms and soles	Fever for 10 days

COMPLICATIONS	PREDISPOSING FACTORS
Dehydration Rare: meningitis, encephalitis, and paralytic disease	Coxsackie A16 or Enterovirus 71
Periorbital swelling	Sensitizing agent such as Rhus plant, nickel, other allergens
Secondary bacterial infection	Insect bites (delayed hypersensitivity)
Secondary bacterial infections Cerebellar ataxia Encephalitis	Varicella-zoster virus
Immunocompromised children have risk of viremia	Varicella-zoster virus reactivation
Bacterial superinfection Iatrogenic complications from misdiagnosis as paronychia	Oral vesicles that child self-inoculated onto finger
Dehydration Pain Recurrent erythema multiforme Disseminated intravascular coagulation (DIC) Meningitis High mortality without early recognition	HSV-1 and HSV-2 (HHV-1 and HHV-2), oral and skin usually type 1 and genital and neonatal usually type 2
Mortality rate of 30%	Variola (pox virus, VARV) Vaccinia

- Acropustulosis of infancy

- Incontinentia pigmentii

- Pemphigus

- Scabies

SUGGESTED READINGS

Centers for Disease Control and Prevention. Secondary and tertiary transfer of vaccinia virus among U.S. military personnel—United States and world-wide, 2002–2004. *MMWR*. 2004;53:103–105.

Cohen BA. *Pediatric dermatology*. 3rd ed. Philadelphia: Elsevier Mosby; 2005:101–117,115.

Eichenfield LF, Frieden IJ, Esterly NB. *Textbook of neonatal dermatology*. Philadelphia: WB Saunders; 2001:201–206.

Feigin RD, Cherry JD, Demmler GJ, et al. *Textbook of pediatric infectious diseases*. 5th ed. Philadelphia: WB Saunders; 2004:1791–1792,1884–1892,1962–1969,1972–1977,2005–2011.

Hurwitz S. *Clinical pediatric dermatology*. 2nd ed. Philadelphia: WB Saunders; 1993:318–327,359–364.

Pickering LK, ed. *Red book*. 26th ed. Elk Grove Village: American Academy of Pediatrics, 2003:269–270,344–347,672–673,680–682.

67

WILLIAM R. GRAESSLE

Nonblanching Rashes

APPROACH TO THE PROBLEM

The child who presents with a nonblanching rash requires careful evaluation. Purpuric lesions, including petechiae and ecchymoses, usually result from vascular injury or disorders of hemostasis. The underlying etiology may be trauma, a simple viral infection, or a more serious condition such as leukemia or a bleeding disorder. When a nonblanching rash is seen in association with fever, serious bacterial infection, including meningococcemia, must be considered.

KEY POINTS IN THE HISTORY

- A history of fever makes an infectious etiology more likely.

- Acute presentation of a nonblanching rash would be more concerning than a rash that has been present for more than a couple of weeks.

- The location and pattern of spread may give a clue to the diagnosis: Rocky Mountain spotted fever (RMSF) tends to begin peripherally; Henoch-Schönlein purpura (HSP) tends to primarily involve the lower extremities and buttocks.

- The presence of photophobia, headache, or both in association with a nonblanching rash raises the suspicion for meningococcal or other bacterial meningitis.

- A history of trauma may be the cause of the nonblanching lesions: localized bruising may follow blunt trauma, and petechiae may be seen in areas of friction or scratching.

- Significant ecchymotic lesions in the absence of trauma should raise the suspicion for child physical abuse or a bleeding disorder.

- Forceful coughing or vomiting may cause petechiae, particularly in the face and upper chest.

- Accompanying fatigue may be caused by anemia because of bone marrow suppression or infiltration as seen with leukemia.

- A history of tick bites or opportunity for exposure to ticks by geography or activities should raise suspicion for RMSF or ehrlichiosis.

- Mongolian spots are present from birth and do not undergo color changes over time in contrast to ecchymoses, which change over time and eventually resolve.

- A history of easy bruising or excessive bleeding in the patient or a family history of a bleeding disorder should raise the suspicion for a bleeding disorder such as hemophilia or von Willebrand's disease.

- Familiarity with home remedies, such as coining and cupping, is essential.

KEY POINTS IN THE PHYSICAL EXAMINATION

- Petechiae are nonblanching macules up to 2 mm in diameter caused by extravasation of blood from capillaries. Mucosal bleeding sometimes is referred to as "wet purpura."

- Forceful coughing or vomiting may cause petechiae on the face and chest, above the nipple line.

- Purpura, seen with inflammatory injury to the smaller blood vessels, are elevated, firm, hemorrhagic plaques located predominantly on dependent surfaces.

- Ecchymoses are larger areas of bleeding into the skin. There is a characteristic change in color as they age, changing from red to purple to green to yellow-brown as the heme is degraded.

- Deep bleeding and hemarthroses are seen with clotting factor deficiencies, whereas petechiae are more commonly seen with thrombocytopenia.

- Ecchymoses that are not explained easily by accidental trauma should raise suspicion of child abuse. Ecchymoses, uncommonly caused by infection, usually are indicative of trauma—accidental and nonaccidental—or a bleeding disorder.

- Cupping and coining are practices used by some Asian cultures to treat acute illnesses. Each has a characteristic appearance, and petechiae and ecchymoses may be seen in both.

DIFFERENTIAL DIAGNOSIS

DIAGNOSIS	ICD-9	DISTINGUISHING CHARACTERISTICS	DISTRIBUTION	ASSOCIATED FINDINGS	PREDISPOSING FACTORS
Mongolian Spots	757.33	Blue-gray lesions with indistinct borders present from birth, no color or size changes with time as one would see with ecchymoses	Most commonly in lumbosacral area, but upper back, shoulders, and extremities also commonly affected	No reddened appearance	Congenital Ethnicities with darker skin, including Asians, Hispanics, and those of African descent
Child Physical Abuse	995.54	Ecchymoses in unusual locations or unusual patterns	Anywhere on the body	Retinal hemorrhages, swelling of extremities, unusual skin marks, bucket handle fractures, spiral fractures, multiple rib fractures, subdural hematomas	Teens and single parents, poverty, substance abuse, domestic violence, and parents who were physically abused as children Young and mentally retarded children are at greater risk
Henoch-Schönlein Purpura	287.0	Initially urticarial, progresses to palpable purpura	Typically, buttocks and extensor surfaces of extremities, but any area of body may be involved	Abdominal pain, vomiting, periarticular and joint swelling, scrotal edema Elevated ESR and thrombocytosis	Preceding upper respiratory infection (URI) or other viral syndrome
Rocky Mountain Spotted Fever	082.0	Initially macular, gradually develops petechial, purpuric, and ecchymotic features	Begins around ankles and wrists; progresses to involve the entire body, including palms and soles	Fever, chills, severe headache, myalgias, and GI symptoms (nausea, vomiting and diarrhea)	Tick bite Most commonly eastern and southern United States 90% occur between April and September
Idiopathic Thrombocytopenic Purpura	287.3	Petechiae, ecchymoses, and mucosal bleeding	Generalized petechiae	Child otherwise well-appearing	Preceding viral illness in 50% to 65% of cases Most commonly 1–4 years of age
Purpura Fulminans	286.6	Palpable purpura, undergoes necrosis	Symmetrical distribution Often begins on dependent surfaces	Ill-appearing child with features of septic shock—hypotension, poor perfusion	Commonly caused by meningococcemia, but may be seen with other bacterial causes of sepsis
Coining	782.7	Linear ecchymotic lesions	Usually back or chest	Usually performed on an individual with an acute illness	Vigorous rubbing with coin or spoon after application of a medicated ointment
Cupping	782.7	Petechiae, ecchymoses, and occasionally first-degree and second-degree burns	Cups placed in area of discomfort—back, abdomen	Usually performed on an individual with an acute illness	Cup applied to skin after igniting alcohol to create a vacuum

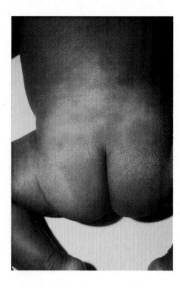

Figure 67-1
Mongolian spots. Blue nevi in the typical sacral area. (Courtesy of Sidney Sussman, MD.)

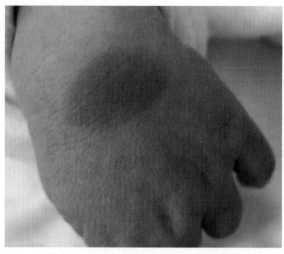

Figure 67-2 Mongolian spot on the hand. (Courtesy of Esther K. Chung, MD.)

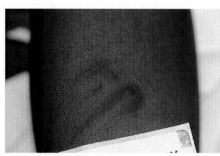

Figure 67-3 Child physical abuse. Curvilinear bruising from a looped cord. (Used with permission from Fleisher GR, Ludwig S, Baskin MN. *Atlas of pediatric emergency medicine.* Philadelphia: Lippincott Williams & Wilkins; 2004:425.)

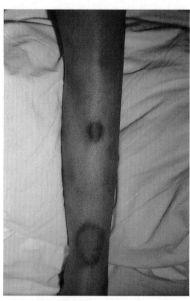

Figure 67-4 Ecchymoses in a patient with hemophilia. (Courtesy of Sidney Sussman, MD.)

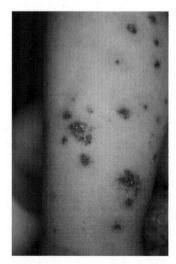

Figure 67-5 Henoch-Schönlein purpura (HSP). Note the palpable purpura on the posterior aspects of this child's leg. (Courtesy of Steven Manders, MD.)

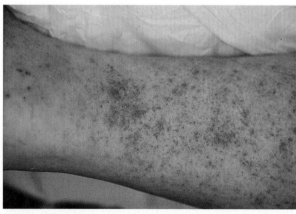

Figure 67-6 Rocky Mountain spotted fever (RMSF). Note the multiple petechial lesions on the forearm. (Courtesy of Steven Manders, MD.)

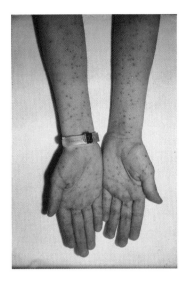

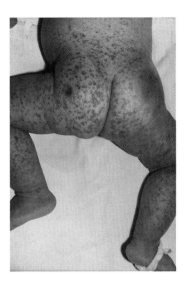

Figure 67-7 Rocky Mountain spotted fever. (Courtesy of Sidney Sussman, MD.)

Figure 67-8 Petechiae and ecchymoses in a patient with idiopathic thrombocytopenic purpura. (Courtesy of Sidney Sussman, MD.)

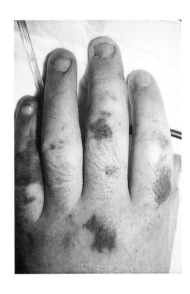

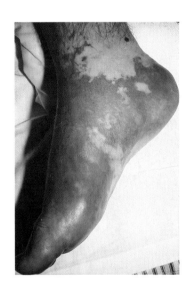

Figure 67-9 Purpura fulminans in a patient with meningococcemia. (Courtesy of Steven Manders, MD.)

Figure 67-10 Purpura fulminans. Purpura on the foot of the same patient in Figure 67.9. (Courtesy of Steven Manders, MD.)

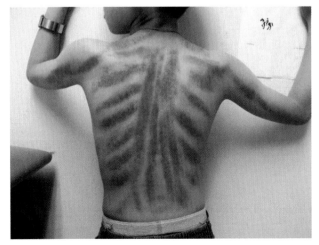

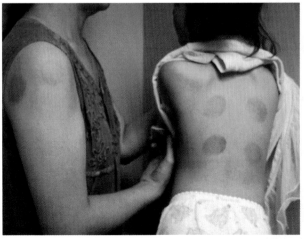

Figure 67-11 Coining. Note the linear petechiae and ecchymoses over the back that are characteristic for this healing practice used by some Asian cultures. (Courtesy of Philip Siu, MD.)

Figure 67-12 Cupping. Note the circular bruises on the mother's arm and the child's back that are the result of cupping, a healing practice used by some Asian cultures. (Courtesy of Philip Siu, MD.)

OTHER
DIAGNOSES TO
CONSIDER

- Leukemia

- Aplastic anemia

- Hemolytic-uremic syndrome

- Systemic lupus erythematosus (SLE)

- Liver disease

- Coagulation disorders

- Drug-induced thrombocytopenia

- Wiskott-Aldrich syndrome

SUGGESTED READINGS

Darmstadt GL. Purpura. In: Long SS ed. *Principles and practice of pediatric infectious diseases.* 2nd ed. New York: Churchill Livingstone; 2003:437–440.
Fleisher GR, Ludwig S, Baskin MN. *Atlas of pediatric emergency medicine.* Philadelphia: Lippincott Williams & Wilkins; 2004:425.
Leung AKC, Chan KW. Evaluating the child with purpura. *Am Fam Physician.* 2001;64(3):419–28.
Mudd SS, Findlay JS. The cutaneous manifestations and common mimickers of physical child abuse. *J Pediatr Health Care.* 2004;18(3):123–129.
Singh-Behl D, LaRosa SP, Tomecki KJ. Tick-borne infections. *Dermatol Clin.* 2003;21(2):237–244.

Scaly Rashes

APPROACH TO THE PROBLEM

The most common scaly rash in pediatrics is atopic dermatitis (eczema), which affects 10% to 15% of the pediatric population. While eczema tends to be chronic in nature, some patients have symptoms primarily during cold and dry weather. Other common causes of scaly rash include pityriasis rosea, tinea corporis, and seborrhea. Psoriasis and ichthyosis are less common. Initial lesions of pityriasis may at times be mistaken for tinea corporis, and ichthyosis may at times be mislabeled as severely dry skin. In general, most dry and scaly rashes tend to be pruritic in nature.

KEY POINTS IN THE HISTORY

- The duration of symptoms will help to distinguish acute and subacute rashes, such as tinea corporis, from more chronic conditions, such as eczema.

- A family history of atopy should raise suspicion for eczema.

- A solitary lesion may suggest tinea corporis or may be the herald patch seen in pityriasis rosea.

- Tinea corporis worsens with topical steroids, whereas eczema generally improves.

- Eczema on the face of young infants may have a circular area of erythema and may be mistaken by less experienced providers for tinea corporis.

- Cold weather generally exacerbates eczema.

- In pityriasis rosea, the rash often starts as a single isolated lesion followed by a more generalized rash occurring 5 to 10 days later.

- In the event a child shares a bed with another individual who denies pruritus or rash, a diagnosis of scabies is unlikely.

- Psoriasis affects 1% to 3% of the population, but it is uncommon in African American populations.

KEY POINTS IN THE PHYSICAL EXAMINATION

- Seborrhea generally stays within the hairline, whereas psoriasis extends beyond the hairline.

- Lesions associated with tinea corporis tend to be round, whereas the herald patch in pityriasis rosea is oval.

- The generalized rash of pityriasis rosea classically runs parallel to the lines of skin cleavage, in a "Christmas-tree" distribution.

- Postinflammatory hypopigmentation commonly occurs following eczema, pityriasis, and tinea. Hypopigmentation can be distressing to families; therefore, discussing this early in the course of the disease may be helpful.

- Patients with eczema often have dry skin, keratosis pilaris, or both.

- Lichenification is pathognomic of chronic atopic dermatitis when it appears in the expected distribution.

- Often, allergic shiners and Dennie-Morgan lines are seen in individuals with atopic dermatitis.

PHOTOGRAPHS OF SELECTED DIAGNOSES

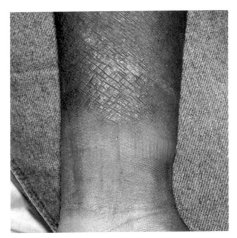

Figure 68-1 Atopic dermatitis. This lesion shows no evidence of active inflammation. Lichenification and postinflammatory hyperpigmentation are apparent. (Used with permission from Goodheart HP. *Goodheart's photoguide to common skin disorders.* 2nd ed. Philadelphia: Lippincott Williams & Wilkins; 2003:44)

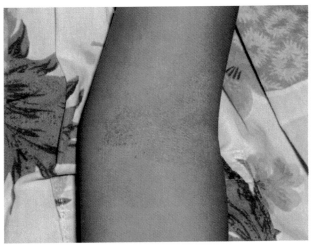

Figure 68-2 Atopic dermatitis. Note the areas of dryness, hypo- and hyperpigmentation and lichenification in the antecubital fossa of this 5-year-old. (Courtesy of Esther K. Chung, MD.)

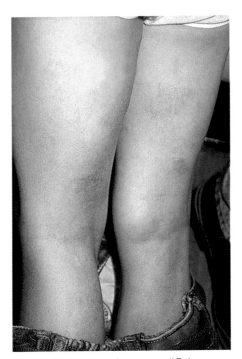

Figure 68-3 Nummular eczema. "Coin-shaped" patches and plaques are located on the legs. (Used with permission from Goodheart HP. *Goodheart's photoguide to common skin disorders.* 2nd ed. Philadelphia: Lippincott Williams & Wilkins; 2003:87)

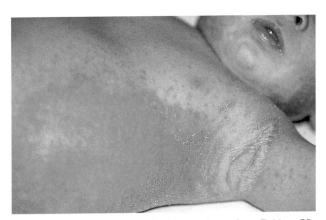

Figure 68-4 Seborrhea. (Used with permission from Fleisher GR, Ludwig S, Baskin MN. *Atlas of pediatric emergency medicine.* Philadelphia: Lippincott Williams & Wilkins; 2004:85)

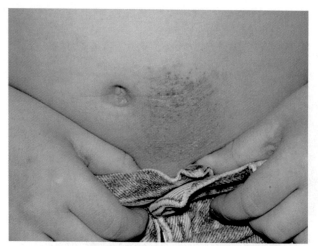

Figure 68-5 Allergic contact dermatitis. This boy developed an eczematous eruption at the site where the nickel snap on his blue jeans contacted his skin. (Used with permission from Goodheart HP. *Goodheart's photoguide to common skin disorders.* 2nd ed. Philadelphia: Lippincott Williams & Wilkins; 2003:67)

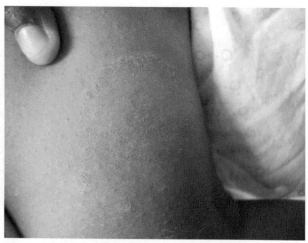

Figure 68-6 Herald patch of pityriasis rosea. (Courtesy of Paul S. Matz, MD.)

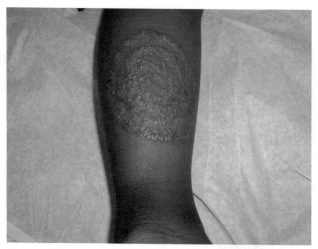

Figure 68-7 Tinea corporis. Note the large size of this lesion that was made worse by the use of topical steroids. (Courtesy of Esther K. Chung, MD.)

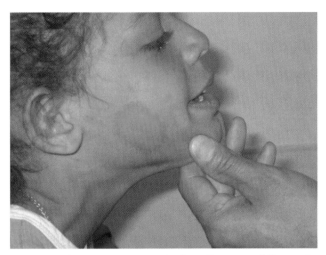

Figure 68-8 Tinea corporis on the face. (Courtesy of George A. Datto, III, MD.)

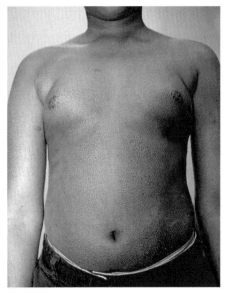

Figure 68-9 Ichthyosis vulgaris. (Courtesy of George A. Datto, III, MD.)

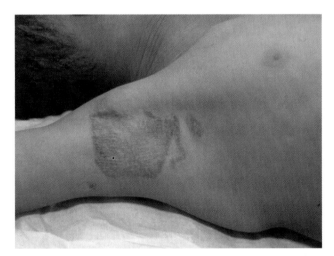

Figure 68-10 Psoriasis. (Courtesy of George A. Datto, III, MD.)

DIFFERENTIAL DIAGNOSIS

DIAGNOSIS	ICD-9	DISTINGUISHING CHARACTERISTICS	DISTRIBUTION
Atopic Dermatitis	691.8	Erythema, papules, vesicles in early infancy Dry, scaly patches in young children Pruritus May present after the newborn period Many individuals only have the condition as young children; some adults are affected	Often begins on the face in young infants Often begins on extensor surfaces and trunk in older infants Antecubital and popliteal fossae, face, and neck in older children and adults Frequently spares the groin
Nummular Eczema	692.9	Starts as vesicles, papules Erythematous, coin-shaped lesions May or may not see pruritus May only occur in the winter months	Extensor surfaces of the extremities
Seborrhea	690.12 (infantile) 690.10 (dermatitis)	Greasy, yellow or salmon-colored Nonpruritic or very mildly pruritic Appears at 1 month of age and disappears at between 8 and 12 months of age. Reappears in adolescence	Scalp (as cradle cap), postauricular areas, cheeks, trunk, extremities, diaper area Intertriginous areas
Contact Dermatitis	692	Focal, mild erythema Resolves shortly after the irritant is removed	Chin, cheeks, extensor surfaces, diaper area
Pityriasis Rosea	696.3	70% to 80% begin with a single patch followed by a general eruption 5–10 days later of smaller, more ovoid lesions Oval shape with flat, pink, brown center with an elevated border that is erythematous with a collarette of fine scales The rash may be more common in young children and in African Americans Peak incidence in adolescence and young adulthood	Trunk, upper arms, neck, and thighs but may occur anywhere on the body
Tinea Corporis	110.5	Round, scaly patches with a papular, vesicular, or pustular border with clear center Most commonly in children, but may be seen in any age group	Predilection for nonhairy areas of the face, trunk, and extremities Asymmetric distribution
Ichthyosis Vulgaris	757.1	Excessive scaling Scales on the tibia may be thick and plate-like Hyperkeratosis Rarely occurs before 3 months of life Scaling on the face is generally limited to childhood and decreases with age	Extensor surfaces Flexural surfaces generally spared May see chapping and accentuation of palmar markings
Psoriasis	696.1	Round, sharply demarcated, deep-red lesion with a silvery scale attached at the center of the lesion Drop-like lesions are seen in guttate psoriasis Unpredictable exacerbations and remissions Prolonged course	Extensor surfaces, scalp, genital regions, and lumbosacral areas Typically, a bilateral, symmetric pattern of lesions

ASSOCIATED FINDINGS	PREDISPOSING FACTORS
Tendency toward dry skin Keratosis pilaris Ichthyosis vulgaris 4% to 12% of patients develop cataracts Cutaneous infection resulting from *S. aureus*, strep Eczema herpeticum (herpes simplex) Eczema vaccinatum (vaccinia)	Worse during the winter months Worsened by frequent bathing Allergenic foods Inhalant allergens Dust mites
N/A	Worse during winter months Manifestation of dry skin (xerosis), ichthyosis (but not necessarily atopy)
N/A	Puberty
N/A	Soaps, detergents Salivary secretions Urine and feces
Prodrome of headache, malaise, pharyngitis may be reported The rash, seen in secondary syphilis, may be similar and should not be overlooked	Associated with preceding viral illness
N/A	Warm, humid climates Contact with an infected individual
Keratosis pilaris	Worse in cold and dry weather Atopy
25% to 50% with nail pits	Stress, trauma, strep infection (such as guttate psoriasis), climate, and certain medications may be precipitating factors in fewer than half of patients

- Scabies

- Letterer-Siwe disease

- Liner's disease

- Acrodermatitis enteropathica (listlessness, diarrhea, failure to thrive, low-serum zinc)

- Wiskott-Aldrich syndrome (diarrhea, purpura, susceptibility to infection)

- Phenylketonuria (mental retardation, seizures, blond hair, eczema)

- Hyper IgE syndrome (recurrent sinopulmonary and cutaneous infections, markedly elevated IgE levels, chronic dermatitis)

- Lichen striatus

- Id reaction

SUGGESTED READINGS
Fleisher GR, Ludwig S, Baskin MN. Atlas of pediatric emergency medicine. Philadelphia: Lippincott Williams & Wilkins; 2004:85.
Goodheart HP. Goodheart's photoguide to common skin disorders. 2nd ed. Philadelphia: Lippincott Williams & Wilkins; 2003:44,67,87.
Hurwitz S. Clinical pediatric dermatology. 2nd ed. Philadelphia: WB Saunders; 1993:45–55,62–63,105–112,122,375–380.
Illi S, von Mutius E, Lau S, et al. The natural course of atopic dermatitis from birth to age 7 years and the association with asthma. J Allergy Clin Immunol. 2004;113(5):925–931.
Larsen S, Hanifin JM. Epidemiology of atopic dermatitis. Immunol Clin North Am. 2002;22:1–24.
Schon MP, Boehncke WH. Psoriasis. N Engl J Med. 2005;352:1899–1912.
Stulberg DL. Pityriasis rosea. Am Fam Physician. 2004;69:87–91.

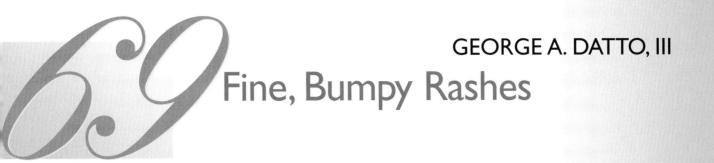

69

GEORGE A. DATTO, III

Fine, Bumpy Rashes

APPROACH TO THE PROBLEM

Small papular rashes that are acute tend to be noticed by parents, but chronic ones tend to go unnoticed or are ignored. These rashes are best appreciated by palpation rather than visual inspection. The distribution and elucidation of other signs will help with the identification of the rash.

KEY POINTS IN THE HISTORY

- A positive family history is present in about half the cases of keratosis pilaris.

- Keratosis pilaris may be associated with insulin resistance that results from obesity.

- Lichen nitidus and keratosis pilaris usually are asymptomatic chronic skin conditions.

- Scarlet fever is associated with fever, sore throat, abdominal pain, headache, and a fine erythematous rash that is typically seen within 12 to 48 hours from the onset of symptoms.

- Stress tends to precipitate dyshidrotic eczema.

KEY POINTS IN THE PHYSICAL EXAMINATION

- The Koebner phenomenon, which describes linear skin lesions appearing in sites of skin trauma, is seen with almost every case of lichen nitidus.

- Keratosis pilaris has visual and physical palpation similarities to that of plucked chicken skin.

- Keratosis pilaris is best appreciated on the lateral surfaces of the upper arms and upper legs.

- Often, the erythema of the scarletiniform rash is underappreciated in dark-skinned individuals, which necessitates bright lighting and palpation of the rash for its identification.

- The scarletiniform rash is accentuated in skin folds and at sites of pressure.

- Fine bumps along the lateral aspects of the fingers or palms and soles are seen in dyshidrotic eczema. After the bumps rupture, there is often irritation, which at times may be misdiagnosed as contact dermatitis.

DIFFERENTIAL DIAGNOSIS

DIAGNOSIS	ICD-9	DISTINGUISHING CHARACTERISTICS	DISTRIBUTION	ASSOCIATED FINDINGS	COMPLICATIONS	PREDISPOSING FACTORS
Scarlet Fever	034.1	Erythematous, "sandpaper" papules	Trunk Skin folds Pressure points	Palatal petechiae Strawberry tongue Pastia's lines Circumoral pallor	Suppurative complications Rheumatic fever Glomerulonephritis	Group A streptococcus
Keratosis Pilaris	701.1	Folliculocentric keratotic 1- to 2-mm papules "Plucked chicken skin"	Upper arms and legs Facial cheeks	None	None	Family history Dry skin Obesity
Lichen Nitidus	687.1	Minute, skin-colored, shiny papules	Forearms Trunk	Koebner phenomenon	None	N/A
Dyshidrotic Eczema (Pompholyx)	705.81	Fine bumps with clear or straw-colored fluid	Palms Soles Lateral aspects of fingers	Burning or itching sensation	None	Stress

PHOTOGRAPHS OF SELECTED DIAGNOSES

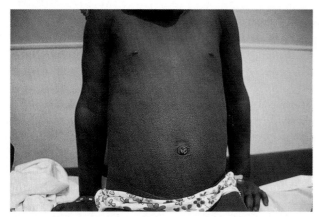

Figure 69-1 Scarlet fever. Fine papules, "sandpaper-like" rash on trunk of child with scarlet fever. (Courtesy of George A. Datto, III, MD.)

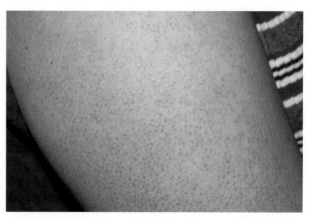

Figure 69-2 Keratosis pilaris. Tiny, rough-textured, follicular papules on lateral upper arms. (Used with permission from Goodheart HP. *Goodhearts photoguide to common skin disorders.* 2nd ed. Philadelphia: Lippincott Williams & Wilkins; 2003:49.)

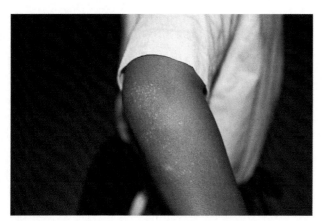

Figure 69-3 Lichen nitidus. Shiny small papules on elbow. (Courtesy of George A. Datto, III, MD.)

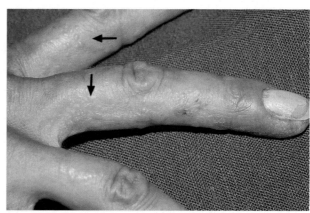

Figure 69-4 Dyshidrotic eczema. Note the fine, fluid-filled bumps on the fingers as depicted by the arrows. (Used with permission from Goodheart HP. *Goodheart's photoguide to common skin disorders.* 2nd ed. Philadelphia: Lippincott Williams & Wilkins; 2003:60.)

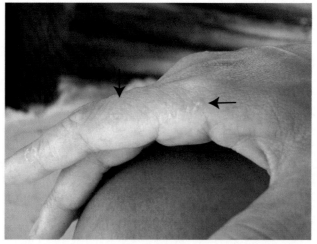

Figure 69-5 Dyshidriotic eczema. Note the fine, fluid filled bumps on the finger (as depicted by the arrows) and the distal area of peeling. (Courtesy of Esther K. Chung, MD.)

OTHER DIAGNOSES TO CONSIDER	• Lichen spinulosis
	• Folliculitis
	• Keratosis follicularis

SUGGESTED READINGS

Bisno AL. Diagnosis and management of group A streptococcal pharyngitis: a practice guideline. *Clin Infect Dis.* 1997;25:574–583.

Garcia-Hidalgo L. Dermatoses in 156 obese adults. *Obes Res.* 1999;7:299–302.

Goodheart HP. *Goodheart's photoguide to common skin disorders.* 2nd ed. Philadelphia: Lippincott Williams & Wilkins; 2003:60.

Hurwitz S. *Clinical pediatric dermatology.* 2nd ed. Philadelphia: WB Saunders; 1993:126–127.

Tilly JT, Drolet BA. Lichneoid eruptions in children. *J Am Acad Dermatol.* 2004;51:606–624.

Hypopigmented Rashes

APPROACH TO THE PROBLEM

Changes in skin pigmentation are often noticed by parents and brought to the attention of clinicians. Hypopigmentation is more easily appreciated in darker-skinned individuals when an increase in color contrast is present between the rash and the normal pigmented skin. Hypopigmentation results from a loss of melanin within the epidermal keratinocytes. Diseases causing hypopigmentation range from benign transient conditions to those that can be associated with significant systemic complications.

KEY POINTS IN THE HISTORY

• It is important to establish whether the hypopigmented lesions are congenital or acquired. Acquired causes of hypopigmentation include vitiligo, pityriasis alba, tinea versicolor, and postinflammatory hypopigmentation.

• Congenital hypopigmentation is often associated with diseases that have systemic manifestations such as tuberous sclerosis, Hypomelanosis of Ito, and Waardenburg syndrome. Affected individuals may have other affected family members.

• A history of any inflammatory skin condition that results in destruction of keratinocytes leads to postinflammatory hypopigmentation.

KEY POINTS IN THE PHYSICAL EXAMINATION

- A Wood's lamp exam may help to distinguish normally pigmented skin from hypopigmented skin, particularly in fair-skinned individuals.

- The hypopigmented lesions in tuberous sclerosis are often described as "ash leaf," "thumbprint," or "confetti."

- The presence of scale in a hypopigmented rash is seen with pityriasis alba and tinea versicolor.

- Differentiating pityriasis alba from tinea versicolor or tinea corporis can be done with a KOH prep, which will be positive in fungal infections.

- Vitiligo often involves skin areas around the face and areas of trauma including the hands, feet, elbows, knees, and ankles.

- Infections due to *Trichophyton tonsurans* and *T. violaceum* do not fluoresce, while infections due to *Microsporum* species and *Malassezia furfur* do.

DIFFERENTIAL DIAGNOSIS

DIAGNOSIS	ICD-9	DISTINGUISHING CHARACTERISTICS	DISTRIBUTION
Postinflammatory Hypopigmentation	709.0	Irregular patches at sites of previous dermatitis	Sites of previous skin inflammation or trauma
Tinea Versicolor	111.0	Macules with fine scale Color depends on contrasting skin pigment	Neck Chest Upper back Upper arms
Pityriasis Alba	696.5	Macules with fine scale	Face Upper trunk Proximal extremities
Vitiligo	709.01	Well-circumscribed macules	Face—eyes and mouth Hands, feet, elbows, knees, and ankles
Tuberous Sclerosis	759.5	Congenital small macules	Posterior trunk Extremities
Hypomelanosis of Ito	709.0	Congenital hypopigmented whorls	Trunk with midline demarcation

ASSOCIATED FINDINGS	COMPLICATIONS	PREDISPOSING FACTORS
None	None	Insect bites Contact dermatitis Atopic dermatitis Seborrheic dermatitis
None	None	*Malassezia furfur*
None	None	Often present in individuals with atopy
None	Autoimmune disorders in adults	Positive family history
Facial angiofibroma Shagreen patch Periungal fibroma	Cardiac rhabdomyomas Seizures Mental retardation	Autosomal dominant 60% new mutations in genes coding for hamartin and tuberin
Strabismus Nystagmus	Seizures	Xp11 mutation

PHOTOGRAPHS OF SELECTED DIAGNOSES

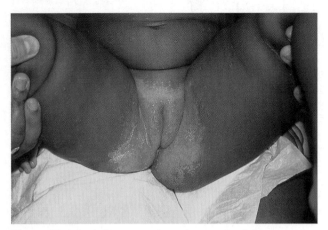

Figure 70-1 Postinflammatory hypopigmentation following a diaper dermatitis. (Courtesy of George A. Datto, III, MD.)

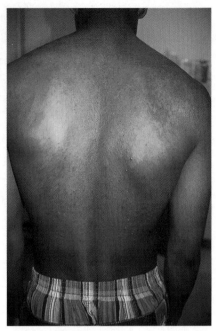

Figure 70-2 Tinea versicolor. Hypopigmented scaly lesions on the back of a darkly pigmented adolescent. (Courtesy of George A. Datto, III, MD.)

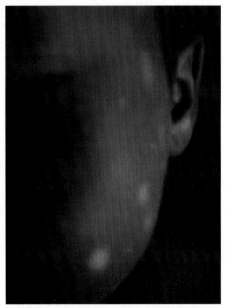

Figure 70-3 Tinea versicolor under Wood's lamp. Note the blue-whitish fluorescence. (Courtesy of Paul S. Matz, MD.)

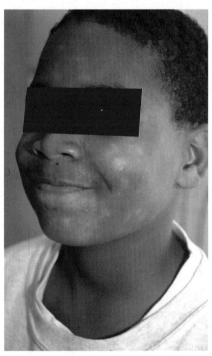

Figure 70-4 Pityriasis alba. (Courtesy of George A. Datto, III, MD.)

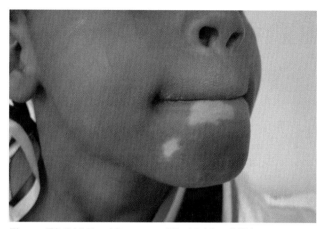

Figure 70-5 Vitiligo. (Courtesy of Paul S. Matz, MD.)

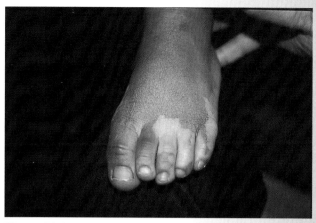

Figure 70-6 Segmental vitiligo on the foot of a child. (Courtesy of George A. Datto, III, MD.)

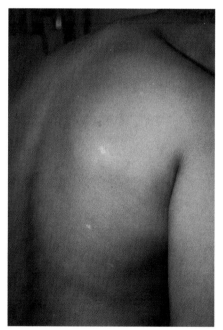

Figure 70-7 Tuberous sclerosis. Hypopigmented "confetti" macules on the back of a child with tuberous sclerosis. (Courtesy of George A. Datto, III, MD.)

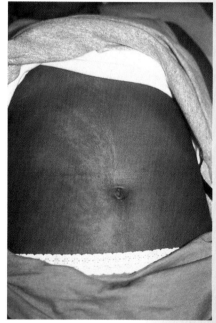

Figure 70-8 Hypomelanosis of Ito. Linear swirl pattern of hypopigmentation on abdomen. (Courtesy of George A. Datto, III, MD.)

OTHER DIAGNOSES TO CONSIDER

- Albinism

- Piebaldism

- Nevus depigmentosus

- Nevus anemicus

SUGGESTED READINGS

Dohil MA, Baugh WP. Vascular and pigmented birthmarks. *Pediatr Clin North Am.* 2000;47(4):783–812.

Hurwitz S. *Clinical pediatric dermatology.* 2nd ed. Philadelphia: WB Saunders; 1993:458–465.

Weston WL, Lane AT, Morelli JG, eds. *Color textbook of pediatric dermatology.* 3rd ed. St. Louis: Mosby; 2002:247–250.

GEORGE A. DATTO, III

Hyperpigmented Rashes

APPROACH TO THE PROBLEM

Increased skin pigmentation (hyperpigmentation) is a clinical problem that is often clinically evident with a careful dermatologic exam. Hyperpigmentation is more noticeable when the underlying patient's skin is light. Increased pigment is the result of increased deposition of melanin in the epidermis. Systemic conditions or focal processes can be the etiologic trigger that results in skin hyperpigmentation.

KEY POINTS IN THE HISTORY

- Focal skin hyperpigmentation in areas of previous skin inflammation, such as bug bites, eczema, or trauma, is best explained by postinflammatory hyperpigmentation.

- Acanthosis nigricans is strongly associated with obesity. The pigment of the lesion often intensifies with increased insulin resistance that may be associated with puberty and increased sugar consumption.

- Patients with acanthosis nigricans are at risk for polycystic ovarian syndrome, type II diabetes mellitus, nonalcoholic steatohepatitis, and sleep apnea.

- It is uncommon to see tinea versicolor in a prepubertal child.

- Café-au-lait (CAL) spots are the cutaneous manifestation of neurofibromatosis but may be associated other diseases. In isolation, CAL spots may be a benign skin finding.

- Freckles, commonly seen in light-skinned individuals, are induced by sun exposure, and they often fade during the winter.

- Pregnancy, oral contraceptive use, and exposure to photosensitizing drugs are predisposing factors for melasma, which has been called the *mask of pregnancy.*

- Most congenital nevi do not undergo much change in childhood; therefore, any lesion that changes rapidly, bleeds, or is described as painful or pruritic should be evaluated by a dermatologist.

KEY POINTS IN
THE PHYSICAL
EXAMINATION

- Epidermal melanin demonstrates increased fluorescence with a Wood's lamp.

- Acanthosis nigricans can be seen in flexural surfaces, armpits, and antecubital fossae, and in the umbilicus. These spots are unusual for postinflammatory changes from contact or atopic dermatitis.

- Five or more CAL spots that are greater than 5 mm in a prepubertal child or six or more greater than 15 mm in a pubertal child should prompt further evaluation for neurofibromatosis.

- Good documentation that may include a photograph of nevi will allow the clinician to determine whether any acute change might raise concern for malignant transformation.

- Multiple small postinflammatory hyperpigmented lesions, particularly in dark-skinned individuals, are found on the distal extremities following insect bites.

- Tinea versicolor may appear more hypopigmented in the summer and hyperpigmented in the winter depending on the underlying skin color.

PHOTOGRAPHS OF SELECTED DIAGNOSES

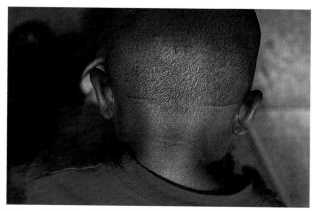

Figure 71-1 Postinflammatory hyperpigmentation. Hyperpigmented linear lesions following skin trauma from a razor. (Courtesy of George A. Datto, III, MD.)

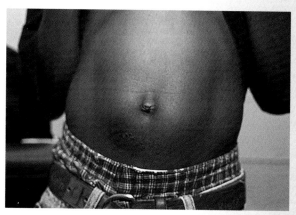

Figure 71-2 Hyperpigmentation resulting from nickel dermatitis. (Courtesy of George A. Datto, III, MD.)

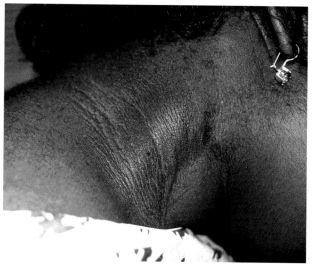

Figure 71-3 Acanthosis nigricans. Thickened, velvety, hyperpigmented epidermis in neck of obese adolescent with type II diabetes mellitus. (Courtesy of George A. Datto, III, MD.)

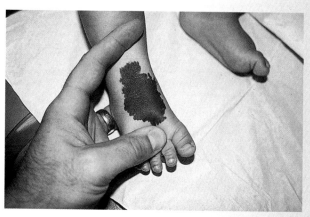

Figure 71-4 Melanotic nevus. A medium-sized, congenital, pigmented nevus on dorsum of foot. (Courtesy of George A. Datto, III, MD.)

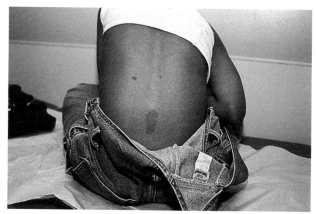

Figure 71-5 Café-au-lait spots. Multiple café au lait spots on back of child. (Courtesy of George A. Datto, III, MD.)

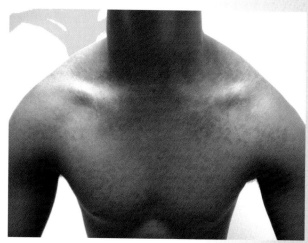

Figure 71-6 Tinea versicolor. While often hypopigmented, this rash may be hyperpigmented as in this individual. (Courtesy of Paul S. Matz, MD.)

DIFFERENTIAL DIAGNOSIS

DIAGNOSIS	ICD-9	DISTINGUISHING CHARACTERISTICS	DISTRIBUTION	ASSOCIATED FINDINGS
Postinflammatory Hyperpigmentation	709.0	Small macules	Sites of previous skin inflammation or trauma	Increased nail bed pigment
Acanthosis Nigricans	701.2	Thickened, velvety, hyperkeratotic lesions	Neck, axillae, antecubital fossae	Skin tags in neck Obesity
Melanotic Nevus	448.1	Acquired—small, flat macules Congenital—macular, papular, verrucous, or nodular	Acquired—diffuse Congenital—trunk, proximal extremities	None
Freckles	709.09	Light to dark brown macules	Sun-exposed areas Face, arms, hands	None
Café-au-Lait Spots	709.09	Macular lesions "coffee with milk" Color depends on underlying skin color: dark skin associated with darker lesions	Diffuse	Neurofibromatosis: Axillary/inguinal freckling Neurofibroma Iris: Lisch nodules Osseous lesions Optic glioma
Tinea Versicolor	111.0	Scaly macules	Neck, upper chest and back, and upper arms	Yellowish-gold or blue-white fluorescence with Wood's lamp KOH prep: "spaghetti and meatballs"
Melasma	709.09	Punctate to confluent macules	Forehead, cheeks, neck	Pregnancy

COMPLICATIONS	PREDISPOSING FACTORS
None	Insect bites Contact dermatitis Atopic dermatitis
Type II diabetes mellitus Sleep apnea Nonalcoholic steatohepatitis	Insulin resistance Hyperinsulinism
Large congenital nevus—melanoma Acquired nevus—melanoma with any significant change in lesion	Acquired—increase in number during adolescence Congenital—none
Risk factor for melanoma independent of melanocytic nevi	Fair-skinned Sun exposure
None, if not associated with systemic disease	N/A
None	*Malassezia furfur*
None	Dark-skinned females Sun exposure Pregnancy Hormonal therapy

• Addison's disease

SUGGESTED READINGS

Cohen BA. *Pediatric dermatology*. London: Mosby; 1999.

Hurwitz S. *Clinical pediatric dermatology*. 2nd ed. Philadelphia: WB Saunders; 1993:470–475.

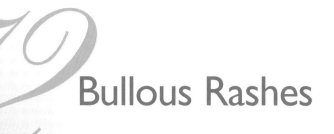

Bullous Rashes

ANGELA ALLEVI

ANGELA ALLEVI

APPROACH TO THE PROBLEM

Blister-associated rashes in children are divided into two groups: *vesicular* rashes and *bullous* rashes. By definition, vesicles are raised, fluid-containing blisters in the skin or mucous membranes that are no more than 0.5 cm in diameter. Bullae are blistering lesions that are greater than 0.5 cm in diameter and may also be seen in the skin or mucous membranes. Vesicles and bullae may be round or have irregular borders. Compared with adult skin, the skin of pediatric patients is very prone to blistering. Vesicular rashes are common in the pediatric population, and are discussed elsewhere. Bullous rashes, on the other hand, are a relatively uncommon class of pediatric skin disorders.

Bullae form secondary to fluid accumulation between cells in the epidermis or between the epidermal and dermal (subepidermal) skin layers. Bullous skin disorders are divided into *congenital* disorders, such as epidermolysis bullosa; *immunologic* disorders, such as Stevens-Johnson syndrome (SJS), toxic epidermal necrolysis (TEN), and photosensitivity rashes; and *infectious* disorders, such as bullous impetigo and staphylococcal scalded skin syndrome (SSSS).

KEY POINTS IN THE HISTORY

- Systemic symptoms, such as fever, fussiness, ill appearance, and diffuse skin involvement are associated with SJS, TEN, and SSSS.

- Congenital blistering diseases, such as epidermolysis bullosa, are often present at birth or during the newborn period.

- Bullae appearing in the first few days or weeks of life may be secondary to epidermolysis bullosa, bullous impetigo of the neonate, or SSSS.

- In epidermolysis bullosa, bullae form at sites of minor skin trauma.

- Because they involve the epidermis only, bullous skin disorders (with the exception of TEN and rarer forms of epidermolysis bullosa) may cause temporary hyperpigmentation and lichenification but tend not to cause permanent scarring.

KEY POINTS IN THE PHYSICAL EXAMINATION

- Bullous impetigo and photosensitivity rashes are seen on exposed parts of the body, primarily the face and extremities.

- Nikolsky's sign—the ability to use gentle traction with a finger to separate the upper epidermis from the underlying skin in bullous lesions—may be seen commonly in systemic bullous disorders (TEN, SSSS, and epidermolysis bullosa).

- Mucous membrane involvement is seen in TEN, SJS, and in epidermolysis bullosa but not in SSSS.

- Bullae are seen on the skin in bullous impetigo, photosensitivity rashes, epidermolysis bullosa and SSSS, but in SJS, they are seen on the mucous membranes of the mouth, nares, the conjunctivae, and the anorectal and perineal mucosae.

- The bullae seen with bullous impetigo are surrounded by an erythematous margin.

PHOTOGRAPHS OF SELECTED DIAGNOSES

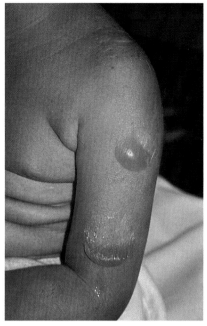

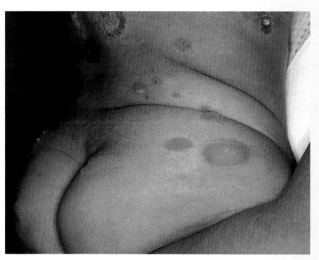

Figure 72-2 Bullous impetigo. (Used with permission from Fleisher GR, Ludwig S, Baskin MN. *Atlas of pediatric emergency medicine.* Philadelphia: Lippincott Williams & Wilkins; 2004:200.)

Figure 72-1 Photosensitivity. Large blisters that developed on the second day following prolonged sun exposure. (Courtesy of George A. Datto, III, MD.)

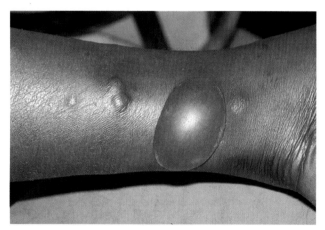

Figure 72-3 Bullous insect bite reaction. (Used with permission from Goodheart HP. *Goodheart's photoguide to common skin disorders.* 2nd ed. Philadelphia: Lippincott Williams & Wilkins; 2003:3.)

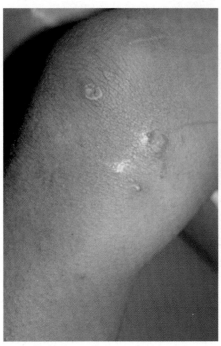

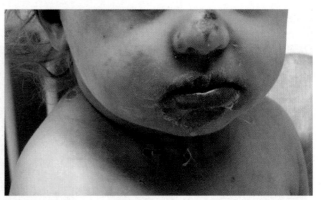

Figure 72-5 Staphylococcal scalded skin syndrome (SSSS) with ruptured bullae. (Courtesy of Gary Marshall, MD.)

Figure 72-4 Blistering rash from streptococcal infection. (Courtesy of George A. Datto, III, MD.)

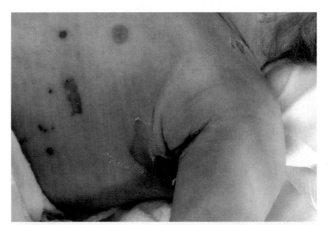

Figure 72-6 Staphylococcal scalded skin syndrome. "Scalded" skin underlying ruptured bulla in SSSS. (Courtesy of Gary Marshall, MD.)

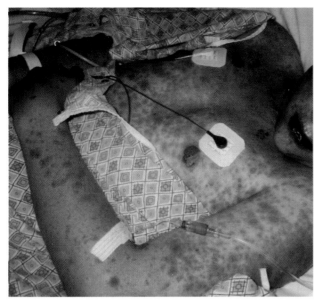

Figure 72-7 Target-like purpuric lesions of Stevens-Johnson syndrome. (Courtesy of Gary Marshall, MD.)

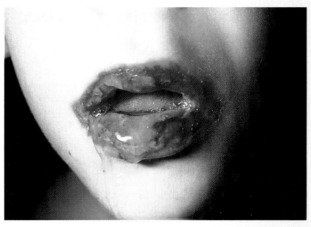

Figure 72-8 Hemorrhagic ulcerative stomatitis in SJS. (Courtesy of Joseph Lopreiato, MD.)

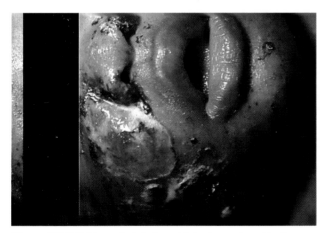

Figure 72-9 Epidermolysis bullosa. Note the ruptured bullous lesion. (Courtesy of Joseph Lopreiato, MD.)

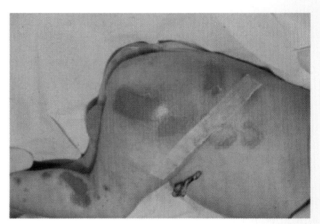

Figure 72-10 Epidermolysis bullosa congenita. (Used with permission from The Benjamin Barankin Dermatology Collection.)

DIFFERENTIAL DIAGNOSIS

DIAGNOSIS	ICD-9	DISTINGUISHING CHARACTERISTICS	DISTRIBUTION
Photosensitivity	692.72	Exaggerated sunburn Occurs in all age groups Sun-exposed areas of skin affected Vesicles and bullae in severe cases Pruritic	Often involves face, upper neck ("V" portion), hands, forearms Covered and shadowed areas of body are spared
Bullous Impetigo	684	More common in infants and young children Child does not appear ill Fluid inside bullae often yellow-brown or purulent and contains *S. aureus* Mucous membranes not involved Bullae surrounded by erythematous margin	Occurs on exposed areas of face and extremities, occasionally in perineal area
Staphylococcal Scalded Skin Syndrome (SSSS)	695.1	More common in neonates (onset 3–7 days of life), but can be seen in children and adults Appears as diffuse erythema that blanches Bullae rupture and leave skin with a "scalded" appearance Mucous membranes not involved Fluid inside bullae are sterile and clear May be clinically indistinguishable from TEN	Often begins as small pustules in diaper area or lower abdomen or as erythema with or without crusting around the mouth, diaper area, or umbilicus Spreads diffusely
Stevens-Johnson Syndrome (SJS)	695.1	Most common in children and young adults Viral-like prodromal symptoms precede cutaneous findings by up to 2 weeks, then rapid development of rash and bullae (24 hours) Bullae found on mucous membranes, but not on skin Rash may have target lesions or nonpalpable purpura and may be generalized or localized <10% of body surface involvement	May be localized to trunk, palms, and soles, or generalized Always involves mucous membranes (mouth, eyes, genitals, perianal, or anorectal area)
Toxic Epidermal Necrolysis (TEN)	695.1	Occurs in all age groups but more common in adults May be clinically indistinguishable from SSSS in neonates Full thickness loss of epidermis >30% of body surface involvement	Begins with mucous membrane involvement similar to SJS, but progresses to diffuse epidermal involvement with full-thickness loss of epidermis
Epidermolysis Bullosa	757.39	Bullae often present at birth Inherited skin disorder Three subtypes: EB simplex, junctional EB, and dystrophic EB	Most commonly involves hands and feet, but also other areas of minor trauma

ASSOCIATED FINDINGS	COMPLICATIONS	PREDISPOSING FACTORS
Pruritus Areas of contact dermatitis	Healing with hyperpigmentation and lichenification May see recurrence even after discontinuation of offending agent	Drug exposure Skin products
Outbreaks in close contacts, such as family members	Recurrent folliculitis Cellulitis from progressive infection	Nasal carriage of group A strep and *S. aureus* increases risk of recurrent impetigo
Fever Fussiness Positive Nikolsky's sign Bullae and underlying skin may be extremely painful	Sepsis Cellulitis Loss of hair and nails Osteomyelitis Pneumonia Fungal or bacterial superinfection Hypovolemia Electrolyte disturbances Mortality approximately 4%, higher with increasing age	Asymptomatic staphylococcal pustulosis
Weakness Lethargy Pneumonia Severe eye involvement in most cases, including conjunctivitis, ulcerations, uveitis Nephritis Ulcerative/hemorrhagic stomatitis from oral lesions	Severe dehydration Secondary infection Respiratory failure Renal failure Gastric perforation Blindness Mortality less than 10%	Infection, including mycoplasma, HSV, and viral upper respiratory infections Drug exposure to anti-epileptics, sulfonamides, penicillin derivatives
Mucous membrane involvement (eyes, mouth) Positive Nikolsky's sign Painful erythematous skin	Fluid and electrolyte imbalance Ocular sequelae in 40% (including blindness) Overwhelming sepsis Mortality up to 30%	Drug exposure, most commonly to analgesics, nonsteroidal anti-inflammatory agents antibacterial and antifungal medications, and antiepileptics
Scarring at previously involved sites Oral involvement Nail dystrophy Palmar and plantar hyperkeratosis	Scarring seen in some forms Hyperpigmentation Superinfection Sepsis Small- and large-joint contractures in severely affected cases	Family history Bullae form at sites of minor trauma

OTHER
DIAGNOSES TO
CONSIDER

- Pemphigus

- Bullous pemphigoid

- Linear IgA bullous dermatosis (LABD)

- Epidermolytic hyperkeratosis (bullous ichthyosis)

- Bullous mastocytosis

- Bullous scabies

SUGGESTED READINGS

Bhumbra NA, McCullough SG. Skin and subcutaneous infections. *Prim Care*. 2003;30(1):1–24.

Fleisher GR, Ludwig S, Baskin MN. *Atlas of pediatric emergency medicine*. Philadelphia: Lippincott Williams & Wilkins; 2004:200.

George A, Rubin G. A systematic review and meta-analysis of treatments for impetigo. *Br J Gen Pract*. 2003;53(491):480–487.

Goodheart HP. Goodheart's photoguide to common skin disorders. 2nd ed. Philadelphia: Lippincott Williams & Wilkins; 2003:3.

McKenna JK, Leiferman KM. Dermatologic drug reactions. *Immunol Allergy Clin North Am*. 2004;24(3):399–423.

Okulicz JF. Epidermolysis bullosa simplex. *Cutis*. 2002;70(1):19–21.

Patel GK. Staphylococcal scalded skin syndrome: diagnosis and management. *Am J Clin Dermatol*. 2003;4(3):165–175.

Spies M, Sanford AP, Low JFA, et al. Treatment of extensive toxic epidermal necrolysis in children. *Pediatrics*. 2001;108(5):162–168.

INDEX

A

abdomen
   enlarged/distended, 213–218
   midline bulge of, 207–212
abdominal distention, 213–218. *see*
      enlarged/distended abdomen
   differential diagnosis/other diagnosis
      and, 216–218
   figures, 215
   imperforate anus and, 384
   historical points, 213–214
   leg asymmetry and, 276
   physical examination, 214
   scrotal swelling and, 365
abdominal mass, discoloration of/around eye
      and, 68
abdominal midline bulge
   differential diagnosis/other diagnosis
      and, 210–212
   figures, 209
   historical points, 207
   physical examination, 208
abdominal tenderness
   differential diagnosis and, 6
   general appearance and, 4
   streptococcal pharyngitis and, 171
abnormal head shape
   differential diagnosis/other diagnosis
      and, 24, 27
   historical points, 22
   physical examination, 23
ABO compatibility, neonatal jaundice and, 397
abscess
   breast swelling/enlargement and, 197
   dermoid cysts and, 121
   focal gum lesions and, f141
   labial, 359–361
   perirectal, f375, 376–377
   peritonsillar, 163–164, 166–167
   pilonidal, 373
abuse. *see* child abuse; sexual abuse
acanthosis nigricans
   hyperpigmented rashes and, 471–472, f473,
      474–476
   obesity and, 217
ACE inhibitors, foot swelling and, 307
achondroplasia, 272, f273
acne
   ear canal findings and, 109
   facial rashes and, 399–400, f401, 404–405
   neonatal, f395, 396–397
acrocephalosyndactyly, 259
acrocyanosis, nail abnormalities and,
      235, 237, f238

acrodermatitis enteropathica, 39
   perianal/buttock redness and, 383
   perineal red rashes and, 350
   scaly rashes and, 458
acropustulosis of infancy
   skin abnormalities in newborns and, 392,
      396–397
   vesicular rashes and, 444
acute abdomen
   associated findings/complications of, 7
   distinguishing characteristics/duration/
      chronicity, 6
   predisposing factors, 7
acute bilateral adenitis, cervical adenitis
      and, 180
acute chest syndrome, dactylitis and, 257
acute endocarditis, septic arthritis and, 257
acute glanular inflammation. *see* balanoposthitis
acute otitis media (AOM), 50
   antibiotics and, 110
   buccal cellulitis and, 43
   external auditory canal (EAC) abnormali-
      ties and, 107
   tympanic membrane abnormalities
      and, 111–112
acute paronychia, fingertip swelling and,
      266–267, f268
acute splenic sequestration, dactylitis
      and, 257
acute tonsillopharyngitis, 163
Addison's disease
   hyperpigmented rashes and, 476
   longitudinal melanonychia/pigmented
      bands, 237
adenoids, 126
adenoma sebaceum, f403, 404–405
adenopathy, lymphangitis and, 422
adenovirus, knee swelling and, 300
adherent lobule of ear, 89, f91
Adie syndrome, pupil abnormalities and, 80
adrenal crisis, 8
albinism, hypopigmented rashes and, 470
alcohol, teeth discoloration and, 145. *see also*
      fetal alcohol syndrome
alkaptonuria, teeth discoloration and, 149
allergic conjunctivitis, f51, 54–55. *see also*
      conjunctivitis
allergic contact dermatitis. *see also* contact
      dermatitis
   foot rashes/lumps and, 317
   scaly rashes and, f454
allergic penile edema, 338
allergic rhinitis, 125–126, f127
allergic shiners, 65, f67, 68–69, 452

allergy conditions/symptoms
   atopic dermatitis and, 457
   contact dermatitis and, 443
   eczema and, 404
   perineal sores/lesions and, 351
   red eye and, 49
alopecia, 23–24, f32. *see also* hair loss
   drug rash and, 411
alopecia areata, 29–30, f32
   nail abnormalities and, 236
alveolar cysts, focal gum lesions and,
      139–140, f141
alveolar lymphangioma, focal gum lesions
      and, 144
ambiguous genitalia
   female genitalia variations and, 321, f325,
      326–327
   penile abnormalities and, 330–333, f335
amblyopia
   capillary hemangiomas of eyelid and, 63
   esotropia and, 83
   exotropia and, 83
   iritis and, 77
   misalignment of the eyes, 79
   nasal hemangioma and, 121
amenorrhea
   ambiguous genitalia and, 321
   imperforate hymen and, 326
amniotocele, swelling of/around the eye and, 57
amyloidosis, nephrotic syndrome and, 311
ANA positivity, juvenile rheumatoid arthritis
      (JRA) and, 299
anasarca, enlarged/distended abdomen and, f215
anemia, 8
   infectious mononucleosis and, 437
   juvenile rheumatoid arthritis (JRA) and, 298
   nonblanching rashes and, 445, 450
   penile edema and, 343
   scleral icterus and, 69
   subgaleal hemorrhages and, 12
aneurysm, arm swelling and, 247
angel's kiss. *see* nevus simplex
angioedema
   swelling of/around the eye and, 57
   viral arthritis and, 257
aniridia, pupil/iris/lens abnormalities and, f73,
      76–77
anisocoria, pupil/iris/lens abnormalities
      and, 76–77
ankle fracture, 308, 310–311
ankle sprain, 307–308, 310–311
ankyloglossia, 150–153, f155
anogenital warts, 373–374, 376–377
anorectal malformation. *see* imperforate anus

anotia, 87

anterior cruciate ligament (ACL), 293

anthrax, cutaneous, 416–417

anti-anxiety medications, diffuse red rashes and, 407

antibiotics
  Candida albicans diaper rash and, 345
  hairy tongue and, 157
  red rashes and, 407, 431
  teeth discoloration and, 145–147, f148
  tongue discoloration/surface changes and, 157

antidepressants, foot swelling and, 307

anti-epileptics, diffuse red rashes and, 407

anti-inflammatory medications, diffuse red rashes and, 407

antimalarial drugs, tongue discoloration/surface changes and, 157

antipsychotics, foot swelling and, 307

Antley Bixler syndrome, craniosynostosis and, 27

anus, imperforate, ear shape/position abnormalities and, 88

anxiety, hair loss and, 28

Apert syndrome
  acrocephalosyndactyly and, 259
  craniosynostosis and, 27
  syndactyly and, 261

aphthous ulcers, 133
  mouth sores/patches and, f136

aplastic anemia, nonblanching rashes and, 450

aplastic crisis, erythema infectiosum and, 405

apnea
  increase of intracranial pressure and, 7
  respiratory failure and, 7
  toxic ingestion and, 7

appendix testis torsion, scrotal swelling and, 365–367, f369

arm displacement
  differential diagnosis/other diagnosis and, 243, 245
  figures, 244
  historical points, 241–242
  physical examination, 242

arm swelling
  historical points, 246
  physical examination, 247

Arnold-Chiari malformation, spina bifida and, 229

arrhythmias, congestive heart failure and, 311

arteriovenous fistulas, leg asymmetry and, 275

arteriovenous malformation, 92

artery malformations, nasal hemangioma and, 121

arthralgias
  erythema infectiosum and, 405
  erythema multiforme (minor) and, 437
  Lyme disease and, 298

arthritis
  arm swelling and, 252
  erythema infectiosum and, 405
  hand swelling and, 253–254

arthrogryposis multiplex
  clubfoot and, 290, 304
  congenital vertical talus and, 271–272

ascites, enlarged/distended abdomen and, 214–216, f215

"ash leaf" lesions
  adenoma sebaceum and, 404
  hypopigmented rashes and, 464

aspiration/respiratory distress, toxic ingestion and, 7

asthma
  discoloration of/around eye and, 65
  eczema and, 404

astigmatism, pterygium and, 63

asymmetric lateral exanthem of childhood, raised red rashes and, 436–437

asymmetric periflexural exanthem. see asymmetric lateral exanthem of childhood

ataxia, cholesteatoma and, 112

ataxia-telangiectasia, craniosynostosis and, 27

atelectasis, f115
  tympanic membrane abnormalities and, 112

atopic dermatitis, 35–37, f239
  allergic rhinitis and, 129
  fine bumpy rashes and, f462
  mouth sores/patches and, 133
  perineal sores/lesions and, 358
  postinflammatory hyperpigmentation and, 472, 475
  postinflammatory hypopigmentation and, 467
  scaly rashes and, 451–452, f453, 456–457

atopy
  allergic conjunctivitis and, 55
  hair loss and, 31

auricular growth. see ears

auricular hematoma, 94–95, f96

auricular sinus, 101, f102

autism, general appearance and, 4

autoimmune diseases. see also human innumodeficiency virus (HIV) infection
  erythema nodosum and, 417
  facial rashes and, 400
  hair loss and, 31
  postinflammatory hypopigmentation and, 467

B

back
  curvature of, 221–226
  midline back pits/skin tags/hair tufts/lesions, 227–231

back dimples, 227–229, f230

bacteremia, buccal cellulitis and, 43

bacterial conjunctivitis, f51, 54–55

bacterial infections
  chronic mycotic otitis externa, 107
  epididymitis and, 367
  hand swelling and, 253
  throat redness and, 169

bacterial meningitis
  associated findings/complications of, 7
  distinguishing characteristics/duration/chronicity, 6
  general appearance and, 4
  predisposing factors, 7

bacterial rhinosinusitis, viral rhinorrhea and, 129

Baker's cyst. see also popliteal cyst
  knee swelling and, f297

balanoposthitis, penile swelling and, 338, f340–341, 342–343

Baller Gerold syndrome, 27

barotrauma, hemotympanum and, 112

barrel chest, abnormal chest shape and, 190–191

Bartholin duct cyst, 359–361

Bartonella henselae, cervical adenitis and, 180

basal cell carcinoma, hair loss and, 31

bathrocephaly, lower extremity abnormalities and, 272

Battle's sign, raccoon eyes and, 68

Beau's lines, nail abnormalities and, 240

Beckwith-Wiedemann syndrome
  ear pits/tags and, 101, 104
  ear shape/position abnormalities and, 87
  leg asymmetry and, 276
  nevus flammeus and, 18
  prune belly syndrome and, 217

Behçet's syndrome, 352, 356–357

benzodiazepines, tongue discoloration/surface changes and, 157

beta-hemolytic streptococcus, throat redness and, 169–171

bezoars, enlarged/distended abdomen and, 213

bifid lobule. see cleft ear-lobe

bifid uvula, 150–153, f155

bilateral periorbital edema, swelling of/around the eye and, 57

biliary atresia, neonatal jaundice and, 397

biliary cirrhosis, xanthogranulomas and, 63

bioterrorism, smallpox and, 440

birth, scalp swelling in newborns and, 11–15

birth control. see also oral contraceptives
  foot swelling and, 307

bismuth, black tongue from, f160

black dot sign, 29–30, f32, 37

black hairy tongue, f161

black heel, foot rashes/lumps and, 317

black tongue. see tongue discoloration/surface changes

black widow spider, 413, 417. see also spider bites

bleeding
  nasal hemangioma and, 121
  tympanic membrane abnormalities and, 115

blepharitis, f52, 54–55
  chalazion and, 63
  hordeolum and, 63

blindness
  cataracts and, 77
  leukocoria and, 77
  Stevens-Johnson syndrome and, 483

blistering distal dactylitis, hand swelling and, 254, f255

Blount disease, leg bowing/knock knees and, 281–282, f283, 284–285

blue nevus, Mongolian spots and, 397

blurred vision, chalazion and, 63

body piercing, ear pits/tags and, 104

Bohn nodules
  focal gum lesions and, 139–140, f141
  swellings in the mouth and, 163–164

bone dysplasias, curvature of the back and, 226

bone lesions, histiocytosis X and, 348

bone tumor, arm swelling and, 247

Borrelia burgdorferi, 299. see also Lyme disease
  erythema migrans and, 417

bottle caries, teeth discoloration and, 146–147, f148

bowels, blood in, 373, 377

bowing of legs. see leg bowing/knock knees; physiologic bowing of legs

Boxer's fracture, hand swelling and, 253, f255

brachial plexus injuries, arm displacement and, 242, f244
brachycephaly, 24, f25
brachydactyly
    abnormal chest shape and, 188
    finger abnormalities and, 259–261, f262
braiding of hair, 28–29, 31
brain abscess
    cholesteatoma and, 110, 112
    dermoid cysts and, 121
    peritonsillar abscess and, 167
branchial cleft cysts, 101, f103
    ear pits/tags and, 100
    neck masses/swelling and, 178–179, f181
branchio-otorenal syndrome, ear pits/tags and, 101, 104
breast asymmetry, breast swelling/enlargement and, 193–195, f196
breast cyst/abscess, breast swelling/enlargement and, 197
breast swelling/enlargement
    differential diagnosis/other diagnosis and, 195, 197
    figures, 196
    historical points, 193
    physical examination, 194
breastfeeding
    mastitis and, 193
    neonatal jaundice and, 397
    oral cleft/other variants and, 150
    rickets and, 201
breech births, lower extremity abnormalities and, 270–274
brown recluse spider, 413, 417. see also spider bites
Brown's syndrome, misalignment of the eyes and, 80
Bruckner test, misalignment of the eyes and, 80
Brushfield spots
    Down syndrome and, 71
    pupil/iris/lens abnormalities and, f75, 76–77
buccal cellulitis, 40–43, f44
bulbar conjunctiva. see eye discoloration
bulla, vesicular rashes and, 439–440
bullous impetigo
    bullous rashes and, f479, 482–483
    sucking blister and, 397
bullous mastocytosis, 484
bullous myringitis, tympanic membrane abnormalities and, 115
bullous pemphigoid, bullous rashes and, 484
bullous rashes
    differential diagnosis/other diagnosis and, 482–484
    figures, 479–481
    historical points, 477
    physical examination, 478
bullous scabies, 484
burns
    cupping and, 447, f449
    palatal and mouth sores/patches, 133
buttock swelling. see perianal/buttock swelling

C
café-au-lait (CAL) spots, f473
    hyperpigmented rashes and, 471–472, 474–476
    leg asymmetry and, 276

callus, f316
    foot deformities and, 302
callus/corn, 313–315
camptodactyly, finger abnormalities and, 259–260
cancer
    anogenital warts and, 377
    testicular, 367
Candida albicans, 345–346, f347
candidal infections, 345–346, f347, 348–349
    white specks in hair and, 37
candidiasis, perianal/buttock redness and, 379–381, f382
capillary hemangiomas
    of eyelid, 57–58, f60
    swelling of/around the eye and, 62–63
caput succedaneum, 11–13, f14
    molding of head and, 13
cardiac abnormalities, ear shape/position abnormalities and, 88
cardiac disease
    abnormal chest shape and, 187
    adenoma sebaceum and, 405
    ascites and, 217
cardiovascular abnormalities, juvenile rheumatoid arthritis (JRA) and, 299
carditis, rheumatic fever and, 298
Carpenter syndrome, 27
    polydactyly/supernumerary digit and, 261
    syndactyly and, 261
Cat Eye syndrome, coloboma and, 77
Cat Scratch disease
    erythema nodosum and, 413
    focal red bumps and, 425, 428–429
    neck masses/swelling and, 177–178, 180, f183
cataracts, 71–72
    aniridia and, 77
    iritis and, 77
    leukocoria and, 77
    pupil/iris/lens abnormalities and, f73, 76–77
caudal regression, 270
cavernous hemangioma, arm swelling and, f251
cavernous sinus thrombosis, buccal cellulitis and, 43
cavus foot, foot deformities and, 306
cellulitis
    bullous impetigo and, 483
    dermoid cysts and, 63
    differential diagnosis of, 95
    ear swelling and, 93, f96
    foot deformities and, 306
    furuncle and, 429
    hordeolum and, 63
    hot tub folliculitis and, 437
    insect bites and, 311
    knee swelling and, f295
    otitis externa and, 104, 107
    peritonsillar abscess and, 171
    red patches/swelling and, 414, f415, 416–417
    staphylococcal scalded skin syndrome (SSSS) and, 483
    swelling of/around the eye and, 58
central punctum, insect bites and, 310
cephalohematoma, 11–13, f14
cerebral agenesis, abnormal head shape and, 27
cerebral palsy
    intoeing and, 292
    nail abnormalities and, 245

cerebrospinal fluid (CSF) rhinorrhea, nasal bridge swelling and, 120–201
cerumen impaction
    external auditory canal (EAC) abnormalities and, 105
    tympanic membrane abnormalities and, 115
cervical adenitis, neck masses/swelling and, 178, 180
cervical adenopathy
    neck masses/swelling and, 178, 180, f182
    streptococcal pharyngitis and, 171
cervical lymphadenopathy
    cat scratches and, 177
    infectious mononucleosis and, 171
    throat redness and, 170
chalazion, swelling of/around the eye and, 57–58, f59, 62–63
CHARGE syndrome
    coloboma and, 71, 77
    ear shape/position abnormalities and, 87
chemosis
    pupil/iris/lens abnormalities and, 72
    red eye and, f53
chest, breast swelling/enlargement, 193–197
chest lumps, 198–203
    differential diagnosis/other diagnosis and, 200–201, 203
    figures, 202
    historical points, 198
    physical examination, 199
chest shape abnormalities, 187–192
    differential diagnosis/other diagnosis and, 190–192
    figures, 189
    historical points, 187
    physical examination, 188
chicken pox (varicella)
    "dew-drop-on-a-rose-petal" lesion and, f441
    vesicular rashes and, 439–440, 442–443
child abuse
    arm swelling and, 246
    chest lumps and, 198–201
    ear swelling and, 94
    nonblanching rashes and, 446–447
    penile trauma and, 343
    sexual abuse, 351–352, f353, 356–357
chlamydia conjunctivitis, f53
choledochal cyst, neonatal jaundice and, 397
cholesteatoma, f114
    ear canal findings and, 109
    hearing loss and, 110
    tympanic membrane abnormalities and, 112
chondrodysplasia, heterozygous achondroplasia and, 270
chordee, penile abnormalities and, 330–333, f335
chromosomal syndromes, ear pits/tags and, 104
chromosome 11q duplication, ear pits/tags and, 101
chromosome 4p deletions, preauricular tags and, 101
chromosome 9q34, adenoma sebaceum and, 405
chronic arthritis, hand swelling and, 253
chronic granulomatous disease, cervical adenopathy and, 180
chronic lung disease, rectal prolapse and, 377
chronic paronychia, fingertip swelling and, 266–267

chronic solitary ulcer, perianal/buttock swelling and, 378
circumcision. see prepubertal/pubertal genitalia
circumoral pallor, scarlet fever and, 404, 461
clavicle anomalies, abnormal chest shape and, 192
clavicular fractures, 198, 200–201
    chest lumps and, f202
cleft earlobe, 87–89, f90
cleft lip/palate, 150–153, f154
    abnormal chest shape and, 190
    sacral agenesis and, 272
cleidocranial dysostosis, abnormal chest shape and, 188, f189, 190–191
clinodactyly, finger abnormalities and, 259–261, f262, f263
cloaca, 385–386, f387
clotting factor deficiencies, nonblanching rashes and, 446
cloverleaf skull, 23, f26
clubfoot
    foot deformities and, 301–302, f303, 304–305
    intoeing and, 287–288, 290–291
CNS tubers, adenoma sebaceum and, 405
coagulation disorders, nonblanching rashes and, 450
Coat disease, leukocoria and, 77
Cobb syndrome, 18
    nevus flammeus and, 18
cocaine, finger abnormalities and, 260
coffee
    hairy tongue and, 157
    teeth discoloration and, 145
coining, f449
    nonblanching rashes and, 446–447
cold sores. see herpes
Colles fracture. see also radius/ulna fractures
    arm swelling and, f250
colobomas
    abnormal head shape and, 24
    ear shape/position abnormalities and, 88
    pupil/iris/lens abnormalities and, 71, f74, 76–77
colonic polyp, perianal/buttock swelling and, 378
compartment syndrome
    arm swelling and, 249, 252
    foot swelling and, 308, 311
concealed penis, 336. see also hidden penis
condyloma lata, 352, f355, 356–357
"confetti," hypopigmented rashes and, 465
congenital
    adrenal hyperplasia, ambiguous genitalia and, 321
    cataracts, 71
    dacryocystocele, swelling of/around the eye and, 57–58, f60, 62–63
    epulis, focal gum lesions and, 144
    heart disease, 190. see also cardiac disease
    hypothyroidism, rectal prolapse and, 377
    lymphedema, penile swelling and, 337–338, f341, 342–343
    malformations, 16, 87, 99–104, 182
    midline nasal masses, 119
    musculoskeletal abnormalities, arm displacement and, 241
    neck masses, 177
    pigmented nevi, heterochromia iridis and, 77
    porphyria, teeth discoloration and, 149
    rubella, congenital cataracts and, 71

torticollis, 22, 177–178, f181
trigger thumb, finger abnormalities and, 264
varicella syndrome, congenital cataracts and, 71
vertical talus (convex pes valgus), 271–272, f273, f303, 306
congestive heart failure (CHF)
    associated findings/complications of, 7
    distinguishing characteristics/duration/chronicity, 6
    foot swelling and, 307–308, 310–311
    hemangiomas and, 417
    predisposing factors, 7
conjunctival nevus, discoloration of/around eye and, 70
conjunctivitis, 49–50, f51–53
    Kawasaki disease and, 432
    molluscum contagiosum and, 405
    scleral epithelial melanosis and, 69
    staphylococcal scalded skin syndrome (SSSS) and, 410
    Stevens-Johnson syndrome and, 483
    throat redness and, 169
    viral pharyngitis and, 171
consanguinity, ambiguous genitalia and, 321
constipation
    enlarged/distended abdomen and, 213–217
    imperforate anus and, 384
    imperforate hymen and, 327
    perirectal skin tag and, 377
    rectal prolapse and, 377
constriction band syndrome
    finger abnormalities and, 264
    leg asymmetry and, 275, f279
contact dermatitis, 345–346, f347, 348–349
    linear red rashes and, 424
    perineal sores/lesions and, 358
    photosensitivity and, 483
    postinflammatory hyperpigmentation and, 472, 475
    postinflammatory hypopigmentation and, 467
    raised red rashes and, 438
    scaly rashes and, 456–457
    vesicular rashes and, 440, 442–443
corn. see callus/corn
corneal abrasion, 54–55
    red eye and, 49, f52
corneal light reflex, misalignment of the eyes and, 80
Cornelia de Lange syndrome
    clinodactyly and, 261
    cutis marmorata and, 397
corticosteroids, oral thrush and, 157
coryza, viral pharyngitis and, 171
Costello syndrome, barrel chest and, 191
costochondral junction, chest lumps and, 199
cough
    mouth sores/patches and, 135
    oral cleft/other variants and, 150
    viral pharyngitis and, 171
cover test, misalignment of the eyes and, 80
coxsackie virus
    hand-foot-mouth disease and, 443
    mouth sores/patches and, 133
    perineal sores/lesions and, 358
    throat redness and, 170
cradle cap. see Seborrhea
cranial meningocele, scalp swelling in newborns and, 15

craniofacial syndromes
    ear pits/tags and, 104
    maldevelopment of ear canal and, 89
craniosynostosis, 22–24, f25
    diseases/syndromes associated with, 27
creased earlobes. see Beckwith-Wiedemann syndrome
crepitus, foot swelling and, 308
cribriform plate fracture, nasal bridge trauma and, 121
Crohn disease
    perianal/buttock swelling and, 373
    perineal sores/lesions and, 358
Crouzon syndrome, 27
cupped ear, f91
cupping, f449
    nonblanching rashes and, 446–447
curvature of the back
    differential diagnosis/other diagnosis and, 224–226
    figures, 223
    historical points, 221
    physical examination, 222
Cushing's disease, longitudinal melanonychia/pigmented bands, 237
Cushing's triad, 6
cutaneous anthrax, red patches/swelling and, 416–417
cutaneous candidiasis, 346, 348–349
cutaneous larva migrans, linear red rashes and, 420, f421, 422–423
cutis aplasia, 30, f33
cutis marmorata (physiologic), skin abnormalities in newborns and, 391, 396–397
cutis marmorata telangiectatica congenita (CMTC), 397
cyanosis
    differential diagnosis and, 6
    skin abnormalities in newborns and, 391
cyclodialysis, iris abnormalities and, 80
Cyrano de Bergerac nose, 120
cystic fibrosis
    nasal polyps and, 129
    rectal prolapse and, 377
cystic hygroma, neck masses/swelling and, 177–178, f182
cystic lesions, swelling of/around the eye and, 57
cystinosis, lens abnormalities and, 80
Cysts. see also lumps on the face
    Baker's (see Baker's cyst)
    Bartholin duct, 359–361
    branchial cleft (see branchial cleft cysts)
    choledochal, 397
    ganglion, 247–249, f250
    lacrimal sac, 57–58
    oral lymphepithelialized, 144
    orbital, 64
    urachal, 207–208, f209, 210–211
cytomegalovirus (CMV)
    cervical adenitis and, 180
    cervical adenopathy and, 180
    enlarged/distended abdomen and, f215
cytopenias, splenomegaly and, 217

D

dacrocystitis, red eye and, 56
dacryocystocele, congenital, 57–58, f60, 62–63

dactylitis
    foot swelling and, 312
    hand swelling and, 254, f255
Dandy-Walker malformation, 22
    abnormal head shape and, 27
deafness, abnormal chest shape and, 190
decreased skin pigmentation. see hypopigment-
    ed rashes
deep vein thrombosis, arm swelling and, 252
deep venous thrombophlebitis
    osteomyelitis and, 257
    viral arthritis and, 257
deer tick. see Borrelia burgdorferi
dehydration
    associated findings/complications of, 7
    distinguishing characteristics/duration/
        chronicity, 6
    mouth sores/patches and, 135
    predisposing factors, 7
Dennie-Morgan lines, scaly rashes and, 452
dental abscesses, focal gum lesions and,
    139–140, f141
dental caries, focal gum lesions and, 142–143
dental discoloration. see teeth discoloration
dental erosion, f148
dentinogenesis imperfecta, teeth discoloration
    and, 149
dependent edema, penile swelling and, 338
depressed sensorium
    respiratory failure and, 7
    toxic ingestion and, 7
dermatitis
    allergic contact, 317, f454
    atopic, 451–452, f453, 456–457
    blepharitis and, 55
    contact, 400, 424, 438, 483
    discoloration of/around eye and, 65
    linear red rashes and, 424
    mouth sores/patches and, 133, f136
    penile edema and, f337
    perianal/buttock redness and, 383
    perineal sores/lesions and, 358
    postinflammatory hyperpigmentation
        and, 472, 475
    postinflammatory hypopigmentation
        and, 467
    raised red rashes and, 438
    rhus, 420, f421, 422–423
    septic arthritis and, 257
    white specks in hair and, 35–36
dermatomyositis, facial rashes and, 406
dermoid cysts
    differential diagnosis/other diagnosis and, 121
    facial lumps and, 40–43
    focal gum lesions and, 144
    nasal bridge swelling and, 119–120, f122
    neck masses/swelling and, 177–178, f181
    orbital tumors and, 57
    swelling of/around the eye and, 62–63
developmental dysplasia of the hip (DDH), 277
    leg asymmetry and, 275
"dew-drop-on-a-rose-petal" lesion, f441
diabetes, see also diabetes mellitus
    nephrotic syndrome and, 311
    obesity and, 217
    xanthogranulomas and, 63
diabetes mellitus
    acanthosis nigricans and, 471, 475
    cutaneous candidiasis and, 349
    perirectal abscesses and, 373

diaper dermatoses, 345–346
    perianal/buttock redness and, 379–381
diarrhea
    asymmetric lateral exanthem of childhood
        and, 437
    rectal prolapse and, 377
    scaly rashes and, 458
    toxic shock syndrome (TSS) and, 410
diastasis recti, abdominal midline bulge and,
    f209, 210–211
diffuse red rashes
    differential diagnosis/other diagnosis and,
        410–412
    figures, 409
    historical points, 407–408
    physical examination, 408
digital clubbing, abnormal chest shape
    and, 190
dimples. see back dimples
diphtheria, throat redness and, 173
diplopia, misalignment of the eyes and, 79
discoid lupus, 30, f33
diskitis, lordosis and, 225
disseminated intravascular coagulation (DIC),
    443
distal limb abnormalities, ear shape/position
    abnormalities and, 88
diuretics, diffuse red rashes and, 407
dizziness
    AOM and, 112
    cholesteatoma and, 112
dolichocephaly, 22, 24, f26
double vision, 65, 79
Down syndrome
    Brushfield spots and, 71
    cutis marmorata and, 397
doxycycline, diffuse red rashes and, 407
drooling, throat redness and, 170
drug exposure/use
    ambiguous genitalia and, 321
    anisocoria and, 77
    diffuse red rashes and, 407–408, f409
    erythema nodosum and, 413
    finger abnormalities and, 259–260
    nail abnormalities and, 235
    nephrotic syndrome and, 311
    photosensitivity and, 483
    raised red rashes and, 438
    Stevens-Johnson syndrome and, 483
    toxic epidermal necrolysis (TEN)
        and, 483
drug rash, diffuse red rashes and, 410–411
drug use, gynecomastia and, 193
Duane syndrome, misalignment of the eyes
    and, 84
dust mites, atopic dermatitis and, 457
dyshidrosis, acropustulosis of infancy
    and, 397
dyshidrotic eczema (pompholyx), 313, 315
    fine bumpy rashes and, 459–461, f462
    foot rashes/lumps, f316
dysphagia
    cat scratch disease and, 180
    mouth sores/patches and, 135
dysplasias
    leg asymmetry and, 275
    skeletal, 270
    dyspnea, congenital heart disease
        and, 311
    dystrophy, lens abnormalities and, 80

E
ear canal findings
    differential diagnosis/other diagnosis and,
        107, 109
    figures, 108
    historical points, 105–106
    physical examination, 106
ear drainage, histiocytosis X and, 348
ear piercing complications, 93, f97
    ear pits/tags and, 104
    eczematous dermatitis and, 106
    perichondritis and, f97
ear popping, OME and, 112
ears
    ear canal findings, 105–109
    ear pits/tags, 99–104
    shape/position abnormalities, 87–92
    swelling of, 93–98
    tympanic membrane abnormalities,
        110–115
ear swelling
    differential diagnosis/other diagnosis and,
        95, 98
    figures, 96–97
    historical points, 93
    physical examination, 94
ecchymoses, 12, f14
    nasal bridge trauma and, 121
ecchymotic discoloration, 68
    discoloration of/around eye and, 66
    leg bowing/knock knees and, 282
    nonblanching rashes and, 446, f448
    penile trauma and, 342
    skin abnormalities in newborns and, 392
ecthyma, focal red bumps and, f427, 428–429
eczema, 37, f38
    dyshidrotic, 459–461, f462
    facial rashes and, 399–400, f401, 404–405
    infantile, 16–18
    postinflammatory hyperpigmentation
        and, 471
    red patches/swelling and, 413
    scaly rashes and, 451–452, f453, 456–457
eczema herpeticum. see herpes simplex
eczema vaccinatum. see vaccinia
eczematous dermatitis
    ear canal findings and, 106, 107
    skin abnormalities in newborns and, 392
edema. see also foot swelling
    acrocyanosis and, 237
    congestive heart failure and, 7
    infected preauricular pits and, 101
    leg asymmetry and, 276
    penile, 337–338, f339–340, 342–343
Edward syndrome
    foot deformities and, f303
    pupil/iris/lens abnormalities and, 71
Ehlers Danlos syndrome
    curvature of the back and, 226
    discoloration of/around eye and, 66
    nail abnormalities and, 245
    rectal prolapse and, 377
ehrlichiosis, nonblanching rashes and, 445. see
    also Rocky Mountain spotted fever
elbow dislocations, arm displacement and,
    241–242
Ellis-van Creveld syndrome
    polydactyly/supernumerary digit and, 261
    postaxial polydactyly and, 259
emesis, bacterial meningitis and, 7

enamel hypoplasia, teeth discoloration and, 149
encephalitis
    cat scratch disease and, 180
    chicken pox (varicella) and, 443
    hand-foot-mouth disease and, 443
    mumps and, 43
encephaloceles
    differential diagnosis/other diagnosis and, 121
    nasal bridge swelling and, 119–120, f122–123
encephalopathy
    cat scratch disease and, 429
    hepatomegaly and, 217
encopresis
    constipation and, 217
    perianal/buttock swelling and, 373
endocrinopathy, penile abnormalities and, 333
enlarged/distended abdomen. see abdominal
        distention
enterocolitis, enlarged/distended abdomen
        and, 218
enterovirus 71, hand-foot-mouth disease
        and, 443
epidermal nevus on ear, 92
epidermoid cysts, 40–43, f44
epidermolysis bullosa
    bullous rashes and, f481, 482–483
    skin abnormalities in newborns and, 391
    sucking blister and, 397
epidermolytic hyperkeratosis (bullous
        ichthyosis), bullous rashes and, 484
epididymitis, scrotal swelling and, 365, 367
epiglottitis, f5
    general appearance and, 4
epignathus, nasal bridge swelling and, 124
epiphora, nasal glioma and, 121
episcleritis/scleritis
    discoloration of/around eye and, 70
    red eye and, 56
epispadias, penile abnormalities and, 336
epistaxis
    nasal bridge swelling and, 121
    nasal glioma and, 121
    nasal polyps and, 129
epithelial inclusion cysts, vulvar swelling/masses
        and, 364
Epstein pearls
    mouth sores/patches and, 133–134, f136
    swellings in the mouth and, 163–164
Epstein-Barr virus (EBV), 180
    cervical adenitis and, 180
    erythema nodosum and, 413
    infectious mononucleosis and, 437
    perineal sores/lesions and, 358
    throat redness and, 169
equinus positioning, foot deformities
        and, 302
eruption cysts, focal gum lesions and,
        139–140, f141
erysipelas, red patches/swelling and, 414, f415,
        416–417
erythema
    breast swelling/enlargement and, 193
    chest lumps and, 199
    diffuse red rashes and, 407–412
    ear pits/tags and, 100, f103
    ear swelling and, 93–95
    hand swelling and, 254
    insect bites and, 310
    neck masses/swelling and, 177
    perianal/buttock redness and, 380

pterygium and, 62
    throat redness and, 169–170
    tympanic membrane abnormalities
        and, 111
erythema infectiosum
    facial rashes and, f403, 404–405
    raised red rashes and, f433, 436–437
erythema marginatum, rheumatic fever
        and, 298
erythema migrans, red patches/swelling and,
        413–414, f415, 416–417
erythema multiforme (minor), raised red
        rashes and, 432, f434, 436–437
erythema nodosum, red patches/swelling and,
        413–414, f415, 416–417
erythema toxicum
    miliaria and, 397
    skin abnormalities in newborns and, 392,
        f393, 396–397
erythematous maculopapules, knee swelling
        and, 294
erythematous oral vesicles, mouth
        sores/patches and, 133–134
erythematous rash. see diffuse red rashes
erythroblastosis fetalis, teeth discoloration
        and, 149
erythrodermic psoriasis, diffuse red rashes
        and, 412
esotropia, 79, f81, 82–83
Ewing sarcoma, knee swelling and, 300
exanthema, diffuse red rashes and, 408
excoriation, infantile eczema and, 18
exercise intolerance, abnormal chest shape
        and, 187
exophthalmos, histiocytosis X and, 348
exotropia, 79, f81, 82–83
external auditory canal (EAC) abnormalities,
        105–106, 107
external auditory canal (EAC) exostosis, ear
        canal findings and, 109
external forces and abnormal head
shape, 22
extremities
    arm displacement, 241–245
    arm swelling, 246–252
    finger abnormalities, 259–264
    fingertip swelling, 265–269
    hand swelling, 253–258
    nail abnormalities, 235–240
extrinsic discoloration of teeth, 145
eye deviation. see eye misalignment
eye discoloration
    differential diagnosis/other diagnosis and,
        68–70
    figures, 67
    historical points, 65–66
    physical examination, 66
eye misalignment
    differential diagnosis/other diagnosis and,
        82–84
    figures, 81
    historical points, 79
    physical examination, 80
eyelid lesions. see swelling of/around the eye
eyes
    discoloration of/around eye, 65–70
    misalignment of the eyes, 79–84
    pupil/iris/lens abnormalities, 71–75
    red eye, 49–56
    swelling of/around the eye, 57–64

F
facial asymmetry, ear shape/position
        abnormalities and, 88, 92
facial deformity
    nasal bridge trauma and, 121
    nasal hemangioma and, 121
facial lesions in newborns
    differential diagnosis/other diagnosis and,
        18, 21
    historical points, 16
    physical examination, 17, f19
facial paralysis
    AOM and, 112
    cholesteotoma and, 112
facial rashes
    differential diagnosis/other diagnosis and,
        404–406
    figures, 401–403
    historical points, 399
    physical examination, 400
facio-auriculo-vertebral spectrum, ear
        shape/position abnormalities and, 87
failure of midline fusion, 351
failure to thrive
    enlarged/distended abdomen and, 213–214
    general appearance and, 8
    oral cleft/other variants and, 150–151
    scaly rashes and, 458
familial hypercholesterolemia, xanthogranulo-
        mas and, 63
familial joint instability syndrome, nail abnor-
        malities and, 245
Farber disease, hand swelling and, 258
farsightedness, misalignment of the eyes and, 79
fat necrosis, 40–43
fatigue
    congenital heart disease and, 311
    Lyme disease and, 298
felon, fingertip swelling and, 266–267, f268
female genitalia variations
    differential diagnosis/other diagnosis and,
        326–327
    figures, 323–325
    historical points, 321–322
    physical examination, 322
femoral torsion, intoeing and, 287–288, f289,
        290–291
femur absence/shortening, leg asymmetry and,
        280
fetal alcohol syndrome, oral cleft/other vari-
        ants and, 156
fever
    AOM and, 112
    arm swelling and, 246
    asymmetric lateral exanthem of childhood
        and, 437
    bullous rashes and, 477
    cat scratch disease and, 429
    cellulitis and, 95, 417
    chicken pox (varicella) and, 442
    cutaneous anthrax and, 417
    drug rash and, 411
    erysipelas and, 417
    erythema migrans and, 417
    erythema nodosum and, 417
    focal gum lesions and, 140
    herpangina and, 171
    infectious mononucleosis and, 171
    juvenile rheumatoid arthritis (JRA) and,
        257, 298

knee swelling and, 293
Ludwig's angina with tongue elevation and, 166
lumps on the face and, 40
Lyme disease and, 298
lymphangitis, 422
mastoiditis, 95
mouth sores/patches and, 133, 135
nonblanching rashes and, 445
pericondritis and, 95
perirectal abscess and, 377
peritonsillar abscess and, 166, 171
preseptal cellulitis and, 55
primary vesicular rashes and, 442
raised red rashes and, 437
red eye and, 49
roseola and, 431
scarlet fever and, 404, 410, 459
septic arthritis and, 256, 298
spider bites and, 417
staphylococcal scalded skin syndrome (SSSS) and, 410, 483
sunburn and, 411
swellings in the mouth and, 163
toxic shock syndrome (TSS) and, 410
fibroadenoma, breast swelling/enlargement and, 197
fibroma, swellings in the mouth and, 168
fibrosarcoma, focal gum lesions and, 144
fibula absence/shortening, leg asymmetry and, 280
Fifth's disease, raised red rashes and, 431
fine bumpy rashes
differential diagnosis/other diagnosis and, 461, 463
figures, 462
historical points, 459
physical examination, 460
finger abnormalities
differential diagnosis/other diagnosis and, 261, 264
figures, 262–263
historical points, 259–260
physical examination, 260
fingertip swelling
differential diagnosis/other diagnosis and, 267, 269
figures, 268
historical points, 265
physical examination, 266
fistulas
focal gum lesions and, 139–140, f141
imperforate anus and, 385–386, f387
flatfeet, foot deformities and, 302
flatus, enlarged/distended abdomen and, 213–217
fluid in ear. see ear canal findings
fluorescein examination, red eye and, 50
fluoride/fluorosis, teeth discoloration and, 145–147, f148
focal gum lesions
differential diagnosis/other diagnosis and, 142–144
figures, 141
historical points, 139
physical examination, 140
focal neurologic signs, increase of intracranial pressure and, 7
focal red bumps, 430
differential diagnosis/other diagnosis and, 428–430

figures, 427
historical points, 425
physical examination, 426
folic acid, spina bifida and, 229
folliculitis
bullous impetigo and, 483
fine bumpy rashes and, 463
furuncle and, 429
perianal/buttock redness and, 379–381, f382
fomites, viral conjunctivitis and, 55
fontanelles, 6
foot deformities
differential diagnosis/other diagnosis and, 304–306
figures, 303
historical points, 301
physical examination, 302
foot progression angle, f289
foot rashes/lumps
differential diagnosis/other diagnosis and, 315, 317
figures, 316
historical points, 313
physical examination, 314
foot sprain, foot deformities and, 306
foot swelling
differential diagnosis/other diagnosis and, 310–312
figures, 309
historical points, 307
physical examination, 308
forceps marks, 18, f19
foreign bodies. see also trauma
external auditory canal (EAC) abnormalities and, 105, 107
foot deformities and, 306
nasal drainage and, 126, f127
tympanic membrane abnormalities and, 115
fourth cranial nerve palsy, misalignment of the eyes and, f81, 82–83
fractures
arm swelling and, 246–249
chest lumps and, 198–201
child abuse and, 199
clavicular, 198, 200–201
fingertip swelling and
foot deformities and, 306
foot swelling and, 308, 310–311
rib, 199–201
freckles, hyperpigmented rashes and, 471, 474–476
fungal infections
ear canal findings and, 106
erythema nodosum and, 413
hypopigmented rashes and, 464
nail abnormalities and, 236
fungal otitis externa, f108
Furstenberg tests
encephaloceles and, 120
nasal glioma and, 121
furuncles
ear canal findings and, 106, 107
focal red bumps and, 426, f427, 428–429
furunculosis, f108
ear canal findings and, 106, 107

G

gait abnormalities, intoeing and, 288, 291
gait unsteadiness, AOM and, 112

galactosemia, enlarged/distended abdomen and, f215
Galeazzi sign, leg asymmetry and, 276, f278
ganglion cyst, arm swelling and, 247–249, f250
Gartner's duct cyst, 359–361
vulvar swelling/masses and, f363
gastroschisis, abdominal midline bulge and, 207–208, f209, 210–211
general appearance
historical points, 3
physical examination, 4
genetic syndromes, oral cleft/other variants and, 152–153
genital herpes, herpetic whitlow and, 265, 267
genital/perineal region
female genitalia variations, 321–327
normal genitalia, 326–327
penile abnormalities, 329–336
penile swelling, 337–343
perineal red rashes, 345–350
perineal sores/lesions, 351–358
scrotal swelling, 365–370
vulvar swelling/masses, 359–364
genital warts, 352, f354, 356–357
genu valgum (knock knees), f283. see also leg bowing/knock knees
intoeing and, 292
leg bowing/knock knees and, 284–285
genu varum (leg bowing), f283. see also leg bowing/knock knees
geographic tongue, 158–159, f161
Gianotti Crosti syndrome, raised red rashes and, 432, f434, 436–437
giant cell granuloma, focal gum lesions and, 144
Gillespie syndrome, aniridia and, 79
gingival abscess, focal gum lesions and, f141
glaucoma
aniridia and, 77
cataracts and, 77
coloboma and, 77
hyphema and, 77
iritis and, 77
photophobia and, 49, 54–55
glomerulonephritis
foot swelling and, 312
scarlet fever and, 411, 437, 461
glomus jugulare tumor, tympanic membrane abnormalities and, 115
glomus tumor, focal red bumps and, 430
glomus tympanicum, tympanic membrane abnormalities and, 115
glossitis, 157–159
Goldenhar syndrome
ear pits/tags and, 99, 104
ear shape/position abnormalities and, 87
gonococcal infection
bacterial conjunctivitis and, 55
ophthalmia, f51
red eye and, 49, 54–55
granuloma gluteale infantum, perianal/buttock redness and, 383
Graves disease, neck masses/swelling and, 184
Greig cephalopolysyndactyly, polydactyly/supernumerary digit and, 261
griseofulvin
diffuse red rashes and, 407
hairy tongue and, 157
group A beta-hemolytic streptococci (GABHS), scarlet fever and, 405, 411

growth failure, congestive heart failure and, 7
growth restriction, leg asymmetry and, 276
grunting, general appearance and, 4
gum abscess. see parulis
gum lesions. see focal gum lesions
gynecomastia
    breast swelling/enlargement and, 193–195,
        f196
    chest lumps and, 198

H
H. influenzae, 50, 55
hair, white specks in, 35–39
hair follicle scarring, traction alopecia and, 31
hair loss. see also hair loss
    differential diagnosis/other diagnosis and,
        30–31, 34
    historical points, 28
    physical examination, 29
hair tufts, 227–231
    midline back and, f230
hairy tongue, 157–159, f161
    tongue discoloration/surface changes and, 157
halitosis
    allergic rhinitis and, 129
    Ludwig's angina with tongue elevation
        and, 166
hand swelling
    differential diagnosis/other diagnosis and,
        256–258
    figures, 255
    historical points, 253
    physical examination, 254
hand-foot-mouth disease, vesicular rashes
        and, 440, f441, 442–443
hands. see also extremities
Hand-Schuller-Christian disease, xanthogranu-
        lomas and, 63
Hashimoto thyroiditis, neck masses/swelling
        and, 184
head
    abnormal head shape, 22–27
head circumference, achondroplasia and, 272
head lice, white specks in hair and, 35
head tilt, misalignment of the eyes and, 80
headaches
    cutaneous anthrax and, 417
    herpangina and, 171
    hot tub folliculitis and, 437
    mouth sores/patches and, 133
    nonblanching rashes and, 445
    pityriasis rosea and, 457
    scarlet fever and, 459
    spider bites and, 417
    sunburn and, 411
hearing loss, 89. see also Ears
    AOM/OME and, 110, 112
    cholesteatoma and, 112
    ear canal findings and, 107
    hemotympanum and, 112
    retraction pockets and, 112
    TM perforation and, 112
    tympanosclerosis and, 112
heart murmur, knee swelling and, 294
helix deformities of ear, 88–89, f90
hemangiomas
    abnormal chest shape and, 190
    arm swelling and, f251
    curvature of the back and, 222

facial lumps and, 40, 42–43, f44
facial rashes and, 406
focal red bumps and, 425–426, f427,
        428–429
hemihypertrophy and, 276
midline back and, 229, f231
mouth sores/patches and, 138
nasal bridge swelling and, 119–121, f123
neck masses/swelling and, 177–178, f182
perineal sores/lesions and, 352, f355,
        356–357
red patches/swelling and, 413–414,
        416–417
swelling of/around the eye and, 57–58, f60
swellings in the mouth and, 168
hemarthroses, nonblanching rashes and, 446
hematemesis, enlarged/distended abdomen
        and, 213
hematocolpos/hematometrocolpos, 322, f325,
        359–361
    vulvar swelling/masses and, f363
hematomas
    arm swelling and, 246–249
    eruption cysts and, 143
    fingertip swelling and, f268
    nasal bridge trauma and, 121
    nasal swelling/discharge/crusting and, 126,
        f127
    neck masses/swelling and, 184
    scalp swelling in newborns and, 11, f14
    vulvar swelling/masses and, 364
hemiatrophy of leg, 277
    leg asymmetry and, f279
hemifacial microsomia, ear pits/tags and, 104
hemihypertrophy, 277
    leg asymmetry and, 275, 276–277, f278
hemolysis, enlarged/distended abdomen and, 213
hemolytic disease, discoloration of/around eye
        and, 66
hemolytic uremic syndrome, nonblanching
        rashes and, 450
hemophilia, nonblanching rashes and, 446
hemorrhagic ulcerative stomatitis in SJS,
        bullous rashes and, f481
hemorrhoids, f375
    perianal/buttock swelling and, 373–374,
        376–377
    perirectal skin tag and, 377
hemotympanum, f115
    ear trauma and, 95
    tympanic membrane abnormalities
        and, 112
Henoch-Schönlein purpura (HSP)
    ear swelling and, 98
    hand swelling and, 258
    knee swelling and, 294
    non blanching rashes and, 447, f448
    scrotal swelling and, 370
    vulvar swelling/masses and, 364
hepatic cirrhosis, foot swelling and, 308
hepatic disease, discoloration of/around eye
        and, 66
hepatic encephalopathy, f5
    general appearance and, 8
hepatic tumor, leg asymmetry and, 276
hepatitis, cat scratch disease and, 429
hepatitis B virus
    Gianotti Crosti syndrome and, 437
    knee swelling and, 300
    viral arthritis and, 256

hepatomegaly
    congenital heart disease and, 311
    enlarged/distended abdomen and, f215
    foot swelling and, 308
    infectious mononucleosis and, 171
    scleral icterus and, 69
hepatospenomegaly
    drug rash and, 411
    enlarged/distended abdomen and, f215
    JRA and, 257
heredity
    cataracts and, 71
    clubfoot and, 301
    intoeing and, 291
    misalignment of the eyes and, 79
hermaphroditism, ambiguous genitalia and,
        326–327
hernia
    abdominal midline bulge and, 212
    inguinal, 359–361, f362, 365–367, f368
    rectal prolapse and, 376
herpangina, f172
    mouth sores/patches and, 134, f136
    throat redness and, 171
herpes
    herpetic whitlow and, 265, 267
    skin abnormalities in newborns and, 391
    sucking blister and, 397
herpes gingivostomatitis, mouth sores/patches
        and, 133–134
herpes keratoconjunctivitis, f52, 54–55
herpes simplex. see also herpes simplex virus
    atopic dermatitis and, 457
    erythema toxicum and, 397
    skin abnormalities in newborns and, 392
    vesicular rashes and, 439–440
herpes simplex virus (HSV), 352, f354,
        356–357
    facial lesions and, 21
herpes zoster iritis, hyphema and, 77
herpes zoster oticus
    ear swelling and, 98
    perineal sores/lesions and, 358
    vesicular rashes and, 439–440, f441,
        442–443
herpetic whitlow
    fingertip swelling and, 265, 267, f268
    vesicular rashes and, f441, 442–443
heterochromia iridium, pupil/iris/lens abnor-
        malities and, f74, 76–77
heterozygous achondroplasia, 270
hidden penis, penile abnormalities and,
        329–330, 332–333
high-arched foot. see cavus foot
hip dislocation, 270
hip dysplasia, metatarsus adductus and, 304
hip flexion contracture, f273
hip rotation. see intoeing
Hirschberg test, misalignment of the eyes and, 80
Hirschsprung disease
    enlarged/distended abdomen and, 214
    rectal prolapse and, 377
histiocytosis X, 346, f347, 348–349
    perianal/buttock redness and, 383
HLA-B27 positivity, juvenile rheumatoid arthri-
        tis (JRA) and, 299
Hodgkin lymphomas
    lymphomas and, 180
    neck masses/swelling and, 177, f183
Hodgkin's disease, knee swelling and, 300

holoprosencephaly, abnormal head shape and, 24
Holt Oram syndrome
  abnormal chest shape and, 188
  clinodactyly and, 261
homocystinuria
  abnormal chest shape and, 190
  curvature of the back and, 226
  cutis marmorata and, 397
hordeolum, swelling of/around the eye and, 57,
  f57, 62–63
hormones, neonatal acne/sebaceous hyperplasia and, 18
Horner's syndrome
  anisocoria and, 77
  heterochromia iridis and, 77
  pupil abnormalities and, 80
"hot potato voice," peritonsillar abscess
  and, 171
hot tub folliculitis, raised red rashes and, 431,
  436–437
HSV gingivostomatitis, mouth sores/patches
  and, f136
human innumodeficiency virus (HIV) infection
  anal fissures and, 374
  cervical adenopathy and, 180
  hairy tongue and, 157
  lumps on the face and, 40
  mycobacterial cervical adenitis and, 180
  oral thrush/oral hairy leukoplakia, 157
  perirectal abscesses and, 373
human papillomavirus (HPV), anogenital warts
  and, 377
hydrocele, scrotal swelling and, 365–367, f368
hydrocephalus
  abnormal head shape and, 27
  misalignment of the eyes and, 84
  spina bifida and, 229
hydrogen peroxide, hairy tongue and, 157
hydronephrosis, imperforate hymen and, 327
hydrops fetalis, sacrococcygeal teratoma and,
  228–229
hydyrocele of the spermatic cord, scrotal
  swelling and, 365–367
hygiene
  perineal sores/lesions and, 351, 358
  perirectal skin tag and, 377
hygroma, neck masses/swelling and, f182
hymen
  sexual abuse and, 356
  types of, f323
hymenal cysts, vulvar swelling/masses
  and, 364
hyoid bone, thyroglossal duct cysts and, 177
hyper IgE syndrome, scaly rashes and, 458
hypercholesterolemia, nephrotic syndrome
  and, 63
hyperhidrosis
  dyshidrotic eczema (pompholyx) and, 315
  juvenile plantar dermatosis and, 315
hyperinsulinism, acanthosis nigricans and, 475
hyperkeratosis, epidermolysis bullosa
  and, 483
hyperlipedemia, xanthogranulomas and, 63
hyperpigmentation
  foot deformities and, 302
  photosensitivity and, 411
hyperpigmented rashes, f473
  differential diagnosis/other diagnosis and,
    474–476
  figures, 473

historical points, 471
  physical examination, 472
hyperpyrexia, acute otitis media (AOM)
  and, 110
hypertelorism, trigonocephaly and, 24
hypertension, hepatomegaly and, 217
hyperthyroidism, craniosynostosis and, 27
hypertonia, intoeing and, 288
hypertropia, misalignment of the eyes and, 80
hyphemas, pupil/iris/lens abnormalities and,
  71–72, f75, 76–77
hypoalbuminemia
  nephrotic syndrome and, 63
  penile edema and, 343
hypoglycemia, cataracts and, 77
hypokalemia, ambiguous genitalia and, 326–327
hypomelanosis of Ito, 464, 466–467, f469
hypopigmentation, lichen striatus and, 423
hypopigmented rashes
  differential diagnosis/other diagnosis and,
    466–467, 470
  figures, 468–469
  historical points, 464
  physical examination, 465
hypospadias, penile abnormalities and,
  330–333, f335
hypotension
  diffuse red rashes and, 407
  toxic shock syndrome (TSS) and, 410
hypothyroidism
  hemangiomas and, 417
  rectal prolapse and, 377
hypotonia
  achondroplasia and, 272
  intoeing and, 288
hypotropia, misalignment of the eyes and, 80
hypovolemia, staphylococcal scalded skin syndrome (SSSS) and, 483
hypoxia, skin abnormalities in newborns and, 391

I

ichthyosis vulgaris, scaly rashes and, f455,
  456–457
icterus, 68–69
  discoloration of/around eye and, 65, f67
id reaction, scaly rashes and, 458
idiopathic cyclic edema, foot swelling and,
  310–311
idiopathic nephrotic syndrome, swelling
  of/around the eye and, 58, f60
idiopathic neuroma, 45
idiopathic penile edema, f339
  penile abnormalities and, 336
idiopathic thrombocytopenic purpura, nonblanching rashes and, 446–447, f449
ileocecal intussusception, perianal/buttock
  swelling and, 378
ileus, enlarged/distended abdomen and, 214
immune-mediated diseases
  herpes zoster oticus and, 439
  swelling of/around the eye and, 64
impaired vision, nasal bridge trauma and, 121
imperforate anus
  differential diagnosis/other diagnosis and,
    386, 388
  figures, 387
  historical points, 384
  physical examination, 385
  sacral agenesis and, 272

imperforate hymen, 321–322, f324
  female genitalia variations and, 326–327
impetigo, 39
  bullous impetigo and, 482–483
  facial rashes and, 399–400, f402, 404–405
  focal red bumps and, 425–426, 428–429
  nasal swelling/discharge/crusting and,
    125–126
  perineal sores/lesions and, 358
incarceration, umbilical hernia and, 211
incontinence
  imperforate anus and, 384
  perirectal abscess and, 377
incontinentia pigmenti, vesicular rashes
  and, 444
increased intracranial pressure
  associated findings/complications of, 7
  distinguishing characteristics/duration/
    chronicity, 6
  predisposing factors, 7
increased skin pigmentation. see hyperpigmented rashes
induration of the hands, 254
infantile eczema, 16–18, f19
infantile physiologic bowing, leg bowing/knock
  knees and, 281
infantile tibia bowing, leg bowing/knock knees
  and, f283, 284–285
infected cysts, focal red bumps and, 430
infections
  fingertip swelling and, 265
  foot deformities and, 301
  foot rashes/lumps and, 313
  labial adhesions and, 327
  leg bowing/knock knees and, 281–282
  nephrotic syndrome and, 311
infectious mononucleosis
  raised red rashes and, 431–432, f434,
    436–437
  throat redness and, 169–171
infertility, ambiguous genitalia and, 321
inflammatory bowel disease (IBD)
  anal fissures and, 374
  erythema nodosum and, 413
  perianal/buttock redness and, 383
  perirectal abscesses and, 373
influenza, perineal sores/lesions and, 358
inguinal hernia
  scrotal swelling and, 365–367, f368
  vulvar swelling/masses and, 359–361, f362
inguinal lymphadenopathy, scrotal swelling
  and, 370
injuries, abnormal chest shape and, 192
insect bites. see also spider bites
  bullous rashes and, f479
  cockroach in external ear canal, f108
  differential diagnosis of, 95
  ear swelling and, 93–94, f96
  focal red bumps and, 426, f427, 428–429
  foot swelling and, 307, f309, 310–311
  hyperpigmented rashes and, 471–472
  knee swelling (Lyme disease) and,
    293, 299
  nonblanching rashes and, 445
  papular urticaria and, 440, 443
  postinflammatory hyperpigmentation and,
    471, 475
  postinflammatory hypopigmentation
    and, 467
  red patches/swelling and, 416–417

insect bites (*Continued*)
  Rocky Mountain spotted fever (RMSF) and, 445, 447, f448–449
  swelling of/around the eye and, 58, f59, 62–63
intoeing
  differential diagnosis/other diagnosis and, 290–292
  figures, 289
  historical points, 287
  physical examination, 288
intracranial extension, buccal cellulitis and, 43
intracranial infection
  AOM and, 112
  nasal bridge trauma and, 121
intracranial pressure, third nerve palsy and, 83
intraocular pressure
  glaucoma and, 55
  misalignment of the eyes and, 80
intraperitoneal hemorrhage, scrotal swelling and, 370
intrauterine fibroids, abnormal head shape and, 22
intrauterine pressure
  abnormal chest shape and, 187
  ear abnormalities, 92
intussusception, enlarged/distended abdomen and, 218
iridis, see heterochromia iridium
iridocyclitis
  conjunctivitis with KD, 55
  JRA and, 257
  red eye and, 56
iridodialysis, iris abnormalities and, 80
iris, 474. see also pupil/iris/lens abnormalities
iritis
  pupil/iris/lens abnormalities and, 72, f74, 76–77
  red eye and, 50, 56
iron, teeth discoloration and, 145–147
irritability, general appearance and, 4
itching, genital, 352

J

jaundice
  discoloration of/around eye and, 66, 68
  drug rash and, 411
  ecchymoses and, 12
  enlarged/distended abdomen and, 213
  infectious mononucleosis and, 171
junctional nevus, f239
juvenile plantar dermatosis, foot rashes/lumps, f316
juvenile rheumatoid arthritis (JRA)
  arm swelling and, 246, 252
  hand swelling and, 254, f255
  knee swelling and, 293–294, f296, 298–299

K

Kaiser-Fleischer rings, pupil/iris/lens abnormalities and, 72, f75, 76–77
Kallmann syndrome, oral cleft/other variants and, 156
Kasabach Merritt syndrome, hemangiomas and, 43, 429
Kawasaki disease (KD)
  conjunctivitis and, 49, f52, 54–55
  foot swelling and, f309, 312
  hand swelling and, 254, f255
  neck masses/swelling and, 184
  perianal/buttock redness and, 380–381

perineal red rashes and, 350
  raised red rashes and, 432, f433, 436–437
keloids, ear swelling and, 93, 95, f97
keratitis, red eye and, 50, 56
keratosis follicularis, fine bumpy rashes and, 463
keratosis pilaris, 461
  atopic dermatitis and, 457
  fine bumpy rashes and, 459–461
  ichthyosis vulgaris and, 457
kerion, 31, f32, 37
  tinea capitis and, 31
kernicterus, scleral icterus and, 69
Kernig/Brudzinski signs, bacterial meningitis and, 7
Klinefelter syndrome, clinodactyly and, 261
Klippel-Trenaunay syndrome, 18
Klippel-Trenaunay-Weber syndrome
  leg asymmetry and, 276
  macrodactyly and, 261
knee cellulitis, knee swelling and, f295
knee effusion, knee swelling and, 294, f295
knee swelling
  differential diagnosis/other diagnosis and, 298–300
  figures, 295–297
  historical points, 293
  physical examination, 294
knock knees. see leg bowing/knock knees
Koebner phenomenon
  lichen nitidus and, 461
  linear red rashes and, 420, f421, 422–423
koilonychia/nail spooning, f239
Koplik spots. see also measles
  mouth sores/patches and, 134, f136
  raised red rashes and, 431
kyphosis, 221–222, f223, 224–225

L

labial abscess, 359–361
labial adhesions
  female genitalia variations and, 321–322, f325, 326–327
  perineal sores/lesions and, 358
labial agglutination, perineal sores/lesions and, 358
labial hematoma, vulvar swelling/masses and, 364
labial hypertrophy, 361
  vulvar swelling/masses and, f362
lacrimal sac cyst, swelling of/around the eye and, 57–58
lactose intolerance, flatus and, 217
lambdoid synostosis, f25
Larsen syndrome, nail abnormalities and, 245
Laurence-Moon-Biedl syndrome, polydactyly/supernumerary digit and, 261
leg asymmetry
  differential diagnosis/other diagnosis and, 277, 280
  figures, 278–279
  historical points, 275
  physical examination, 276
leg bowing/knock knees
  differential diagnosis/other diagnosis and, 284–286
  figures, 283
  historical points, 281–282
  physical examination, 282
leg length, 277. see also leg asymmetry
  juvenile rheumatoid arthritis (JRA) and, 299

Legg-Calves-Perthes disease, 277
lens. see pupil/iris/lens abnormalities
lens subluxation, lens abnormalities and, 80
lenticular myopia, lens abnormalities and, 80
lethargy
  cutaneous anthrax and, 417
  differential diagnosis and, 6
  Stevens-Johnson syndrome and, 483
  toxic shock syndrome (TSS) and, 410
Letterer-Siwe disease, 39
  scaly rashes and, 458
leukemia
  erythema nodosum and, 413
  hand swelling and, 258
  knee swelling and, 300
  neck masses/swelling and, 184
  nonblanching rashes and, 450
leukemic infiltration, scrotal swelling and, 370
leukocoria, pupil/iris/lens abnormalities and, 72, f74, 76–77
leukocytosis, juvenile rheumatoid arthritis (JRA) and, 298
leukonychia striata, f239
  nail abnormalities and, 236
leukoplakia
  HIV and, 157
  mouth sores/patches and, 138
  oral hairy, f161
Levy-Hollister syndrome, ear shape/position abnormalities and, 87
lice. see head lice
lichenification
  scaly rashes and, 452
  white specks in hair and, 37
lichen nitidus, fine bumpy rashes and, 459, 461, f462
lichen planus
  Koebner phenomenon and, 423
  nail abnormalities and, 240
  tongue discoloration/surface changes and, 157
lichen sclerosus et atrophicus, 352, f355, 356–357
lichen spinulosis, fine bumpy rashes and, 463
lichen striatus
  linear red rashes and, 419–420, f421, 422–423
  scaly rashes and, 458
linear epidermal nevus, linear red rashes and, f421, 422–423
linear IgA bullous dermatosis (LABD), bullous rashes and, 484
linear morphea, linear red rashes and, 424
linear red rashes
  differential diagnosis/other diagnosis and, 422–424
  figures, 421
  historical points, 419
  physical examination, 420
Liner's disease, scaly rashes and, 458
lipid metabolism, abnormal, xanthelasma and, 63
lipomas
  facial rashes and, 406
  midline back and, 228
  vulvar swelling/masses and, 364
lipomatosis, leg asymmetry and, 276
lipoprotein abnormalities, xanthogranulomas and, 63
Lisch nodules, café-au-lait (CAL) spots and, 474

liver disease
  ascites and, 217
  hepatomegaly and, 217
  Kaiser-Fleischer rings and, 77
  nonblanching rashes and, 450
  xanthogranulomas and, 63
longitudinal melanonychia, nail abnormalities
      and, 235, f238
longitudinal ridging of nails, f239
lopped ear, f91
lordosis, 221–222, f223, 224–225
lower extremity abnormalities
  differential diagnosis/other diagnosis and,
      272, 274
  figures, 273
  foot deformities, 301–306
  foot rashes/lumps, 313–317
  foot swelling, 307–312
  historical points, 270
  intoeing, 287–292
  knee swelling, 293–300
  leg asymmetry, 275–280
  leg bowing/knock knees, 281–286
  physical examination, 271
  breech births, 272
low-set ears, 87, 92
Ludwig's angina with tongue elevation, f165
  swellings in the mouth and, 164, 166–167
lumps on the face
  differential diagnosis/other diagnosis and,
      42–43, 45
  historical points, 40
  physical examination, 41
lung deformities, abnormal chest shape and, 187
Lyme disease. see also erythema migrans
  knee swelling and, 293–294, 298–299
lymph nodes (swollen), throat redness
      and, 169
lymphadenopathy
  asymmetric lateral exanthem of childhood
      and, 437
  drug rash and, 411
  histiocytosis X and, 348
  juvenile rheumatoid arthritis (JRA)
      and, 298
lymphangioma
  swelling of/around the eye and, 58, f60
  swellings in the mouth and, 168
  vulvar swelling/masses and, 364
lymphangitis, linear red rashes and, 420, f421,
      422–423
lymphedema
  foot swelling and, 312
  leg asymmetry and, f279
  lower extremity, 277
lymphepithelialized cyst, focal gum lesions
      and, 144
lymphocytoma cutis, 45
lymphomas
  ascites and, 217
  erythema nodosum and, 413
  knee swelling and, 300
  neck masses/swelling and, 178, 180

M
macrodactyly, finger abnormalities and,
      259, 261
macroglossia, hemihypertrophy and, 276
macular edema, iritis and, 77

malabsorption, enlarged/distended abdomen
      and, 214
malaise
  arm swelling and, 246
  cellulitis and, 417
  drug rash and, 411
  erysipelas and, 417
  erythema migrans and, 417
  erythema multiforme (minor) and, 437
  hot tub folliculitis and, 437
  Lyme disease and, 298
  mouth sores/patches and, 135
  pityriasis rosea and, 457
  postseptal cellulitis and, 55
  staphylococcal scalded skin syndrome
      (SSSS) and, 410
  sunburn and, 411
Malassezia furfur
  hypopigmented rashes and, 464, 467
  tinea versicolor and, 475
malignancies
  arm swelling and, 249
  cervical adenopathy and, 180
  chest lumps and, 199
  curvature of the back and, 221
  enlarged/distended abdomen and, 214
  foot deformities and, 301
  hand swelling and, 253
  knee swelling and, 294, 300
  leg bowing/knock knees and, 281–282
  nail abnormalities and, 235
  nephrotic syndrome and, 311
malignant, 177
  neck masses/swelling, 177–178
  otitis externa, 109
malignant histiocytosis, knee swelling and, 300
malignant melanoma, nail abnormalities and, 235
malnutrition
  foot swelling and, 307
  nephrotic syndrome and, 311
  rectal prolapse and, 377
mammary hyperplasia/hypertrophy, breast
      swelling/enlargement and, 193
Marfan syndrome
  abnormal chest shape and, 188, 190
  curvature of the back and, 226
  discoloration of/around eye and, 66
  nail abnormalities and, 245
mask of pregnancy. see melasma
masses. see also nasal bridge swelling
mastitis, breast swelling/enlargement and,
      193–195, f196
mastoiditis, 94
  AOM and, 112
  differential diagnosis of, 95
  ear swelling and, f96
  tympanic membrane abnormalities and, 115
maternal use of drugs, finger abnormalities
      and, 259–260
measles, raised red rashes and, 431–432, f435,
      436–437
meatal atresia, 88–89, f91
meconium, imperforate anus and,
      384–386, f387
meconium aspiration syndrome, barrel chest
      and, 191
meconium peritonitis, meconium sequestration
      and, 367
meconium sequestration, scrotal swelling
      and, 367

medial collateral ligament laxity, leg
      bowing/knock knees and, 282
mediastinitis
  Ludwig's angina with tongue elevation
      and, 167
  peritonsillar abscess and, 167
Mees' lines, nail abnormalities and, 240
melanoma
  freckles and, 475
  melanotic nevus and, 475
melanosis oculi, discoloration of/around eye
      and, 66
melanotic nevus, f473
  hyperpigmented rashes and, 471–472,
      474–476
melasma, hyperpigmented rashes and, 474–476
melena, enlarged/distended abdomen and, 213
Melnick Fraser syndrome, ear pits/tags and, 104
meningitis, f5
  buccal cellulitis and, 43
  cholesteatoma and, 112
  dermoid cysts and, 43, 121
  general appearance and, 4
  hand-foot-mouth disease and, 443
  nasal bridge encephalocele and, 121
  nasal glioma and, 121
  peritonsillar abscess and, 167
  septic arthritis and, 257
meningocele, midline back and, f231
meningomyelocele
  congenital vertical talus and, 272
  sacral agenesis and, 272
Menkes syndrome, 34
menstrual cycle, foot swelling and, 307
mental retardation
  abnormal head shape and, 24
  craniosynostosis and, 24
  tuberous sclerosis and, 467
mesenteric cysts, enlarged/distended abdomen
      and, 218
metabolic disorders, leg bowing/knock knees
      and, 282
metabolic errors, general appearance and, 8
metabolic joint disease, hand swelling and, 253
metastatic neuroblastoma, 68–69
  discoloration of/around eye and, 66
metatarsus adductus
  foot deformities and, 301–302, f303,
      304–305
  intoeing and, 287–288, 290–291
metopic synostosis, f25
microcephaly, sacral agenesis and, 272
micro-ear, 87, 89
micropenis, penile abnormalities and,
      330–333, f335
Microsporum, 29
Microsporum species, hypopigmented rashes
      and, 464
microtia, 87–89, f90
  protrusion of external ear, 89
middle ear effusion (MEE), cholesteotoma
      and, 110
midline back pits, 227–231
midline bulge. see abdominal midline bulge
midline fusion failure, f354, 356–357
migraines, misalignment of the eyes and, 80
milia
  sebaceous hyperplasia and, 17, 21
  skin abnormalities in newborns and, 392,
      f394, 396–397

miliaria
    erythema toxicum and, 397
    skin abnormalities in newborns and, 392,
        f395, 396–397
miliaria rubra, facial lesions and, 21
Möbius syndrome, misalignment of the eyes
    and, 84
molding, 13, f14
    abnormal head shape and, 22
molluscum contagiosum, 352, 356–357
    facial rashes and, 400, f402, 404–405
    Koebner phenomenon and, 423
Mongolian spots
    nonblanching rashes and, 446–447, f448
    skin abnormalities in newborns and,
        391–392, f393, 396–397
monilethrix, 34
mononucleosis, throat redness and, 169–171
mottling, congestive heart failure and, 7
mouth
    focal gum lesions, 139–144
    mouth sores/patches, 133–138
    oral cleft/other variants, 150–156
    swellings in the, 163–168
    teeth discoloration, 145–149
    tongue discoloration/surface changes,
        157–161
mouth sores/patches
    differential diagnosis/other diagnosis and,
        135, 138
    figures, 136–137
    historical points, 133
    physical examination, 134
mucocele
    mouth sores/patches and, 138
    swelling of/around the eye and, 57
    swellings in the mouth and, 163–164, f165,
        166–167
mucoepidermoid carcinoma, focal gum lesions
    and, 144
mucohydrocolpos, 322
mucopolysaccharidoses
    craniosynostosis and, 27
    oral cleft/other variants and, 156
mucus membranes, general appearance and, 4
Muehrcke's lines, nail abnormalities and, 240
multiple enchondromas, arm swelling
    and, 249
multiple mucosal neuromas (MEN IIB), 45
multiple myeloma
    Kaiser-Fleischer rings and, 77
    nephrotic syndrome and, 311
mumps, 40–43
    knee swelling and, 300
    parotitis and, 43
myalgia
    erythema migrans and, 417
    toxic shock syndrome (TSS) and, 410
myasthenia gravis, misalignment of the eyes
    and, 79, 84
mycobacterial cervical adenitis, neck
    masses/swelling and, 178, 180
Mycoplasma pneumoniae, pharyngitis from, 173
Mycoplasma tuberculosis, 180
mycotic otitis externa, ear canal findings
    and, 107
myeloma
    Kaiser-Fleischer rings and, 77
    xanthogranulomas and, 63
myelomeningocoele, midline back and, 228

myopia
    cataracts and, 77
    leukocoria and, 77
myringosclerosis. see tympanosclerosis

N

nail abnormalities
    differential diagnosis/other diagnosis and,
        237, 240
    figures, 237–239
    historical points, 235
    physical examination, 236
nail clubbing
    enlarged/distended abdomen and, 214
    nail abnormalities and, 236–237
nail dystrophy, f239
nasal bridge broadness, pseudostrabismus and,
    80, 82–83
nasal bridge encephalocele, differential diagno-
    sis/other diagnosis and, 121
nasal bridge swelling
    differential diagnosis/other diagnosis and,
        121, 124
    figures, 122–123
    historical points, 119
    physical examination, 120
nasal bridge trauma, differential diagnosis/other
    diagnosis and, 121
nasal dermoid cysts, 119–120
nasal fractures, 120
nasal glioma, 120
    differential diagnosis/other diagnosis and, 121
    nasal bridge swelling and, f123
nasal hemangioma, differential diagnosis/other
    diagnosis and, 121
nasal polyps, f127
    recurring infections and, 125–126
nasal swelling/discharge/crusting
    differential diagnosis/other diagnosis and,
        128–129
    figures, 127
    historical points, 125
    physical examination, 126
nasolacrimal duct injury, nasal bridge trauma
    and, 121
nasolacrimal duct obstruction, swelling
    of/around the eye and, 57
nasopharyngeal teratoma, nasal bridge swelling
    and, 124
natal teeth present at birth, focal gum lesions
    and, 140, f141
nausea
    glaucoma and, 55
    scrotal swelling and, 365
    spider bites and, 417
    sunburn and, 411
neck, throat redness, 169–173
neck masses/swelling
    differential diagnosis/other diagnosis and,
        179–180, 184
    figures, 181–183
    historical points, 177
    physical examination, 178
neck stiffness, Lyme disease and, 298
necrotizing enterocolitis, enlarged/distended
    abdomen and, 218
neglect, general appearance and, 4
Neisseria gonorrhoeae, septic arthritis
    and, 256

nematode exposure, cutaneous larval migrans
    and, 423
neonatal acne
    facial lesions and, 16, 18, f19
    skin abnormalities in newborns and, 392
neonatal death, congenital adrenal hyperplasia
    (CAH) and, 321
neonatal herpes, vesicular rashes and, f441
neonatal jaundice (physiologic), skin abnormali-
    ties in newborns and, f394, 396–397
neonatal vesicular rash, vesicular rashes and,
    442–443
neoplasms, general appearance and, 8
nephritis, Stevens-Johnson syndrome and, 483
nephrotic syndrome, 57–58, f60
    foot swelling and, 307–308, 310–311
    scrotal swelling and, f369
    swelling of/around the eye and, 57
nerve palsies, misalignment of the eyes and,
    80, f81
neuroblastoma
    discoloration of/around eye and, 66
    knee swelling and, 300
    neck masses/swelling and, 177
neurofibromatosis
    café-au-lait (CAL) spots and, 276, 471, 474
    macrodactyly and, 261
neurologic abnormalities, juvenile rheumatoid
    arthritis (JRA) and, 299
neurologic symptoms, infectious mononucleo-
    sis and, 437
neuromuscular disorders, curvature of the
    back and, 226
neuromuscular problems
    intoeing and, 292
    lordosis and, 225
neutrophil dysfunction, perirectal abscesses
    and, 373
nevus
    heterochromia iridis and, 77
    linear epidermal, f421, 422–423
nevus anemicus, hypopigmented rashes
    and, 470
nevus depigmentosus, hypopigmented rashes
    and, 470
nevus flammeus, 16–18, f19
nevus of Ota, discoloration of/around eye and,
    66, f67
nevus simplex, 16–18, f19
newborns
    abnormal head shape and, 22–27
    capillary hemangiomas of eyelid in, 57
    clavicular fractures in, 198
    facial lesions, 16–21
    lower extremity abnormalities in, 270–274
    nasolacrimal duct obstruction and, 57
    red eye and, 49
    scalp swelling in, 11–15
nickel allergy, dyshidrotic eczema (pompholyx)
    and, 315
Nikolsky's sign
    bullous rashes and, 478
    diffuse red rashes and, 408
    staphylococcal scalded skin syndrome
        (SSSS) and, 483
nipples, supernumerary, 199–201
nits. see head lice
nocturia, congenital heart disease and, 311
nonalcoholic steatohepatitis, acanthosis
    nigricans and, 475

nonblanching rashes
    differential diagnosis/other diagnosis and,
        447, 450
    figures, 448–449
    historical points, 445–446
    physical examination, 446
non-Hodgkin lymphomas
    lymphomas and, 180
    neck masses/swelling and, 177
nonimmune fetal hydrops, erythema infectio-
    sum and, 437
Noonan syndrome
    abnormal chest shape and, 188, 190
    ear shape/position abnormalities and, 87
    penile abnormalities and, 329
nose
    nasal bridge swelling, 119–124
    nasal swelling/discharge/crusting and,
        125–129
NSAIDSs, diffuse red rashes and, 407
nuchal rigidity, bacterial meningitis and, 7
nummular eczema, scaly rashes and, f453,
    456–457
nursemaid's elbow, arm displacement and,
    241, f244
nutrition
    leg bowing/knock knees and, 281–282
    teeth discoloration and, 145–146
nystagmus, aniridia and, 77

O

obesity
    acanthosis nigricans and, 471, 474
    breast swelling/enlargement and, 194
    enlarged/distended abdomen and, f215
    keratosis pilaris and, 461
    lordosis and, 225
    pilonidal sinus/cyst and, 229
obsessive-compulsive behavior, hair loss and, 28
obstructive sleep apnea, obesity and, 217
occipital lymphadenopathy, 36
occipital plagiocephaly, f25
occult bacteremia, general appearance and, 4
occult foot fracture, foot deformities
    and, 306
occult spinal pathology, 227, 229
ocular abnormalities, nasal hemangioma
    and, 121
ocular albinism, iris abnormalities and, 80
ocular misalignment. see eye misalignment
ocular symptoms, allergic rhinitis and, 129
oculoauriculovertebral syndromes
    ear pits/tags and, f102, 104
    preauricular tags and, 101
olanzapine, foot swelling and, 307
oleoresin. see rhus dermatitis
oligohydramnios, leg asymmetry and, 275
Ollier disease, arm swelling and, 249
omphalocele
    abdominal midline bulge and, 207–208, f209,
        210–211
    hemihypertrophy and, 276
omphalomesenteric cyst, abdominal midline
    bulge and, 212
onychomycosis, 237
    nail abnormalities and, 237, f238
    tinea pedis and, 315
Opitz syndrome, penile abnormalities and, 329
optic glioma, café-au-lait (CAL) spots and, 474

oral cleft/other variants
    differential diagnosis/other diagnosis and,
        152–153, 156
    figures, 154–155
    historical points, 150
    physical examination, 151
oral contraceptives
    cutaneous candidiasis and, 349
    diffuse red rashes and, 407
    foot swelling and, 307
    melasma and, 471
oral hairy leukoplakia, 157–159, f161
oral herpes, herpetic whitlow and, 265, 267
oral lesions. see focal gum lesions
oral lymphepithelialized cyst, focal gum lesions
    and, 144
oral thrush
    candidal infections and, 348
    HIV and, 157
orbital cellulitis, 50, f53, 54–55
    dermoid cysts and, 121
orbital cyst, swelling of/around the eye and, 64
orbital tumors
    discoloration of/around eye and, 70
    hyphema and, 77
organomegaly, enlarged/distended abdomen
    and, 214
orofacial-digital syndrome
    milia and, 397
    oral cleft/other variants and, 156
orthopnea
    congenital heart disease and, 311
    differential diagnosis and, 6
orthostatic edema, foot swelling and,
    310–311
Osgood-Schlatter disease, knee swelling and,
    294, f296–297, 300
osseous lesions, café-au-lait (CAL) spots
    and, 474
ossicular damage, TM perforation and, 112
osteochondritis dissecans, knee swelling
    and, 300
osteogenesis imperfecta, curvature of the back
    and, 226
osteogenic sarcoma
    focal gum lesions and, 144
    knee swelling and, 300
osteomyelitis
    ear canal findings and, 109
    dermoid cysts and, 121
    foot deformities and, 301, 306
    hand swelling and, 253, f255
    knee swelling and, 300
    peritonsillar abscess and, 167
    septic arthritis and, 257
    staphylococcal scalded skin syndrome
        (SSSS) and, 483
osteoporosis
    curvature of the back and, 226
    kyphosis and, 225
osteosarcoma
    arm swelling and, 252
    foot deformities and, 306
otalgia
    acute otitis media (AOM) and, 110, 112
otitis externa, 104, f108
    cellulitis of the auricle and, 93
    external auditory canal (EAC) abnormali-
        ties and, 105–106, 107
    malignant, 98

otitis media
    bacterial conjunctivitis and, 55
    external auditory canal (EAC) abnormali-
        ties and, 105
    mastoiditis, 95
    otitis externa and, 107
otitis media-conjunctivitis syndrome, 50
otitis media with effusion (OME), f113
    acute otitis media (AOM) and, 110–112
otomastoiditis, mycobacterial cervical adenitis
    and, 180
otorrhea, f108
    cholesteatoma and, 112
    mastoiditis, 95
otosclerosis, tympanic membrane abnormali-
    ties and, 115
ovarian failure, breast swelling/enlargement
    and, 193
ovarian pathology, ascites and, 217

P

pain
    cellulitis and, 417
    chest lumps and, 198
    dental abscesses and, 139, 143
    ear swelling and, 93
    erysipelas and, 417
    erythema migrans and, 417
    female genitalia variations and, 321
    foot swelling and, 308
    general appearance and, 4
    glaucoma and, 55
    hemorrhoids and, 376
    hemotympanum and, 112
    knee swelling and, 294
    leg bowing/knock knees and, 281
    lordosis and, 225
    lymphangitis and, 422
    mouth sores/patches and, 135
    ocular, 49
    perianal/buttock swelling and, 373
    perineal sores/lesions and, 351–352
    peritonsillar abscess and, 166
    plantar wart and, 315
    precision of children's description of, 105
    preseptal cellulitis, 55
    primary vesicular rashes and, 443
    red eye and, 54–55
    scarlet fever and, 459
    scoliosis and, 221
    septic arthritis and, 256
    sinusitis and, 126
    spider bites and, 417
    sprains/fractures, 310
    streptococcal pharyngitis and, 171
    swellings in the mouth and, 163
    testicular torsion and, 365
    throat redness and, 169
    vulvar swelling/masses and, 359
painful urination, tinea cruris and, 348
pallor, enlarged/distended abdomen
    and, 214
palmar erythema, 254
    diffuse red rashes and, f409
pancreatic pseudocyst, enlarged/distended
    abdomen and, 218
panniculitis, 40–43, f44
papular urticaria, vesicular rashes and,
    439–440, f441, 442–443

papulovesicles on hands/feet, viral pharyngitis and, 171
paramyxovirus, measles and, 437
paraphimosis, penile abnormalities and, 332–333, f334
parasympathetic lesions, anisocoria and, 77
paraurethral duct cyst, 359–361
    vulvar swelling/masses and, f362
Parinaud's oculoglandular syndrome, cat scratch disease and, 180
parotid swelling, 40, f44
parulis, swellings in the mouth and, 168
parvovirus
    erythema infectiosum and, 405
    knee swelling and, 300
Pastia's lines, scarlet fever and, 461
Patau syndrome, foot deformities and, f303
patent urachus, abdominal midline bulge and, 207–208, 212
patent vitelline/omphalomesenteric fistula, abdominal midline bulge and, 212
pectoralis muscle absence. see Poland syndrome
pectus carinatum, abnormal chest shape and, 190–191
pectus excavatum, 187–188, f189, 190–191
pediculosis capitis, f38. see also head lice
pemphigus
    bullous rashes and, 484
    vesicular rashes and, 444
penile abnormalities
    differential diagnosis/other diagnosis and, 332–333, 336
    figures, 334–335
    historical points, 329–330
    physical examination, 330–331
penile adhesions, penile abnormalities and, 329–330, 332–333, f334
penile edema, penile swelling and, 337–338, f339–340, 342–343
penile skin bridging, penile abnormalities and, 336
penile swelling
    differential diagnosis/other diagnosis and, 342–343
    figures, 339–341
    historical points, 338
    physical examination, 338
penile torsion, penile abnormalities and, 330–333, f335
penile trauma, penile swelling and, 338, f340, 342–343
penoscrotal transposition, penile abnormalities and, f335
pentalogy of Cantrell, abnormal chest shape and, 190
perborate, hairy tongue and, 157
perforated tympanic membrane. see TM perforation
perfusion
    congestive heart failure and, 7
    dehydration and, 7
perianal/buttock redness
    differential diagnosis/other diagnosis and, 381, 383
    figures, 382
    historical points, 379
    physical examination, 380
perianal/buttock swelling
    differential diagnosis/other diagnosis and, 376–378
    figures, 375

historical points, 373–374
    physical examination, 374
perianal skin tag, 375
pericarditis, juvenile rheumatoid arthritis (JRA) and, 257, 298
perichondritis, ear swelling and, 94, 95, f97
perinatal infections, leg asymmetry and, 275
perineal fistula, f387
perineal red rashes
    differential diagnosis/other diagnosis and, 348–350
    figures, 347
    historical points, 345
    physical examination, 346
perineal sores/lesions
    differential diagnosis/other diagnosis and, 356–358
    figures, 353–355
    historical points, 351–352
    physical examination, 352
periorbital cellulitis, f53, 54–55
periorbital edema, raised red rashes and, 432
periorbital swelling, discoloration of/around eye and, 68
periosteal abscess, osteomyelitis and, 257
peripheral cyanosis, dehydration and, 7
peripheral giant cell granuloma, focal gum lesions and, 144
perirectal abscess, f375
    perianal/buttock swelling and, 376–377
perirectal skin tag, perianal/buttock swelling and, f375, 376–377
peritoneal irritation, general appearance and, 4
peritonitis
    ascites and, 217
    enlarged/distended abdomen and, 213–214
    intestinal obstruction and, 217
peritonsillar abscess, f172
    swellings in the mouth and, 163–164, 166–167
    throat redness and, 169–171
pernicious anemia, longitudinal melanonychia/pigmented bands, 237
persistent hyperplastic primary vitreous (PHPV), leukocoria and, 77
pes calcaneovalgus, 272
pes planus, foot deformities and, 301–302, f303, 304–305
petechiae
    bacterial meningitis and, 7
    nonblanching rashes and, 446, f449
    scarlet fever and, 410
Peutz Jeghers syndrome, longitudinal melanonychia/pigmented bands, 237
PHACE syndrome, hemangiomas and, 43
pharyngitis, f172
    pityriasis rosea and, 457
    red eye and, 50
    scarlet fever and, 404
    throat redness and, 173
phenothiazines
    diffuse red rashes and, 407
    tongue discoloration/surface changes and, 157
phenylketonuria, scaly rashes and, 458
phenytoin, tongue discoloration/surface changes and, 157
phimosis
    penile abnormalities and, 329–330, 332–333, f334

penile edema and, 343
    posthitis and, 343
phlyctenule, discoloration of/around eye and, 70
photodermatitis, diffuse red rashes and, 407
photophobia, 49, 54–55
    allergic conjunctivitis and, 55
    aniridia and, 77
    nonblanching rashes and, 445
    pupil/iris/lens abnormalities and, 72
photosensitivity
    bullous rashes and, 478, f479, 482–483
    diffuse red rashes and, 407–408, f409, 410–411
physical abuse. see child abuse
physiologic bowing of legs, 272, f273
phytotoxins, diffuse red rashes and, 407
piebaldism
    heterochromia iridium and, 77
    hypopigmented rashes and, 470
piercing
    breast swelling/enlargement and, 194
    ear pits/tags and, 104
Pierre-Robin syndrome, oral cleft/other variants and, 156
pigmentation around eye. see eye discoloration
pili torti, 34
pilomatrixoma, 45
pilonidal abscesses, perianal/buttock swelling and, 373–374
pilonidal sinus/cyst, 228, 229, f230
ping pong ball sensation, leg bowing/knock knees and, 282
pingueculae, swelling of/around the eye and, 57
pink eye. see red eye
Pinocchio nose, 120
pinworms, 379–381
pitted keratolysis, foot rashes/lumps and, 317
pitting, penile swelling and, 338
pityriasis, scaly rashes and, 452, f454
pityriasis alba, 464–467, f468
    facial rashes and, 399–400, f403, 404–405
pityriasis rosea, scaly rashes and, 451, 456–457
plagiocephaly, 23–24
    scalp swelling in newborns and, 15
plane xanthoma. see xanthogranulomas
plantar corns/warts, 313–315
    foot rashes/lumps, f316
pleuritis, juvenile rheumatoid arthritis (JRA) and, 298
pneumatic otoscopy, 110, 111
pneumonia
    dactylitis and, 257
    enlarged/distended abdomen and, 213
    staphylococcal scalded skin syndrome (SSSS) and, 483
    Stevens-Johnson syndrome and, 483
poison ivy. see rhus dermatitis
Poland syndrome
    abnormal chest shape and, 188, f189, 190–191
    brachydactyly and, 261
    syndactyly and, 259, 261
polyarthritis, knee swelling and, 293
polychondritis, ear swelling and, 98
polycystic ovarian syndrome, acanthosis nigricans and, 471
polydactyly/supernumerary digit, finger abnormalities and, 259, 261, f262

pompholyx. *see* dyshidrotic eczema
popliteal cyst, knee swelling and, 294
popsicle panniculitis, 40–43, f44
porencephalic/leptomeningeal cyst, scalp
    swelling in newborns and, 15
portal hypertension, enlarged/distended
    abdomen and, 213
port-wine stain. *see* nevus flammeus
positional plagiocephaly, 22, f25
posterior fossa abnormalities, nasal
    hemangioma and, 121
posthitis, penile swelling and, 338, f341,
    342–343
postinflammatory hyperpigmentation, 471–472,
    474–476
postinflammatory hypopigmentation, 464,
    466–467, f468
postseptal cellulitis, 54–55
Prader Willi syndrome, penile abnormalities
    and, 329
preauricular abcess, f103
preauricular node, conjunctivitis and, 50
preauricular pits, 99–104, f102
preauricular sinus, f103
preauricular tags, 101, f102, f103
pregnancy
    cutaneous candidiasis and, 349
    enlarged/distended abdomen and, 214
    foot swelling and, 312
    melasma and, 471, 474–475
premature thelarche, breast swelling/enlargement
    and, 193, 195
premature tooth eruption, histiocytosis X
    and, 348
prematurity, abnormal head shape and, 22
prenatal alcohol/drug use, misalignment of the
    eyes and, 79, 83
prepatellar bursitis, knee swelling and, 294
prepubertal/pubertal genitalia, f323–324
    penile abnormalities, 329–336
    penile swelling, 337–343
preputial inflammation. *see* posthitis
preseptal cellulitis. *see* periorbital cellulitis
preterm birth, misalignment of the eyes and,
    79, 83
primary irritant diaper dermatitis, perianal/
    buttock redness and, 379–381, f382
primary vesicular rash, 442–443
proboscis lateralis, nasal bridge swelling
    and, 124
prolapsed ureterocele, 359–361
prolonged standing, foot swelling and, 307
pronation of feet, intoeing and, 292
proptosis
    dermoid cysts and, 63
    discoloration of/around eye and, 66, 68
    swelling of/around the eye and, 57–58
proteinuria, nephrotic syndrome and, 63
Proteus syndrome, leg asymmetry and, f278
protruding colonic polyp, perianal/buttock
    swelling and, 378
protruding ileocecal intussusception,
    perianal/buttock swelling and, 378
protrusion of external ear, 87–89
Prune Belly syndrome, enlarged/distended
    abdomen and, f215
pruritus
    acropustulosis of infancy and, 392
    asymmetric lateral exanthem of childhood
    and, 437

contact dermatitis and, 442
    drug rash and, 410
    ear swelling and, f96
    eczema and, 404
    erythema and, 413
    foot rashes/lumps and, 314
    furuncles and, 426
    infantile eczema and, 18
    insect bites and, 310, 417
    linear red rashes and, 419–420
    papular urticaria and, 442
    perirectal abscesses and, 373
    perirectal skin tag and, 377
    photosensitivity and, 483
    red eye and, 49
    red patches/swelling and, 413
    scarlet fever and, 410
    seborrhea and, 404
    urticaria and, 417
pseudoarthrosis of clavicle, chest lumps and,
    200–201, f202
pseudogynecomastia, breast swelling/enlarge-
    ment and, 194
pseudohypoparathyroidism, brachydactyly
    and, 261
pseudomonas infections, ear canal findings and,
    106
Pseudomonas aeruginosa, hot tub folliculitis
    and, 437
pseudostrabismus, misalignment of the eyes
    and, 80, f81, 82–83
psoriasis, 39, f347, 348–349
    Koebner phenomenon and, 423
    perianal/buttock redness and, 380
    scaly rashes and, 451, f455, 456–457
psoriatic dermatitis
    ear canal findings and, 106
    otitis externa and, 107
    perineal sores/lesions and, 358
psoriatic nail pitting, nail abnormalities
    and, f238
psychiatric disorders
    general appearance and, 4
    hair loss and, 31
psychologic distress, constipation and, 217
psychotropic agents, tongue discoloration/
    surface changes and, 157
pterygium, swelling of/around the eye and, f61,
    62–63
ptosis, capillary hemangiomas of eyelid and, 63
puberty, seborrhea and, 457
pulmonary atelectasis, rickets and, 201
pulmonary disease
    abnormal chest shape and, 187
    chronic cervical lymphadenitis and, 177
pupil/iris/lens abnormalities
    differential diagnosis/other diagnosis and,
    76–78
    figures, 73–75
    historical points, 71
    physical examination, 72
purpura, facial rashes and, 406
purpura fulminans, f449
    nonblanching rashes and, 447
pustular melanosis, skin abnormalities in new-
    borns and, 392, f393, 396–397
pustular psoriasis, foot rashes/lumps and, 317
pyogenic granuloma, 40, 42–43, f44
    focal red bumps and, 425–426, f427,
    428–429

pyriform sinuses/cysts, neck masses/swelling
    and, 184
pyuria, epididymitis and, 367

R
raccoon eyes, 68–69
"rachitic rosary"
    chest lumps and, 199
    leg bowing/knock knees and, 282
radial head subluxation, arm displacement and,
    241–242
radiation, breast swelling/enlargement
    and, 193
radioulnar synostosis, nail abnormalities
    and, 245
radius/ulna fractures, arm swelling and,
    246–249, f250
raised red rashes
    differential diagnosis/other diagnosis and,
    436–438
    figures, 433–435
    historical points, 431
    physical examination, 432
Ramsay Hunt syndrome, ear swelling and,
    f97, 98
range of motion, kyphosis/lordosis and,
    222, 225
ranula, swellings in the mouth and, 163–164,
    f165, 166–167
rashes. *see also* skin
    bullous rashes, 477–484
    diffuse red rashes, 407–412
    facial, 399–406
    fine bumpy rashes, 459–463
    focal red bumps and, 425–430
    hyperpigmented rashes, 471–476
    hypopigmented rashes, 464–470
    juvenile rheumatoid arthritis (JRA) and,
    257, 298
    knee swelling and, 293
    linear red rashes, 419–424
    Lyme disease and, 298
    nonblanching rashes, 445–450
    perianal/buttock redness and, 379–383
    perineal red rashes, 345–350
    raised red rashes, 431–438
    red patches/swelling, 413–417
    scaly rashes, 451–458
    vesicular rashes, 439–444
    white specks in hair and, 37
Raynaud's phenomenon, nail abnormalities
    and, 235
rectal atresia, 386
rectal bleeding, perirectal abscess and, 377
rectal prolapse
    perianal/buttock swelling, 373–374,
    376–377
    perirectal abscesses and, f375
rectourethral fistula, 386, f387
rectovestibular fistula, f387
recurrent vesicular rash, 442–443
red eye
    differential diagnosis/other diagnosis and,
    54–56
    figures, 51–53
    historical points, 49
    physical examination, 50
"Red Man syndrome," diffuse red rashes
    and, 407

red patches/swelling
  differential diagnosis/other diagnosis and, 416–417
  figures, 415
  historical points, 413
  physical examination, 414
red reflex test, misalignment of the eyes and, 80
red streaking, cellulitis and, 95
red-cell aplasia, erythema infectiosum and, 437
reflexes, tympanic membrane abnormalities and, 111
renal anomalies, sacral agenesis and, 272
renal disease
  ear position and, 89
  hepatomegaly and, 217
  nephrotic syndrome, 63
  Prune Belly syndrome and, 217
  Stevens-Johnson syndrome and, 483
renal ultrasonography, ear pits/tags and, 99
respiratory distress
  congestive heart failure and, 7
  dermoid cysts and, 63
  diffuse red rashes and, 407
  general appearance and, 4
  Ludwig's angina with tongue elevation and, 167
  nasal hemangioma and, 121
  Stevens-Johnson syndrome and, 483
  toxic ingestion and, 7
respiratory failure
  associated findings/complications of, 7
  distinguishing characteristics/duration/chronicity, 6
  general appearance and, 4
  predisposing factors, 7
respiratory infections, rickets and, 201
retinal detachment
  coloboma and, 77
  leukocoria and, 77
retinoblastoma, leukocoria and, 77
retraction pockets, f115
  tympanic membrane abnormalities and, 111–112
retropharyngeal cellulitis, throat redness and, 170
retropharyngeal process, general appearance and, 4
Rh incompatibility, neonatal jaundice and, 397
rhabdomyoma
  adenoma sebaceum and, 405
  tuberous sclerosis and, 467
rhabdomyosarcoma
  focal gum lesions and, 144
  knee swelling and, 300
  neck masses/swelling and, 184
  swelling of/around the eye and, 64
rheumatic fever
  knee swelling and, 293–294, 298–299
  scarlet fever and, 411, 437, 461
  streptococcal pharyngitis and, 171
rhinitis
  allergic, 125–126
  discoloration of/around eye and, 65, 69
rhinorrhea, 125–126, f127
  throat redness and, 169
rhus dermatitis
  Koebner phenomenon and, 423
  linear red rashes and, f421, 422–423

rib anomalies
  abnormal chest shape and, 192
  chest lumps and, 198–199
rib fractures, chest lumps and, 199–201
RICE (rest, ice, compression, and elevation), wrist sprain and, 249
rickets
  arm swelling and, f251, 252
  chest lumps and, 198–201
  curvature of the back and, 226
  leg bowing/knock knees and, 281–282, 284–285
Rieger syndrome, coloboma and, 77
Robinow syndrome
  oral cleft/other variants and, 156
  penile abnormalities and, 329
rockerbottom foot. see congenital vertical talus
Rocky Mountain spotted fever (RMSF), nonblanching rashes and, 445, 447, f448
rosacea, blepharitis and, 55
roseola, raised red rashes and, 431–432, f433, 436–437
rubella
  knee swelling and, 300
  viral arthritis and, 256
Rubinstein Taybi syndrome, polydactyly/supernumerary digit and, 261
ruptured globe, discoloration of/around eye and, 70

S

sacral agenesis, 271–272, f273
  clubfoot and, 290, 304
  imperforate anus and, 388
sacral dimple/pit, 229, f230
sacrococcygeal teratoma, midline back and, 227–229, f231
sagittal synostosis, f26
salmon patch. see nevus simplex
Salmonella infections, dactylitis and, 257
sarcoma botryoides, 360–361
  vulvar swelling/masses and, f363
Sarcopetes scabiei, 423, 437. see also scabies
scabies
  acropustulosis of infancy and, 397
  bullous, 484
  linear red rashes and, 419–420, 422–423
  raised red rashes and, 432, f435, 436–437
  scaly rashes and, 458
  vesicular rashes and, 444
scalp ecchymoses, caput succedaneum and, 13. see also ecchymoses
scalp eczema, 37, f38
scalp swelling in newborns
  differential diagnosis/other diagnosis and, 13, 15
  historical points, 11
  physical examination, 12
scaly rashes
  differential diagnosis/other diagnosis and, 456–458
  figures, 453–455
  historical points, 451
  physical examination, 452
scaphocephaly, f25–26
scarlet fever
  diffuse red rashes and, 408, f409, 410–411
  facial rashes and, 400, 404–405
  fine bumpy rashes and, 459, 461, f462

perineal red rashes and, 350
  raised red rashes and, 432, f433, 436–437
scarring
  of external ear canal, 107
  hair loss and, 31
Schamroth's sign, nail abnormalities and, 236
Scheurman's disease, kyphosis, 225
Schwartze's sign, tympanic membrane abnormalities and, 115
scleral epithelial melanosis, 68–69
  discoloration of/around eye and, 66, f67
scleral icterus. see icterus
scleral rupture, pupil/iris/lens abnormalities and, 72
scoliosis
  abnormal chest shape and, 190
  curvature of the back, 221, f223, 224–225
scrotal swelling
  differential diagnosis/other diagnosis and, 367, 370
  figures, 368–369
  historical points, 365
  physical examination, 366
seasonal allergic rhinitis, 125
sebaceous hyperplasia, f19
sebaceous nevus of Jadassohn, 30, f33
seborrhea, f19, f38, 346, f347, 348–349
  ear canal findings and, 106, 107
  facial lesions and, 16–18
  facial rashes and, 400, 404–405
  hair loss and, 29
  perineal sores/lesions and, 358
  postinflammatory hypopigmentation and, 467
  scaly rashes and, 452, f453, 456–457
  skin abnormalities in newborns and, 392, f395, 396–397
seborrheic dermatitis, 35–37
  blepharitis and, 55
  perianal/buttock redness and, 383
secondary phimosis, penile abnormalities and, 336
seizures
  adenoma sebaceum and, 405
  bacterial meningitis and, 7
  herpes keratoconjunctivitis and, 55
  hypomelanosis of Ito and, 467
  roseola and, 437
  scaly rashes and, 458
  tuberous sclerosis and, 467
selective serotonin reuptake inhibitors (SSRIs), tongue discoloration/surface changes and, 157
sensorium
  differential diagnosis and, 6–7
  general appearance and, 4
sentinel skin tag, perianal/buttock swelling and, 373
sepsis
  herpes keratoconjunctivitis and, 55
  staphylococcal scalded skin syndrome (SSSS) and, 483
  vesicular rashes and, 442–443
septal hematomas, nasal swelling/discharge/crusting and, 126, f127
septal necrosis, nasal bridge trauma and, 121
septic arthritis
  arm swelling and, 252
  hand swelling and, 253–254
  knee swelling and, 293–294, 298–299

serum hyperbilirubinemia, scleral icterus and, 69
serum sickness
    hand swelling and, 258
    knee swelling and, 300
sexual abuse, 351–352, f353, 356–357
    anogenital warts and, 377
    molluscum contagiosum and, 405
    perianal/buttock redness and, 383
    perianal condylomata and, f375
    sexually transmitted disease (STD), 357
Shagreen patch, adenoma sebaceum and, 404
shield chest, abnormal chest shape and,
        190–191
shock
    general appearance and, 4, 8
    toxic shock syndrome (TSS), 407, 410–411
short bowel syndrome, gastroschisis and, 211
short digits. see brachydactyly
shoulder dislocations, arm displacement and,
        241–242
sickle cell disease
    craniosynostosis and, 27
    hand swelling and, 253–254
sinus cysts. see also dermoid cysts
    enteric cyst, abdominal midline bulge and, 207
sinusitis
    mycobacterial cervical adenitis and, 180
    pain and, 126
sixth nerve palsy, 82–83
    misalignment of the eyes and, 80, f81
skin
    diffuse red rashes, 407–412
    facial rashes, 399–406
    focal red bumps, 425–430
    general appearance and, 4
    linear red rashes, 419–424
    overlying sternal cleft, 188
    raised red rashes, 431–438
    red patches/swelling, 413–417
    skin abnormalities in newborns, 391–397
skin abnormalities in newborns
    differential diagnosis/other diagnosis and,
        396–397
    figures, 393–395
    historical points, 391
    physical examination, 392
skin lesions, impetigo and, 129
skin lines
    foot rashes/lumps and, 314
    thigh folds and, f278
skin pigmentation. see hypopigmented rashes
skin tag, 227–231
    acanthosis nigricans and, 474
    leg asymmetry and, 276
    midline back and, 229, f230
    at nasal vestibule, f127
    perianal/buttock swelling and, 373–374, f375
skull fracture
    cephalohematoma and, 11
    forceps marks and, 18
    raccoon eyes and, 68–69
    scalp swelling in newborns and, 15
"slapped cheeks," raised red rashes and, 431
sleep apnea
    acanthosis nigricans and, 471, 475
    obesity and, 217
slipped capital femoral epiphysis, 277
small-bowel obstruction, enlarged/distended
        abdomen and, 213
smallpox, vesicular rashes and, 439–440, 442–443

Smith-Lemli-Opitz syndrome
    ear shape/position abnormalities and, 87
    polydactyly/supernumerary digit and, 261
Smith-McCort dysplasia, barrel chest and, 191
sodium peroxide, hairy tongue and, 157
soft-tissue tumors, hand swelling and, 258
solitary ulcer, perianal/buttock swelling and, 378
spasticity, intoeing and, 292
speech delays/difficulties, 107. see also ears
    muffled "hot potato" voice and, 164
    OME and, 112
    oral cleft/other variants and, 151, 153
    ranulas and, 167
spermatocele, scrotal swelling and, 365, 367
spider bites, red patches/swelling and,
        413–414, f415, 416–417
spina bifida
    clubfoot and, 290, 304
    midline back and, 227–229
spinal cord defects, dermoid cyst and, 43
spinal dysraphism
    curvature of the back and, 222
    leg asymmetry and, 276
    midline back and, 228
spinal muscular atrophy, clubfoot and, 290, 304
spinal tumors, curvature of the back and, 226
splenic rupture
    infectious mononucleosis and, 171, 437
    splenomegaly and, 217
splenomegaly
    infectious mononucleosis and, 171
    splenic rupture, 217
spondyloepiphyseal dysplasia, barrel chest
        and, 191
spondylolisthesis
    curvature of the back and, 226
    lordosis and, 225
sports participation, scoliosis and, 221
Sprengel deformity, arm displacement and, 242
staphylococcal scalded skin syndrome (SSSS)
    bullous rashes and, 477–478, f480, 482–483
    diffuse red rashes and, 407–408, f409,
        410–411
staphylococcus
    ear pits/tags and, 100
    erythema toxicum and, 397
    pustular melanosis and, 397
    scarlet fever and, 405
Staphylococcus aureus
    cervical adenitis and, 180
    focal red bumps and, 426
    hand swelling and, 253
    hordeolum, 62
    impetigo and, 429
    neck masses/swelling, f182
    osteomyelitis and, 256
    septic arthritis and, 256
    suppurative parotitis and, 40
steatohepatitis, acanthosis nigricans and, 471
Steinert myotonic dystrophy, lower extremity
        abnormalities and, 274
sternal cleft, abnormal chest shape and, 188,
        190–191
Stevens-Johnson syndrome (SJS), f5
    bullous rashes and, 477–478, f481, 482–483
    perineal sores/lesions and, 358
stigmatism, capillary hemangiomas of eyelid
        and, 63
stomatitis
    bullous rashes and, f481

Stevens-Johnson syndrome and, 483
    throat redness and, 170
stork bite. see nevus simplex
strabismus. see also eye misalignment
    cataracts and, 77
straddle injury, 351–352, f353, 356–357
strawberry lesions. see hemangiomas
strawberry tongue
    scarlet fever and, 404, 410, 461
streptococcal dermatitis, perianal/buttock
        redness and, 379–381, f382
streptococcal infections
    atopic dermatitis and, 457
    ear pits/tags and, 100
    knee swelling and, 293–294
    lymphangitis and, 423
    osteomyelitis and, 256
    perianal/buttock redness and, 379–381
    perineal sores/lesions and, 358
    psoriasis and, 457
    red patches/swelling and, 413
    rheumatic fever and, 299
    scarlet fever and, 461
streptococcal pharyngitis, f172
    throat redness and, 169–171
striae, linear red rashes and, 424
stridor, 6
Sturge Weber syndrome, nevus flammeus
        and, 18
stye of the eye. see hordeolum
subconjunctival hemorrhage, f51, 54–55
subcutaneous nodules, rheumatic fever and, 298
subgaleal hemorrhage, 11–13, f14
subungual hematoma, fingertip swelling and, f268
sucking blister, skin abnormalities in newborns
        and, 391, f394, 396–397
sulfonamides, diffuse red rashes and, 407
sunburn, diffuse red rashes and, 407, f409,
        410–411
sundowning, increase of intracranial pressure
        and, 7
superior vena cava syndrome, lymphomas
        and, 180
supernumerary nipples, chest lumps and,
        199–201, f202
suppuration, cat scratch disease and, 180
suppurative parotitis, 40–41
supracondylar fracture, f5
swelling of/around the eye
    differential diagnosis/other diagnosis and,
        62–64
    figures, 59–61
    historical points, 57
    physical examination, 58
swellings in the mouth
    differential diagnosis/other diagnosis and,
        166–168
    figures, 165
    historical points, 163
    physical examination, 164
swimmer's ear, 106
Sydenham chorea, rheumatic fever and, 298
syndactyly
    abnormal chest shape and, 188, 190
    finger abnormalities and, 259–261, f262
synovitis
    hand swelling and, 254
    Lyme disease and, 294
syphilis
    anal fissures and, 374

syphilis (*Continued*)
    condyloma lata and, 357
    perineal sores/lesions and, 351
    pityriasis rosea and, 457
    raised red rashes and, 432
    tongue discoloration/surface changes and, 157
systemic disease
    arm swelling and, 246
    clubbing and, 237
    hair loss and, 28–29
    hand swelling and, 253
    hypopigmented rashes and, 464
    linear red rashes and, 419
    nail abnormalities and, 235–236
    sixth nerve palsy and, 83
    spider bites and, 414
    swellings in the mouth and, 163
    teeth discoloration and, 146
systemic lupus erythematosus (SLE)
    diffuse red rashes and, 412
    hand swelling and, 258
    knee swelling and, 300
    nephrotic syndrome and, 311
    nonblanching rashes and, 450
systemic vasculitis, hand swelling and, 253–254

T

tachypnea
    acute abdomen and, 7
    differential diagnosis and, 6
    toxic ingestion and, 7
tampon use, diffuse red rashes and, 408
Tanner stages
    breast swelling/enlargement and,
        194–195, f196
    female genitalia, variations and, 321
tarsal coalition, foot deformities and, 302
tea
    hairy tongue and, 157
    teeth discoloration and, 145
teeth abnormalities/deformities
    cleft lip and, 153
    cleidocranial dysotosis, 190
teeth discoloration
    differential diagnosis/other diagnosis and,
        147, 149
    figures, 148
    historical points, 145
    physical examination, 146
telangiectasia, facial lesions and, 21
telogen effluvium, 28–30
tenosynovium, hand swelling and, 254
teratogens, oral cleft and, 150, 153
teratomas, focal gum lesions and, 144
testicular cancer, scrotal swelling and,
        366–367, f369
testicular torsion, scrotal swelling and,
        365–367, f368
tethered cord
    leg asymmetry and, 276
    midline back and, 227, f231
tetracycline, teeth discoloration and,
        145–147, f148
thalassemia major, craniosynostosis and, 27
thalidomide, brachydactyly and, 259
thigh folds, leg asymmetry and, f278
third cranial nerve palsy, 82–83
    misalignment of the eyes and, 80, f81
    pupil abnormalities and, 80

throat redness
    differential diagnosis/other diagnosis and,
        171, 173
    figures, 172
    historical points, 169
    physical examination, 170
thrombocytopenia, nonblanching rashes and,
        446, f449, 450
thrombocytopenia absent radius syndrome
        (TAR), brachydactyly and, 261
thrombosed capillaries, 314
thrush
    focal gum lesions and, 139
    HIV and, 157
    mouth sores/patches and, 133–134,
        f136–137
    oral, 157–159
"thumbprint," hypopigmented rashes and, 464
thyroglossal duct cysts, neck masses/swelling
        and, 177–178, f181
tibia absence/shortening, leg asymmetry and, 280
tibia vara. see Blount disease
tibial torsion
    intoeing and, 287–288, f289, 290–291
    leg bowing/knock knees and, 282
tick bite, f448. see also insect bites
tinea capitis, 28–30, f32, 35–37, f38
tinea corporis, scaly rashes and, 452, f454–455,
        456–457
tinea cruris, 345–346, 348–349
tinea pedis, foot rashes/lumps, 313–315, f316
tinea versicolor, hyperpigmented rashes and,
        464–467, f468, 471–472, f473, 474–476
TM perforation, f113
    ear trauma and, 95
    tympanic membrane abnormalities and,
        110–112
tobacco
    hairy tongue and, 157
    teeth discoloration and, 145
tongue discoloration/surface changes
    differential diagnosis/other diagnosis and,
        159, 160–161
    historical points, 157
    physical examination, 158
tongue tie. see ankyloglossia
tonsillopharyngitis, 163
torticollis, 22
    general appearance and, 4
    lower extremity abnormalities and, 272
toxic epidermal necrolysis (TEN), bullous rash-
        es and, 477–478, 482–483
toxic shock syndrome (TSS)
    diffuse red rashes and, 407, 410–411
    general appearance and, 4, 8
toxicity, mastoiditis and, 95
toxocariasis, leukocoria and, 77
toxoplasmosis, neck masses/swelling and, 184
trachyonychia, nail abnormalities and, 236
traction alopecia, 28, f32
trauma
    abnormal chest shape and, 192
    abnormal head shape and, 22
    acrocyanosis and, 237
    arm displacement and, 241–243
    arm swelling and, 246–249
    auricular hematoma and, 94–95, f96
    breast swelling/enlargement and, 193
    chest lumps and, 198

corneal abrasion and, 55
discoloration of/around eye and, 65, f67
epidermolysis bullosa and, 483
external auditory canal (EAC) abnormali-
        ties and, 105, 107
fingertip swelling and, 265
focal red bumps and, 430
foot swelling and, 307
furuncle and, 429
hand swelling and, 253
hemotympanum and, 112
heterochromia iridis and, 77
hyphema and, 77
knee swelling and, 293–294, 298–299
leg bowing/knock knees and, 281–282
lumps on the face and, 40
misalignment of the eyes and, 80
mucoceles and, 167
nail abnormalities and, 235–236
nasal bridge swelling and, 121
newborn facial lesions and, 16
nonblanching rashes and, 445, 446
penile swelling and, 338, f340, 342–343
pilonidal sinus/cyst and, 229
plantar wart and, 315
postinflammatory hyperpigmentation
        and, 471
psoriasis and, 457
pupil/iris/lens abnormalities and, 71–72
pyogenic granuloma and, 43, 429
raccoon eyes and, 68
ranulas and, 167
red eye and, 49, 55
rib fractures and, 201
septal hematomas and, 126
subconjunctival hemorrhage and, 55
teeth discoloration and, 149
tympanic membrane abnormalities and, 115
Treacher Collins syndrome, ear shape/position
        abnormalities and, 87
trichodysplasia, milia and, 397
trichoepithelioma, 45
trichophagy, trichotrillomania and, 31
Trichophyton Species
    hair loss and, 29
    hypopigmented rashes and, 465
trichorrhexis nodosa, 34
trichotrillomania, 30–31, f33
Trichuriasis infestations, rectal prolapse
        and, 377
tricyclic antidepressants, foot swelling and, 307
trigonocephaly, 24, f25–26
tripod position, 4, f5
trismus
    peritonsillar abscess and, 171
    swellings in the mouth and, 164
Trisomy 13
    coloboma and, 77
    polydactyly/supernumerary digit and, 261
Trisomy 18
    coloboma and, 77
    congenital vertical talus and, 272
    ear shape/position abnormalities and, 87
    penile abnormalities and, 329
Trisomy 21
    Brushfield spots and, 77
    cataracts and, 77
    clinodactyly and, 261
Trisomy 28, clinodactyly and, 261

tropical regions, pterygium and, 63
tuberculosis
    erythema nodosum and, 413
    mycobacterial cervical adenitis and, 180
tuberculosis adenitis, neck masses/swelling and, f183
tuberous sclerosis, 464–467, f469
    facial rashes and, 399–400, f403
tularemia, erythema nodosum and, 413
tumors
    hand swelling and, 258
    leg asymmetry and, 275–276
Turner syndrome
    abnormal chest shape and, 188, 190
    brachydactyly and, 261
    clinodactyly and, 261
    pupil/iris/lens abnormalities and, 71
tympanic membrane abnormalities
    differential diagnosis/other diagnosis and, 112, 115
    figures, 113–115
    historical points, 110
    physical examination, 111
tympanosclerosis, f113
    hearing loss and, 110–112

U
ulceration, nasal hemangioma and, 121
umbilical granuloma, abdominal midline bulge and, 207, f209, 210–211
umbilical hernia, abdominal midline bulge and, 207–208, f209, 210–211
unilateral conjunctivitis, 50
unilateral laterothoracic exanthema, raised red rashes and, f435
upper respiratory infection (URI)
    AOM/OME and, 110
    neck masses/swelling and, 177
    postseptal cellulitis and, 55
    septic arthritis and, 257
    Stevens-Johnson syndrome (SJS) and, 483
    throat redness and, 169
urachal carcinoma, urachal cysts and, 211
urachal cysts, abdominal midline bulge and, 207–208, f209, 210–211
uremia, general appearance and, 8
urethral caruncle, 360–361
    vulvar swelling/masses and, f363
urethral discharge, epididymitis and, 367
urethral polyps, vulvar swelling/masses and, 364
urethral prolapse, 359–361
urinary tract abnormalities, 365
    abnormal head shape and, 24
urinary tract infections (UTI)
    erythema infectiosum and, 404
    labial adhesions and, 327
    penile abnormalities and, 333
    pinworms and, 381
urticaria, f5
    diffuse red rashes and, 407
    raised red rashes and, 438
    red patches/swelling and, f415, 416–417
    viral arthritis and, 257
urticarial wheals, knee swelling and, 294
uveitis
    conjunctivitis with KD, 55
    discoloration of/around eye and, 70

juvenile rheumatoid arthritis (JRA) and, 257, 298–299
    red eye and, 50, 56
    Stevens-Johnson syndrome (SJS) and, 483

V
vaccinia
    atopic dermatitis and, 457
    smallpox and, 443
VACTERL (VATER with cardiac/limb anomalies), imperforate anus and, 388
vacuum extraction, scalp swelling in newborns and, 11
vacuum suctioning
    caput succedaneum and, 13
    cephalohematoma and, 13
    subgaleal hematoma and, 13
vaginal web, 321
Valsalva maneuvers, encephaloceles and, 120
valvulitis, rheumatic fever and, 299
vancomycin, diffuse red rashes and, 407
varicella, 443
    herpes zoster and, 443
    knee swelling and, 300
    vesicular rashes and, f441
varicella-induced ulcerations, perineal sores/lesions and, 358
varicocele, scrotal swelling and, 365–367, f368
variola, smallpox and, 443
vascular congestion of the conjunctiva.
        see red eye
vascular diseases, cutis marmorata and, 397
vascular ischemia, leg asymmetry and, 275
vascular lesions, swelling of/around the eye and, 57
VATER (vertebral defects, anal atresia, tracheoesophageal fistula with esophageal atresia, radial/renal dysplasia)
    brachydactyly and, 261
    imperforate anus and, 388
vertebral anomalies
    curvature of the back and, 222
    lordosis and, 225
vertex delivery, caput succedaneum and, 13
vertigo
    OME and, 112
    TM perforation and, 112
vesicular lesions, red eye and, 50
vesicular rashes. see also bullous rashes
    differential diagnosis/other diagnosis and, 442–444
    figures, 441
    historical points, 439–440
    physical examination, 440
vertebral deformities, abnormal chest shape and, 192
viral arthritis
    hand swelling and, 253–254
    knee swelling and, 300
viral conjunctivitis, f51, 54–55
viral pharyngitis, 169–170, f172. see also throat redness
viral syndrome, viral conjunctivitis and, 55
viremia, chicken pox (varicella) and, 443
vision loss, juvenile rheumatoid arthritis (JRA) and, 299
vitamin D deficiency
    leg bowing/knock knees and, 281–282

rickets and, 198, f251
    wrist swelling and, 246
vitiligo, 464–467, f469
volvulus, enlarged/distended abdomen and, 218
vomiting
    abnormal head shape and, 22
    acute abdomen and, 7
    asymmetric lateral exanthem of childhood and, 437
    congenital adrenal hyperplasia (CAH) and, 321
    enlarged/distended abdomen and, 213
    glaucoma and, 55
    petechiae and, 445–446
    respiratory failure and, 7
    spider bites and, 417
    toxic ingestion and, 7
    toxic shock syndrome (TSS) and, 410
Von Willebrand's disease, nonblanching rashes and, 446
vulvar swelling/masses
    differential diagnosis/other diagnosis and, 361, 364
    figures, 362–363
    historical points, 359
    physical examination, 360
vulvovaginitis, 345, 351–352

W
Waardenburg syndrome
    heterochromia iridis and, 77
    hypopigmented rashes and, 464
WAGR syndrome
    aniridia and, 77
    Wilms tumor and, 217
warts
    anogenital warts and, 377
    genital, 352, f354, 356–357
    Koebner phenomenon and, 423
webbing. see syndactyly
weight gain
    congenital heart disease and, 311
    idiopathic cyclic edema and, 311
    nephrotic syndrome and, 311
weight loss, malignancies and, 177
Werdnig-Hoffman disease, lower extremity abnormalities and, 274
wheezing, 6
whipworms, rectal prolapse and, 377
white pupillary reflex, pupil/iris/lens abnormalities and, 72
white specks in hair
    differential diagnosis/other diagnosis and, 37, 39
    historical points, 35
    physical examination, 36
white sponge nevus, mouth sores/patches and, 138
Wilms tumor
    legrasymmetry and, 276
    WAGR syndrome, 217
Wilson disease, Kaiser-Fleischer rings and, 77
Wiskott Aldrich syndrome, 39
    nonblanching rashes and, 450
    scaly rashes and, 458
Wolf-Hirschhorn, coloboma and, 77

Wood's lamp examination
    hair loss and, 29
    hyperpigmented rashes and, 472
    hypopigmented rashes and, 464
    tinea versicolor and, 474
    white specks in hair and, 36
wrist dislocations, arm displacement and, 241

X

xanthelasma, swelling of/around the eye and, 62–63
xanthogranuloma, f61
xanthogranulomatosis, hyphema and, 77
xanthomatosis, ear swelling and, 98
Xp11 mutation, hypomelanosis of Ito and, 467

xyphoid process, chest lumps and, 198, 200–201, f202

Z

zinc deficiency, perianal/buttock redness and, 383